Health Issues Related to Alcohol Consumption

Paulus M. Verschuren

Executive Editor

ILSI Europe

ILSI Press
1126 Sixteenth Street, N.W.
Washington, D.C. 20036

ILSI Europe
Avenue E. Mounier 83, Box 6
B-1200 BRUSSELS
Belgium

Printed in the United States of America

ISBN 0-944398-17-0

Health Issues Related to Alcohol Consumption

Contents

Authors

Prof. E.L. Abel
C.S. Mott Center
275 East Hancock Avenue
Detroit, Michigan 48201, USA

Prof. D.P. Agarwal
University of Hamburg Medical School
Institute for Human Genetics
32 Butenfeld
D-2000 Hamburg 54, Germany

Dr. A. Algra
Rijksuniversiteit te Utrecht
Klinische Epidemiologie RUU/AZU
Huispostnr. X 00.123, Postbus 85500
NL-3508 GA Utrecht, The Netherlands

Prof. H. Begleiter
State University of New York
Health Sciences Center at Brooklyn
Neurodynamics Laboratory
Department of Psychiatry
450 Clarkson Avenue, Box 1203
Brooklyn, New York 11203, USA

Dr. K. Butterworth
BIBRA Toxicology International
Woodmansterne Road
Carshalton, Surrey SM5 4DS, United
  Kingdom

Prof. D. Conning
The British Nutrition Foundation
High Holburn House
5354 High Holburn
London WC1V 6RQ, United Kingdom

Prof. P. Couzigou
Hôpital Haut Lévêque
Laboratoire de Génétique
Avenue de Magellan
F-33604 Pessac, France

Prof. M.H. Criqui
University of Calfornia
San Diego School of Medicine
Mail Code 0607
La Jolla, California 92093, USA

Prof. G. Debry
University of Nancy
Centre de Nutrition Humaine
40, rue Lyonnais
F-54000 Nancy, France

Sir R. Doll
University of Oxford
Clinical Trial Services and
  ICRF Cancer Studies Unit
Radcliffe Infirmary
Oxford OX2 6HE, United Kingdom

Dr. E. Engelsman
Kevergerb 50
NL-1082 BE Amsterdam, The
  Netherlands

Dr. G. Farchi
Laboratorio de Epidemiologia e
  Biostatistica
Istituto Superiore di Sanita
Viale regina Elena 299
I-0016 Rome, Italy

Dr. D. Forman
University of Oxford
ICRF Cancer Epidemiology Unit
Gibson Laboratory
Radcliffe Infirmary
Oxford OX2 6HE, United Kingdom

Prof. D.E. Grobbee
Erasmus University Medical School
Department of Epidemiology and
  Biostatistics
P.O. Box 1738
EE24 Rm 63c
3000-DR Rotterdam, The Netherlands

Prof. C. Guerri
Fundacion Valenciana de Investigaciones
  Biomedicas
Instituto de Investigaciones Citologicas
Amadeo de Saboya 4
E-46010 Valencia, Spain

Prof. U. Keil
Herzog-Ludwigestraße, 55
D-8011 Zorneding, Germany

Dr. K. Kiianmaa
Biomedical Research Center
Alko Ltd.
Box 350
SF-00101 Helsinki, Finland

Dr. C. La Vecchia
Istituto di Ricerche Farmacologiche
  "Mario Negri"
Via Eritrea 62
I-20157 Milan, Italy

Prof. I. Macdonald
University of London
Hillside
Fountain Drive
London SE19 1UP, United Kingdom

Prof. K. McPherson
London School of Hygiene and Tropical
  Medicine
University of London
Health Promotion Sciences Unit
Department of Public Health and Policy
Keppel Street, Gower Street
London WC1E 7HT, United Kingdom

Dr. M. Plant
Edinburgh University
Alcohol Research Group
Department of Psychiatry
Royal Edinburgh Hospital
Morningside Park
Edinburgh EH10 5HF, United Kingdom

Prof. S. Renaud
INSERM
Unit 63
22, Ave. Doyen L'Espine
F-69675 Bron Cedex, France

Prof. J. Rodés
Hospital Clinico i Provincial de Barcelona
Servico de Hepatologia
Villarroel 170
E-08036 Barcelona, Spain

Prof. M. Salaspuro
University of Helsinki
Research Unit of Alcohol Diseases
Tukholmankatu 8F
SF-00290 Helsinki, Finland

Prof. T.I.A. Sorensen
Copenhagen Health Services
Institute of Preventive Medicine
Kommunehosptalet
DK-1399 Copenhagen, Denmark

Dr. M.J. Stampfer
Harvard Medical School
Channing Laboratories
180 Longwood Avenue
Boston, Massachusetts 02115, USA

Dr. F.M. Sullivan
St. Thomas's Hospital
United Medical and Dental Schools
Department of Pharmacology and
  Toxicology
Lambeth Palace Road
London SE1 7EH, United Kingdom

Prof. J.D. Swales
University of Leicester
School of Medicine
Leicester Royal Infirmary
P.O. Box 65
Leicester LE2 7LX, United Kingdom

Prof J. van Gijn
University of Utrecht
Department of Neurology
Postbus 85500
NL-3508 GA Utrecht, The Netherlands

Dr. J. Veenstra
TNO Institute
Postbus 360
NL-3700 AJ Zeist, The Netherlands

Dr. K. Westerterp
University of Limberg
Department of Human Biology
P.O. Box 616
NL-6200 MD Maastricht, The
  Netherlands

Dr. C. Wolfe
Guy's and St. Thomas's United Medical
  and Dental School
Department of Public Health Medicine
Lambeth Palace Road
London SE1 7EH, United Kingdom

Dr. R. Woutersen
TNO Toxicology and Nutrition Institute
Department of Biological Toxicology
Postbus 360
NL-3700 AJ Zeist, The Netherlands

Foreword

This publication results from a project organised by the International Life Sciences Institute-ILSI Europe. ILSI is a non profit, worldwide foundation established in 1978 to advance the understanding of scientific issues relating to nutrition, food safety, toxicology, and environmental safety. ILSI's standards, the quality of the research it supports, and the worldwide as well as regional meetings and symposia it sponsors are recognised by the scientific community throughout the world. Additionally, ILSI is affiliated with the World Health Organization as a nongovernmental organisation of international significance and has specialised consultative status with the Food and Agriculture Organization of the United Nations. ISLI receives its funding from member company dues, governmental projects, and publication sales.

Although alcohol has been one of the most studied and researched substances consumed by man, there are few sources one can consult for an objective review of the current state of scientific knowledge in this very broad area. While recognising that not every possible issue concerning alcohol and health could be examined in a single project, ILSI Europe, through its Task Force on Alcohol, organised nine panels consisting of leading scientists to critically and objectively review nine important alcohol-related issues: hypertension, stroke, coronary heart disease, digestive tract cancer, liver disease, breast cancer, pregnancy, overweight, and genetics as a factor in alcoholism.

This book, which has been submitted to the Commission of the European Communities (Directorate General V), comprises the reports of the nine panels and is preceded by an overview summary. These reports, which were peer reviewed by independent experts before publication, reflect a tremendous work effort that deserves recognition. The outcome identifies areas of scientific consensus, gaps in the current state of knowledge, methodological problems in the existing research, and areas for future research activities that should make a lasting contribution to work in this area.

Paulus M. Verschuren
Scientific Director
ILSI Europe

Overview of the Biomedical Project on Alcohol and Health

K. Butterworth
BIBRA, United Kingdom

Introduction

The role of beverages containing alcohol has been a prominent feature of life in many societies. For as long as alcohol has been consumed, and that is millennia, the relationships between drinking and various aspects of health have been explored.

Through the auspices of the International Life Sciences Institute-ILSI Europe, leading scientists were invited to critically and objectively review the current state of information available on the relationship between alcohol consumption and nine important health issues. This group of scientists included epidemiologists, clinicians, toxicologists, and other biomedical researchers. The task assigned was to appraise what we know and, equally important, what we do not know about alcohol as it pertains to a wide range of biomedical considerations.

Nine panels were formed, each with its own chairman. Each panel was asked to address the relationship between alcohol consumption and one of the following subject areas: hypertension, stroke, coronary heart disease, digestive tract cancers, liver diseases, breast cancer, pregnancy, overweight, and genetics. All but the genetics panel were asked the following:

(1)   To list possible associations between specific biomedical conditions and the consumption of alcohol.

(2)   For each possible association or hypothesis, to assess the progress reached in achieving a scientific consensus, including whether a consensus exists, the specific content of the consensus, and the body of research that allows the consensus to form. The panels were also asked to address whether the consensus reached far enough to cover a relationship between biomedical consequences and a particular dose or range of dosage, and whether the intakes are consistent across the population.

(3)   To identify issues where a scientific consensus does not exist and, in such cases, to identify the gaps in knowledge or contradictory results that preclude such a consensus, and to specify research tasks necessary for shifting each possibility to a thorough consensus, confirmation, or dismissal.

(4)   To determine whether there are cases:
  (a)   where a hypothesis is supported by epidemiological findings that demonstrate a relationship between alcohol con-

sumption and a biomedical effect, but where a causal relationship cannot be confirmed because of the absence of clinical, laboratory, or animal research defining a mechanism;

(b) where the findings are too dependent on a particular piece of research to permit consensus; or

(c) where it is recommended that increased attention be paid to contrary evidence.

The genetics panel was asked to conduct a critical review of the epidemiological and biochemical data relating to whether there is a genetic basis for alcoholism. The genetics panel was also asked to assess the quality of research in this area, the availability of new technologies, and the length of time it might take to determine a specific genetic profile for alcoholism, if such a profile is possible.

This overview is intended to summarize the reports of the nine panels; readers interested in the details can refer to the full report. The overview is organised by related topics: (1) those concerning the cardiovascular system, (2) those concerning the gastrointestinal tract and related systems, and (3) other topics.

The reader will note that different panels have used differing measurements of the amounts of alcohol consumed by subjects in medical research. This reflects differences in the measurements employed in the studies themselves. A number of the panel reports measure consumption in grams of pure ethanol consumed. In most countries, a standard serving of beer, wine, or spirits equals approximately 8 to 12 grams of ethanol.

Moreover, several of the panels have noted serious methodological problems in the consumption measurements employed in the currently available studies reviewed by the panels, especially those of the nonexperimental observational studies. Measurement of alcohol intake in the studies is usually based on self-reporting by the subjects of the study, and this can result in recall errors. Specifically, people in general, and heavy drinkers in particular, often underreport their intake. In other words, subjects may not recall (or wish to admit) precisely how many grams or millilitres they consumed per day or what concentration of a mixed drink consumed consisted of alcohol. Because of this underreporting, the threshold amounts of alcohol consumption associated with certain health risks may in fact be higher than those indicated in the existing studies. Alternatively, persons reporting as teetotallers may have been former heavy drinkers, and indeed self-styled abstainers have been found to have alcohol in their urine. Here again, such misclassification may cast doubt on the precise consumption figures shown in the research literature.

Additional methodological problems are presented by a number of "confounding factors," such as age, sex, body mass index, diet, physical activity, smoking, coffee consumption, educational attainment, Type A/B behaviour, socioeconomic status, and medical history, that may be factors in particular health problems in persons who have been the subjects of the reported studies. For example, a generally poor nutritional condition could possibly play a significant role in various health problems associated with heavy drinkers. In most of the investigations, adjustments could be made for many of these confounding factors, but for some this was not possible because the relevant information was not available or assessment was too difficult.

It bears noting that the ILSI Europe panels did not address every aspect of alcohol and health or every system of the human body. The panels were charged with considering nine specific issues, with an emphasis on the health effects of moderate consumption. For example, some topics involving the neuropathological consequences of alcohol consumption, such as the psychiatric effects of alcohol abuse and injuries from drinking and driving, have not been addressed by the panels.

The Cardiovascular System

Three panels addressed the effects of alcohol on the cardiovascular system: (1) hypertension, (2) stroke, and (3) coronary heart disease.

Alcohol Intake and its Relationship to Hypertension

A possible relationship between alcohol intake and blood pressure has been investigated in cross-sectional, prospective cohort and intervention studies. The hypertension panel concluded that there is a causal association between the chronic intake of alcohol and risk of hypertension. There is less certainty, however, as to the precise cutoff level above which the effect of alcohol becomes apparent on the exact shape of the association. Still, it seems likely that a threshold exists at about 30–60 g/day of alcohol, above which the risk of hypertension increases. Chronic consumption at or above these levels may be the second most important nongenetic factor for hypertension, coming closely behind obesity as a well-established risk factor. Focusing on the population attributable risk percentage, it has been calculated from several studies that 7–11% of hypertension in men is due to alcohol intake of

40 g/day or more. The panel reports that the threshold for women is at the lower end of this 30–60 g/day range, probably because of differences in the way that men and women metabolize alcohol.

The role of chronic alcohol consumption above certain levels in causing hypertension is best evidenced by studies that have tested the effect of alcohol withdrawal on blood pressure. These studies have reported a fall in the blood pressure of heavy drinkers who abstained or severely restricted their alcohol intake for purposes of the study.

The precise effect of chronic ingestion of alcohol in causing increased blood pressure is poorly understood, but it is extremely unlikely that a single mechanism accounts for the effects observed. It appears that neural, humoral, and direct vascular mechanisms are possible causes of the alcohol–blood pressure association, but the role of each of these mechanisms is unclear.

The hypertension panel recommended that further research concentrate on obtaining a much more accurate assessment of alcohol intake by the subjects of studies, including detailed information on lifetime specific use, in order to develop a more precise delineation of the alcohol–blood pressure association and to better pinpoint the threshold levels of alcohol consumption that can lead to hypertension.

The Association Between Alcohol and Stroke

A stroke can be either ischaemic, due to an embolism or thrombosis (85% of all strokes); or haemorrhagic, due to intracerebral or subarachnoid bleeding (10% and 5% of all strokes, respectively).

At least 19 prospective epidemiological studies, with an aggregate of nearly two million person-years of observation, have been reported. It has been shown that there is little association between habitual alcohol consumption and risk of total stroke, except for a possible modest increase in risk at higher levels of alcohol intake.[1] The dose range where some adverse effect may be present is unclear, but it appears to be several drinks a day. When the data were segregated according to the two broad categories of stroke type, however, more consistent patterns emerged. There is substantial evidence for an association between habitual high-level alcohol consumption and risk of haemorrhagic stroke (15% of stroke cases), with typically about a threefold excess risk for the higher levels of alcohol consumption.

---

[1]In this report, moderate alcohol consumption is classified as less than 60 grams of ethanol per day, and higher levels of consumption as drinking more than this amount.

In contrast, there was equally strong evidence against any material adverse association between even high levels of alcohol consumption and the risk of ischaemic stroke (85% of stroke cases).

From case-control epidemiological studies, moderate drinkers appeared to have an equal or modestly elevated risk from total stroke compared with nondrinkers. In fact, there is some evidence of a "J-shaped curve" association between the level of alcohol intake and total stroke in white populations, with reduced risk for those reporting light drinking as compared to nondrinkers.[2] All studies specifically addressing ischaemic stroke risk found no association with alcohol intake. For haemorrhagic stroke, an increased risk was found in chronic high alcohol drinkers that was independent of chronic hypertension.

Some studies on "binge drinking" of alcohol, using case-control studies, suggested a positive relationship between the ingestion of large quantities of alcohol over a short time span and overall stroke. The value of these studies is diminished, however, by methodological problems and by the failure to adjust adequately for confounding variables such as smoking.

One of the weaknesses in many studies is the fact that stroke is not always unequivocally diagnosed. Cerebral haemorrhages and cerebral infarctions are immediately recognizable by computerized tomography (CT) scans. CT scanning also allows most other conditions to be excluded from the diagnosis.

Alcohol Drinking and Coronary Heart Disease

According to studies of both morbidity and mortality resulting from coronary heart disease, a moderate intake of alcohol in the form of beer, wine, or spirits appears to provide protection against coronary heart disease over nondrinkers by a factor of 10–70%. These results are consistent across ecological, case-control, and prospective studies. Particular confidence can be given to the results of the most recent cohort studies, which involved more than 500,000 subjects over a period of 2–12 years. All of these recent studies have confirmed that the coronary heart disease risk was lowest in moderate drinkers.

The studies also show that at alcohol intake levels of 10–20 g/day, even mortality from all causes was significantly decreased as compared to nondrinkers. It is therefore becoming generally agreed among

---

[2]Studies that identify U-shaped or J-shaped curves refer to research results that show that the health effect being considered is elevated at zero alcohol consumption, declines at certain levels of consumption, and increases again at certain higher levels of consumption.

medical scientists that there is either a U-shaped or J-shaped curve relationship between the level of alcohol intake and total mortality, with nondrinkers and heavier drinkers showing relative increases in deaths from different causes, including total cardiovascular disease. The protective effect of alcohol seems to be present at all ages, in women as well as in men, whatever the length of follow-up (2–22 years), and with other risk factors taken into consideration in addition to alcohol.

The panel rejected the criticism reported in some medical literature that the observed U-shaped curve might be the consequence of including former heavy drinkers who have developed heart problems with nondrinkers. Several studies addressed this issue directly by separating the lifetime abstainers from the former drinkers. These studies found that the risk of coronary heart disease in the former heavy drinkers was equal to or greater than the risk among the lifetime abstainers, and that the risk for both was greater than for moderate drinkers.

The partial inhibitory effect of alcohol on atherosclerosis seems to be due to an increase in the reverse transport of cholesterol through the level of high density lipoprotein (HDL), consistently enhanced, in a dose-related manner, by alcohol drinking. As a confirmation of the only partially protective effect of the raised level of HDL, multivariate analysis of epidemiological data indicates that HDL would explain only 50% of the preventive effect of alcohol on coronary heart disease.

An additional effect of alcohol, especially at low dosage, may be protection from myocardial infarction (i.e., coronary thrombosis). Since alcohol consumption can predispose to cerebral haemorrhage, part of the mechanism could be through haemostatic functions. Blood platelets, the primary factor involved in thrombosis, have been shown to have their aggregability decreased by alcohol—in vitro, ex vivo, and in epidemiological studies—after acute and long-term alcohol ingestion in man and animals. Effects of moderate alcohol consumption on the fibrinolytic system have also been reported.

The final confirmation of the protective effect of moderate alcohol consumption could only be achieved by a randomized intervention trial study, which may be impossible due to methodological difficulties.

Diseases of the Gastrointestinal Tract and Related Organs

Two of the nine panels reviewed the medical literature concerning the effects of alcohol on various aspects of the gastrointestinal tract and related organs: (1) the possible effects of alcohol on cancer of the digestive tract and larynx, and (2) the effects of alcohol on the liver.

Alcoholic Beverages and Cancers of the Digestive Tract and Larynx

Ethanol is not a carcinogen by standard laboratory tests. Animal experiments suggest, however, that, given by mouth, it may act as a cocarcinogen in the production of cancers in the oesophagus and possibly also in the nonglandular (fore)stomach, but not in the glandular stomach or pancreas. The evidence relating to the production of colorectal cancer is conflicting, and no conclusion can be drawn from it.

Epidemiological evidence shows that the consumption of alcoholic beverages increases the risk of developing cancers of the mouth (other than the salivary glands), pharynx (other than the nasopharynx), and larynx; that the risks are principally due to the presence of ethanol and increase with the amount consumed; that the risks are increased by increased smoking, each agent approximately multiplying the effect of the other; and that, in the absence of smoking, the risks in developed countries are small unless consumption is exceptionally heavy. The risks may be diminished by a diet rich in fruit and green vegetables, but the evidence is inconclusive. Whether the cocarcinogenic effects of different alcoholic beverages depend solely on the presence of ethanol and are unaffected by its concentration or by the presence of congeners (other constituents in alcoholic beverages) is uncertain.

The epidemiological evidence also suggests that there may be some direct relationship between the consumption of alcohol and colorectal cancer. The apparent relationship is quantitatively moderate, and even with heavy consumption a doubling of the relative risk can be excluded. No apparent difference exists between the susceptibility of men and women or of the two sites (colon and rectum), or between the effect of different types of alcoholic beverage. The nature of the observed relationship remains in doubt: it may be causal, it may be due to confounding between the consumption of alcoholic beverages and some other dietary factor that increases the risk of the disease, and it may be due, at least in part, to the selective publication of positive results. Research aimed at discovering whether the association can be explained by confounding with dietary habits should be encouraged.

The balance of the evidence suggests that alcoholic beverages do not cause cancers of the stomach or pancreas, but it does not rule out the possibility altogether. Alcohol may contribute specifically to the production of cancer of the gastric cardia and, indirectly through the production of chronic (calcifying) pancreatitis, to cancer of the pancreas; but the evidence is insufficient for any conclusion to be reached.

Alcohol and Liver Diseases

There is strong evidence for a direct relationship between the toxicity of alcohol and liver damage. The liver plays a major role in the metabolism of alcohol. By the action of alcohol dehydrogenase, alcohol is transformed to acetaldehyde, which in turn is rapidly oxidized in the liver to acetate by aldehyde dehydrogenase. Acetaldehyde is a very potent and reactive compound, and it has been suggested that it is one of the major factors in the pathogenesis of alcoholic liver disease.

There is a firm consensus about the association between chronic alcohol consumption at excessive amounts and the development of fatty liver, perivenular fibrosis, acute alcoholic hepatitis, and hepatic cirrhosis. The potential for developing these conditions is higher in individuals who, for a period of time, have had a daily excessive intake of alcohol. Whereas the consensus about the qualitative association between excessive alcohol consumption and the development of the above-mentioned hepatic lesions is well established, there is much uncertainty about the dose-effect relationship.

The key mechanism in the genesis of fatty liver is due to the alcohol-induced change in the redox state of the liver. Excessive alcohol intake may produce liver damage by other mechanisms, such as promotion of lipid peroxidation and toxicity associated with an activation of the microsomal alcohol oxidizing system. Although there is some evidence that both mechanisms may play a role in the development of alcoholic injury of the liver, further studies are required to reach a definite consensus. Nutritional studies have also been implicated, but data is insufficient to establish a critical role.

It is considered that chronic alcoholism constitutes a significant public health problem. Four prospective studies have assessed the relationship between daily consumption reported at the start of the study and subsequent cirrhosis mortality during long-term follow up. In one study it was found that, among persons reporting minimum consumption of 50 g/day, the number of persons who develop cirrhosis after 10–15 years was about 2% per year. Many studies have demonstrated a very close correlation between total consumption in populations and mortality from cirrhosis. Although the incidence of heavy drinkers is higher among males, females are more sensitive to the development

of liver injury. Individuals drinking intermittently had a lower incidence of liver damage. Abstinence will reverse, improve, or delay progression of alcoholic liver disease depending on the stage of the lesion,
which also indicates that alcohol is responsible for the liver damage.

The fact that only a minor portion of individuals who consume
excessive amounts of alcohol develop the most severe forms of liver
damage, cirrhosis in particular, indicates that other causal factors may
be involved. Despite years of research, no consensus has been reached
on any one such factor. Current research focuses on genetic factors,
viral infections, and specific nutritional disturbances.

Other Topics Studied

Other topics considered by the panels include the possible effects
of alcohol on (1) the risk of breast cancer, (2) pregnancy, and (3) body
weight. A final panel considered the subject of whether there is a genetic link to alcoholism and related problems.

Breast Cancer

There is currently insufficient evidence to support any general
causative relationship between alcohol and breast cancer. Several studies have found a weak positive association, but this was not found
consistently. No specific relationship emerged, except for the possibility that the association was strongest for large amounts of daily alcohol consumption and for premenopausal breast cancer. With such a
weak association and a relatively poor understanding of the aetiology
of breast cancer, it is therefore impossible to exclude the likelihood
that the association is explained by other confounding risk factors.
The most likely confounding factors are some aspects of the diet, but
there are many other possible factors, including age at menopause,
marital status, age at first full-term pregnancy, family history of breast
cancer, oestrogen use, socioeconomic status, and body mass. Certain
aspects of the diet, particularly in relation to dietary fat, have been
shown to be associated with the risk of breast cancer.

Since experimental studies where confounding factors could be
minimized are unlikely, resolution of this question must await the
ability to better adjust for dietary and other confounding factors by
knowing more about their roles as primary risk factors for breast cancer. This will involve prospective studies in which the consequences
of contemporary dietary patterns are observed. In the meantime, any

recommendation that women should limit their alcohol consumption specifically to reduce their risk of breast cancer cannot be justified on existing epidemiological grounds.

Alcohol and Pregnancy

Foetal alcohol syndrome (FAS) is characterized by a cluster of anomalies occurring in children of alcohol-dependent women. This pattern of anomalies consists of defects in each of the following categories:

(1) prenatal and/or postnatal growth deficiency, including intrauterine growth retardation, small-for-dates, failure to thrive, and continuing growth below the tenth percentile for gestational age;

(2) morphological anomalies, including a specific cluster of facial features giving a distinctive appearance; and

(3) central nervous system dysfunction, which includes cognitive disabilities, the most serious being mental retardation.

Only alcohol-dependent women are at risk of giving birth to children with FAS, although even in alcohol-dependent women it is not inevitable that this damage will occur. In fact, most alcohol-dependent mothers do not give birth to FAS babies. No particular patterns and levels of alcohol consumption have been shown consistently to characterize this condition, but this is probably because estimates of alcohol intake are based on unreliable self-reported data. Alcohol-dependent women also have an increased risk of spontaneous abortions.

Although high doses of alcohol are necessary to cause FAS, a number of other factors are also typically present. These include low socioeconomic status, poverty, poor maternal health care, poor diet, problematic past obstetric history, older age, greater parity, smoking, and illicit drug use. The contribution of these factors to FAS needs to be clarified. It is also possible that some alcohol-related birth defects may be male-mediated. In most cases, fathers of FAS children are also either heavy drinkers or alcohol-dependent.

Current evidence does not support any clear-cut relationship between lower levels of maternal alcohol consumption and adverse effects in the foetus or child. The lower the level of alcohol consumption, the greater the influence of confounding factors. In contrast to studies on smoking in pregnancy, where reduced birth weight is obtained in almost all studies, reduced birth weight is only found occasionally in studies of moderate alcohol consumption during pregnancy.

Moreover, such a large number of confounding variables are involved in low birth weight (e.g., nutrition, tobacco smoking, and maternal health) that it is likely that the contribution from moderate alcohol intake is low.

Animal models, in a variety of species, have provided evidence for the teratogenic effects of alcohol. Such studies have shown that the presence of specific anomalies depends on the amount of alcohol consumed and the stage of pregnancy at which this occurs. An important use of animal studies is that confounding factors can be both investigated and controlled.

With regard to future research, one area that needs to be examined is the risk of psychopathological behaviour resulting from prenatal exposure to alcohol. Further epidemiological studies are also needed to determine the effects, if any, of low levels of maternal alcohol intake on the behavioral development of the child. Further long-term longitudinal studies should be undertaken in affected children, with follow-up extending well into school age, in order to identify which effects are permanent and which are transient. Here environmental factors could well confound the issue. In all future epidemiological studies, adequate measurements of alcohol consumption should be a prerequisite.

Alcohol and Overweight

Alcohol constitutes on average approximately 4–6% of the energy intake in the Western diet, but obviously alcohol intake is not equally distributed over the total population. The majority of people in a "drinking population," however, will be moderate drinkers. In this review, the focus is on the effect of alcohol consumption on energy balance in moderate drinkers, defined as subjects with an average consumption of 15–45 g/day of alcohol.

From an epidemiological standpoint, establishing a relationship between moderate alcohol intake and body weight is difficult, and the results of studies are conflicting. Correlation between moderate alcohol consumption and body mass index (BMI) has been reported as positive, negative, or nonexistent. The surveys are difficult to interpret because of the many uncontrolled confounding factors such as smoking, personality patterns and life-styles, socioeconomic status, level of education, and physical activity. Accordingly, only studies that take these confounding factors into account should be considered.

In contrast to the survey types of studies are intervention studies, ideally with a crossover design, in which the effect of alcohol consumption in subjects has been studied by dividing the subjects into groups with and without the addition of moderate amounts of alcohol to the diet. From five such studies, under strictly controlled conditions in a metabolic ward, it has been shown that moderate alcohol consumption had no measurable effect, in men of normal body weight, on energy balance and body weight over intervals of up to 4 weeks. Even 4 weeks of heavy drinking under these strictly controlled conditions resulted in a slight negative energy balance (i.e., intake of fewer calories than expended as energy). Investigations have failed to identify a mechanism for increased metabolism or energy deposition after alcohol ingestion, but suggest that, at moderate levels, alcohol is efficiently used as a fuel by the liver.

It thus appears that alcohol tends to supplement rather than displace macronutrient energy, though there are some alterations in the dietary pattern. Individuals who consume alcohol but are not alcohol-dependent, appear to add the energy from alcohol to their normal intake rather than replace food with alcohol. Further research is needed to provide evidence of how the energy from ingested alcohol disappears. Most studies comparing the effect of alcohol on body weight of men and women have found no difference between the sexes. Others, however, have indicated an inverse relationship between alcohol consumption and body mass in women but not in men. This reported difference between the sexes may be due to different lifestyles that have not been controlled for in all the studies.

In studying the relationship between alcohol intake and the distribution of body fat, a negative correlation was found between alcohol consumption and waist-hip ratio in women in some studies, while other studies showed a positive correlation. Studies in men also produced conflicting results. In view of the possible significance of waist-hip ratio as a predictor of cardiovascular disease, there could be further investigations of the body fat distribution associated with alcohol consumption.

Genetics and Alcohol

Genes have long been suspected of playing a role in the aetiology of alcoholism, and now there is considerable evidence amassing for a strong genetic influence. The fact that alcoholism often runs in families does not necessarily imply a hereditary factor, but it is possible that a genetic factor is implicated. Although it is unlikely that a single gene could account for the transmission of such a complex disorder as alcoholism, it is theoretically possible that different genes could affect different aspects of alcoholism and alcohol-related diseases. In an attempt to disentangle genetic and environmental effects, twin and adoption studies, as well as a wide range of animal experiments, have been undertaken.

Twin studies are one way to assess the relative effects of genetic and environmental components of alcohol-related problems. If there is a greater concordance among monozygotic (MZ) twins than dizygotic (DZ) twins for a particular trait, then there is evidence for that trait to be under genetic control. It has been shown that values for both amount and frequency of alcohol drinking in MZ twins indicate the presence of a genetic factor. The concordance for alcoholism was consistently higher in MZ than DZ twin pairs. This was true for both men and women.

While twin studies are a powerful tool, they do not completely exclude effects of the environment. Living together increases the similarity in alcohol intake among both types of twin pairs. Even when these influences were factored out, however, there remained a higher concordance for MZ than DZ twins.

Adoption studies allow genetic and environmental factors to be assessed independently. It has been found that sons of alcoholic parents had a nearly fourfold higher alcoholism rate than adopted sons whose biological parents were nonalcoholic, whether they were raised by nonalcoholic foster parents or by their own biological parents. Adopted sons of alcoholics were found to be more likely to be alcoholic at an earlier age than their peers.

Both twin and adoption studies can be subject to bias introduced by the practice of adoption agencies that match the adoptees to the adopting parents. Nevertheless, there is sufficient evidence for a genetic role in alcoholism.

Much knowledge concerning the role of heredity in ethanol abuse is derived from animal studies. Various inbred strains of mice differ widely in their voluntary intake of ethanol. This demonstration of significant strain differences is evidence of genotype involvement in ethanol preference. Animal experiments can also study reinforcement, learned behavioral disorder, blocking of reinforcement, alcohol resistance, relapse, binge drinking, and satiety.

The development of alcoholism for some individuals depends on the presence of genetically influenced predisposing factors interacting with environmentally determined precipitating factors. Alcoholism is clinically heterogeneous; it may develop at variable ages, it may develop from additive effects of more than one gene, and single mutations at different genetic loci may result in clinically indistinguishable disease states. Not every individual who inherits the genes will develop the disorder, thus reflecting the complex genetic interactions. A substantial number of individuals without a disease genotype manifest alcoholism resulting from nongenetic causes.

The search for predisposing biological markers associated with genetic factors for alcoholism must be conducted in accordance with a specific set of criteria. Some of the most widely studied biological markers include the event-related potential P300, the Al allele of D2 dopamine receptor, monoamine oxidase activity in platelets, and adenylate cyclase activity. While the presence of these trait markers may identify individuals who are at risk of developing alcoholism, there are other trait markers, such as aldehyde dehydrogenase 2 deficiency, whose presence may denote protection against alcoholism.

Research has already made it possible to identify individuals, especially in Oriental populations, with a particularly low risk for alcoholism, and it seems very likely that in the future markers will be found for a high risk of alcoholism. The markers could be genotypic or phenotypic. A single "alcoholism gene," however, is very unlikely. Current evidence in animals and humans instead points toward polygenic control, probably with several genes having substantial influences but a very large number of genes still having some effect. Although the influences are generally imagined as additive, more complex interactions are possible.

The ethical problems raised by the likely discovery of such markers are already being considered. Educational strategies need to be determined to allow identified high-risk subjects to change their lifestyle most effectively.

Conclusion

Taken together, the panel reports suggest that there are significant health effects associated with alcohol consumption. Alcohol is and has been one of the most intensively studied and researched substances consumed by man. There is an abundance of medical literature addressing the health effects of excessive consumption, but there is less written about the effects of light to moderate consumption.

The panels identified common problems in virtually all of the existing biomedical research discussed in the reports, including:

(1) methodological problems in calculating the amounts of alcohol actually consumed by subjects, including difficulties in recalling the precise amount of alcohol consumed, underreporting of consumption by subjects of the studies, and the presence in studies of former alcoholics who report themselves as "nondrinkers;" and

(2) difficulties in accounting for confounding factors in studies, such as tobacco smoking, nutrition and diet, and other lifestyle factors.

For example, final confirmation of the effects—positive or negative—of alcohol consumption shown in epidemiological studies can only be achieved by randomized intervention trial studies, which may be impossible in some cases due to methodological difficulties.

The panels recommended several areas for further research studies on the effects of drinking on health.

2

Alcohol Intake and its Relation to Hypertension

U. Keil
Ruhr-University Bochum, Germany

J.D. Swales
University of Leicester, United Kingdom

D.E. Grobbee
Erasmus University Medical School, The Netherlands

Abstract

A relationship between alcohol intake and blood pressure has been noted since 1915. A large number of cross-sectional studies, a smaller number of prospective cohort studies, and a number of intervention studies have addressed the nature of this relationship in the last 25 years. Although a number of questions—such as the validity of measurement of alcohol intake, shape of the alcohol–blood pressure relationship, threshold dose for hypertension, and plausible pathophysiologic mechanisms—have not yet been answered satisfactorily, it is clear that a causal association exists between chronic intake of $\geq$ 30–60 g/day of alcohol and blood pressure elevation in men and women. To call the alcohol–blood pressure relationship causal is justified because chance and to a large degree bias and confounding have been ruled out as plausible explanations in most epidemiological studies. More importantly, the intervention studies support the observational studies. This indicates that confounding factors are not responsible for the observed alcohol–blood pressure relationship, even where these have not been specifically controlled for in observational studies. The intervention studies show a remarkable consistency in demonstrating a potentially valuable fall in blood pressure when heavy drinkers abstain or restrict their alcohol intake. The fall in blood pressure induced in these studies is of similar magnitude to that which would be predicted from the observational associations if these represented a causal effect. Taken in conjunction, therefore, the observational and intervention studies create a powerful case for alcohol as an important life-style factor in elevated blood pressure. From observational and intervention studies, a rule of thumb can be derived: above 30 g/day of alcohol intake, an increment of 10 g/day of alcohol increases systolic blood pressure on average by 1–2 mmHg, and diastolic blood pressure by 1 mmHg. Focusing on the population-attributable risk percent, it has been calculated from several studies that about 7–11% of hypertension ($\geq$ 160/95 mmHg) in men in the community is due to alcohol intake of $\geq$ 40 g/day. In women this percentage is much smaller because of their much lower alcohol intake. The pressor effect of chronic ingestion of alcohol is still poorly understood. At present, neural, humoral, and direct vascular mechanisms are seen as possible mediators of the alcohol–blood pressure association. The role of each of these mechanisms is still unclear. Today, alcohol intake of more than 30–60 g/day is seen as the second most important acquired determinant of hypertension, closely behind the risk factor overweight (obesity).

Aims and Objectives

A relationship between alcohol consumption and blood pressure elevation was first suggested by Lian in 1915, who noted that French servicemen drinking 2.5 litres of wine or more per day had increased prevalence of hypertension (Lian 1915). Since 1967, attention shifted to the question of whether an association exists between alcohol consumption and blood pressure in populations not selected on the basis of alcohol intake. A large number of cross-sectional studies, a smaller number of prospective cohort studies, and a few experimental studies have addressed this question. Most studies have reported a positive association between alcohol consumption and blood pressure (MacMahon 1987).

The following questions and aspects of the alcohol–blood pressure relationship will be addressed in this report:

(1) To what extent does alcohol consumption contribute to the prevalence of hypertension in the population?
(2) What are the effects on blood pressure of modification of alcohol intake?
(3) Is the alcohol-blood pressure relationship linear, J-shaped, or U-shaped?
(4) Is there a threshold dose for hypertension risk?
(5) What are the difficulties in measuring alcohol consumption in population studies?
(6) What are the major putative confounders of the alcohol–blood pressure relationship?
(7) What are the physiologic mechanisms for the alcohol–blood pressure link?
(8) How must observational studies be improved to better understand the alcohol–blood pressure relationship?

Observational and Experimental Studies Concerning Alcohol and Hypertension

Cross-Sectional Studies

The alcohol–blood pressure association has been investigated worldwide in at least 32 cross-sectional studies: 10 in Europe

(Gyntelberg and Meyer 1974, Kozarevic et al. 1980, Milon et al. 1982, Salonen et al. 1983, Cairns et al. 1984, Kornhuber et al. 1985, Kromhout et al. 1985, Keil et al. 1989, Bulpitt et al. 1987, Keil et al. 1991), 12 in North America (Clark et al. 1967, Dyer et al. 1977, Klatsky et al. 1977, Harburg et al. 1980, Criqui et al. 1981, Kagan et al. 1981, Fortmann et al. 1983, Gordon and Kannel 1983, Coates et al. 1985, Gruchow et al. 1985, Klatsky et al. 1986, Gordon and Doyle 1986), six in Australia (Mitchell et al. 1980, Baghurst and Dwyer 1981, Cooke et al. 1982, Arkwright et al. 1982, Savdie et al. 1984, MacMahon et al. 1984), two in New Zealand (Paulin et al. 1985, Jackson et al. 1985) and two in Japan (Ueshima et al. 1984, Kondo and Ebihara 1984).

All of the European studies found evidence of an alcohol–blood pressure association independent of a number of putative confounding factors such as age, weight (body mass index = BMI = kg/m^2), physical activity, smoking, coffee consumption, educational attainment, and Type A/B behaviour. Dietary intake was not assessed in most studies.

In the Munich Blood Pressure Study (MBS) (Cairns et al. 1984) and the Lübeck Blood Pressure Study (LBS) (Keil et al. 1989), generally the blood pressures of nondrinkers were either greater than or no different from those of persons consuming 10–20 g/day of alcohol. In the LBS, blood pressure was greater in drinkers than it was in nondrinkers at consumption levels of ≥ 40 g/day of alcohol. In the MBS, the respective alcohol consumption level was ≥ 60 g/day for men and ≥ 40 g/day for women.

The MONICA Augsburg Survey 1984/85 (Keil et al. 1991) confirmed the MBS results in that blood pressure was clearly greater in drinkers than in nondrinkers at alcohol consumption levels of ≥ 60 g/day in men and ≥ 40 g/day in women. Among the three studies performed in Germany with the same methodology, a clear J-shaped curve was found for the alcohol–systolic blood pressure relationship only in LBS men (Keil et al. 1989).

In the three studies performed in Germany, a strong interaction between alcohol consumption and smoking was found in older women; in the MONICA Augsburg Survey this interaction was found in men and women (Cairns et al. 1984, Keil et al. 1989, Keil et al. 1991). Obviously, smoking can act as an effect modifier on the alcohol–blood pressure relationship, i.e., Augsburg men who consume ≥ 60 g/day of alcohol and are smokers have 2–8 mmHg higher systolic and/or diastolic blood pressure values compared to nonsmokers. In LBS and Augsburg women ages 45–69 years, this alcohol-smoking interaction was seen at alcohol levels of ≥ 20 g/day. A physiological interpretation of this newly found interaction is not yet available.

With the exception of the Canada Health Study (Coates et al. 1985), all of the 12 North American studies have reported a statistically significant positive association of alcohol and blood pressure. In the first Kaiser Permanente Study (Klatsky et al. 1977), only a small difference was found in systolic or diastolic blood pressure between nondrinking men and those consuming 10–20 g/day of alcohol. In women, systolic and diastolic blood pressures were greater in nondrinkers than in women consuming 10–20 g/day of alcohol. Thus, a J-shaped relationship was found in women. The findings of this study suggested that there might be a threshold effect of 30 g/day of alcohol for blood pressure elevation in men and women and in all racial groups. Many more subsequent North American studies confirmed these findings (Criqui et al. 1981).

With the exception of one study (Baghurst and Dwyer 1981), the six Australian and the two New Zealand studies found linear, J-shaped, and U-shaped associations between alcohol and blood pressure. In the National Heart Foundation of Australia Risk Factor Prevalence Study (MacMahon et al. 1984) and the Auckland Study (Jackson et al. 1985), there was evidence of greater blood pressure values in drinkers than in nondrinkers at consumption levels of ≥ 30 g/day. Both Japanese studies (Ueshima et al. 1984, Kondo and Ebihara 1984) reported independent linear associations of alcohol with blood pressure.

Prospective Cohort Studies

There are at least seven prospective cohort studies of the alcohol–blood pressure association (Kromhout et al. 1985, Dyer et al. 1977, Gordon and Kannel 1983, Gordon and Doyle 1986, Dyer et al. 1981, Reed et al. 1982, Witteman et al. 1989). The results of all but the Honolulu Heart Study (Reed et al. 1982) are consistent with those of the cross-sectional studies and indicate a positive alcohol–blood pressure association. The prospective association of alcohol with blood pressure has been investigated over 4 years in the Framingham Study (Gordon and Kannel 1983). In both men and women, an increase in alcohol consumption over 4 years was associated with a significant increase in blood pressure, whereas a decrease in alcohol consumption was associated with a significant decrease in blood pressure. Recently results from the Nurses Health Study have been published (Witteman et al. 1989). From a cohort of 58,000 U.S. nurses free of diagnosed hypertension, 3,275 reported an initial diagnosis of elevated blood pressure during a 4-year follow-up period. When compared to nondrinkers, women drinking 20–34 g/day of alcohol had an approximate 1.4-fold increased risk of occurrence of hypertension during follow-up. In those drinking 35 grams or more, the relative risk was 1.9.

Table 1 provides an overview of observational studies on the alcohol–blood pressure association. The studies in this table are categorized by the unit of measurement of alcohol intake.

Intervention Trials on Blood Pressure and Alcohol Intake

Acute Withdrawal

Blood pressure rises when alcohol is acutely withdrawn from very heavy drinkers. This response is associated with clinical evidence of sympathetic nervous system activation (tachycardia and sweating) and raised plasma catecholamines, renin activity, aldosterone, and cortisol (Bannan et al. 1984, Eisenhofer et al. 1985). One detailed clinical study demonstrated that the pressor response was maximal the day after admission to hospital for detoxication in alcoholics but then fell progressively over the next few days (Bannan et al. 1984). Withdrawal of alcohol in hypertensives may also give rise to postural hypotension. In some but not all patients who show this effect, the catecholamine response to standing is inhibited, suggesting impaired cardiovascular reflexes (Eisenhofer et al. 1985).

Chronic Withdrawal

A limited number of investigators have examined the effect of withdrawing alcohol for several days or weeks in moderate to heavy drinkers. To detect blood pressure lowering effects, such studies have to be carefully designed. Withdrawal of alcohol in a group of subjects may produce blood pressure lowering; this might be the result of a placebo response rather than being a direct consequence of alcohol withdrawal. The observational associations suggest that blood pressure changes may be limited to a few millimetres of mercury. Thus, group size has to be adequate to ensure a sufficient statistical power to demonstrate an effect. Finally, advice to reduce alcohol intake may be unsuccessful or may be associated with other dietary changes that may have an important influence on blood pressure. Thus, reduction in body mass or increase in physical activity may produce significant blood pressure lowering effects that may wrongly be attributed to alcohol withdrawal.

For the above reasons, the largest study of nonpharmacological manoeuvres aimed at lowering blood pressure does not throw light

Table 1

**Overview of observational studies on the alcohol-blood pressure associa-
tion. Examples of differences in blood pressure between categories with
highest and lowest alcohol intake. In general, lowest category pertains to
abstainers, although sometimes low alcohol users have also been included.
Studies are categorized by the unit of measurement of alcohol intake.**

Study by first author	M/F	Category with highest alcohol consumption	SBP (mmHg)	DBP (mmHg)
Studies reporting alcohol use by "unit"				
Gyntelberg 1974	M	6–10 units/day	8.1	4.8
Kozarevic 1982	M	≥ 1 unit/day	7.7	4.3
Coates 1985	M, age 20–34 yr	≥ 2.14 units/day	1.9	0.4
	M, age 35–49 yr	≥ 2.14 units/day	2.9	4.0
	M, age ≥ 60 yr	≥ 2.14 units/day	−3.4	−0.5
	F, age 20–34 yr	≥ 2.14 units/day	1.8	−0.1
	F, age 35–49 yr	≥ 2.14 units/day	−2.4	−5.4
	F, age ≥ 60 yr	≥ 2.14 units/day	−5.7	−2.1
Bulpitt 1987	M	> 10 units/day	20.0	7.3
	F	> 10 units/day	5.5	3.4
Lang 1987	M	> 5 units/day	8.9	5.3
	F	> 5 units/day	14.3	6.1
Weissfeld 1988	M, age 18–39 yr	> 2 units/day	3.3	3.7
	M, age 40–59 yr	> 2 units/day	0.7	1.9
	M, age ≥ 60 yr	> 2 units/day	2.4	4.5
	F, age 18–39 yr	> 2 units/day	8.4	6.9
	F, age 40–59 yr	> 2 units/day	6.1	2.8
	F, age ≥ 60 yr	> 2 units/day	9.7	3.3
Wannamethee 1991	M	> 6 units/day	6.5	4.0
Studies reporting alcohol use in millilitres				
Pincherle 1974	M	≥ 60–90 ml/day	4.3	3.2
Klatsky 1977	M	≥ 72 ml/day	5.4	2.1
	F	≥ 72 ml/day	10.9	4.5
Arkwright 1981	M	> 50 ml/day	5.1	n.s.
Milon 1982	M, age < 40 yr	≥ 12 ml/day	n.s.	n.s.
	M, age 40–49 yr	≥ 12 ml/day	10.6	n.s.
	M, age > 50 yr	≥ 12 ml/day	11.9	n.s.

Table 1. *Continued*

Study by first author	M/F	Category with highest alcohol consumption	SBP (mmHg)	DBP (mmHg)
Studies reporting alcohol use in millilitres *continued*				
Fortmann 1983	M, age 20–34 yr	≥ 30 ml/day	2.6	−1.6
	M, age 35–49 yr	≥ 30 ml/day	3.0	1.2
	M, age 50–74 yr	≥ 30 ml/day	15.4	6.6
	F, age 20–34 yr	≥ 30 ml/day	2.3	0.5
	F, age 35–49 yr	≥ 30 ml/day	−0.4	−0.2
	F, age 50–74 yr	≥ 30 ml/day	12.8	6.5
Gordon 1983	M	≥ 74.7 ml/day	7.3	n.s.
	F	≥ 74.7 ml/day	8.4	n.s.
Elliott 1987	M	> 42.8 ml/day	13.2	5.4
Trevisan 1987	M	> 114 ml/day	3.0	1.0
	F	> 114 ml/day	6.7	0.4
Dyer 1990	M, "white"	> 30 ml/day	2.4	2.0
	M, "black"	> 30 ml/day	2.8	0.9
	F, "white"	> 30 ml/day	1.5	1.5
	F, "black"	> 30 ml/day	−0.3	2.4
Klag 1990	M, "Japanese"	> 58 ml/day	14.1	8.9
	M, "white"	> 30 ml/day	5.6	3.6
Yamada 1991	M	> 58 ml/day	4.9	3.9
Studies reporting alcohol use in grams				
Myrhed 1974	M+F	> 27.4 g/day	9.6	6.7
Dyer 1977	M	"alcoholics"	4.7	n.s.
	M	≥ 25 g/day	9.7	5.9
Marmot 1981	M	> 34 g/day	2.8	2.3
Cooke 1983	M	> 30 g/day	7.7	4.7
	F	> 30 g/day	5.0	3.8
Ueshima 1984	M, "urban"	> 83 g/day	17.4	10.3
	M, "rural"	> 83 g/day	16.9	8.5
Cairns 1984	M	≥ 60 g/day	2.4	1.2
	F	≥ 40 g/day	n.s.	2.4

Table 1. *Continued*

Study by first author	M/F	Category with highest alcohol consumption	SBP (mmHg)	DBP (mmHg)
Studies reporting alcohol use in grams *continued*				
Jackson 1985	M, age > 50 yr	> 34 g/day	1.8	1.7
	F, age > 50 yr	> 34 g/day	10.2	4.5
Paulin 1985	M	≥ 42.8 g/day	9.8	8.9
	F	≥ 42.8 g/day	−6.0	1.0
Simon 1988	M	> 50 g/day	n.s.	n.s.
Keil 1989	M	≥ 40 g/day	5.5	4.5
	F	≥ 20 g/day	9.6	5.2
		(association only in smokers)		
Salvaggio 1991	M	> 60 g/day	3.5	1.8
Keil 1991	M, age 25–34 yr	≥ 80 g/day	4.5	5.1
	M, age 35–44 yr	≥ 80 ml/day	8.2	5.3
	M, age 45–54 yr	≥ 80 ml/day	11.5	6.3
	M, age 55–64 yr	≥ 80 ml/day	2.8	2.2
	F, age 25–34 yr	≥ 40 ml/day	3.0	3.1
	F, age 35–44 yr	≥ 40 ml/day	6.5	4.7
	F, age 45–54 yr	≥ 40 ml/day	6.5	3.0
	F, age 55–64 yr	≥ 40 ml/day	2.1	1.0
Studies reporting alcohol use in ounces				
Harburg 1980	M	≥ 2.27 oz/day	5.8	3.8
	F	≥ 1.98 oz/day	2.0	5.5
Kagan 1981	M	≥ 1.97 oz/day	6.1	3.4
Gordon 1986	M	≥ 2.96 oz/day	7.3	5.6
Studies reporting miscellaneous measures of alcohol intake				
Clark 1967	M	"yes"	1.9	1.6
Hofman 1985	M	"daily alcohol consumption"	2.2	2.7
	F	"daily alcohol consumption"	0.7	1.3
Schnall 1992	M	"regular alcohol consumption"	3.6	2.8

One milliliter (ml) = 0.9 g alcohol
One ounce (oz) = 28 g alcohol

upon the causality of the alcohol–blood pressure relationship. Stamler et al. (1987) adopted a multifactorial approach in a large population by intensive advice on weight control, dietary control of lipids, physical activity, electrolyte intake, and alcohol intake. Significant blood pressure lowering was achieved, and it was possible to reduce antihypertensive medication. The contribution of advice on alcohol reduction cannot be assessed from such an approach; it seems likely that the contribution was small, however, since there was no significant impact of advice on alcohol intake as assessed by self-reporting.

Table 2 provides an overview of a number of randomized trials addressing the changes in alcohol intake and their impact on blood pressure of hypertensive and normotensive subjects.

In a randomized trial, either a parallel group or crossover design can be adopted. In the latter, subjects are randomly assigned to normal or low alcohol intake but then reallocated to the other group for a second intervention period. Using this design, Potter and Beevers (1984) admitted a group of heavy-drinking hypertensive patients to hospital and withdrew alcohol from half of the group for 3 days and maintained the other half on normal alcohol intake. Alcohol was withdrawn from the latter group and given to the former group for the next 4 days. The period of alcohol withdrawal in both groups was associated with significant lowering of blood pressure. Puddey et al. (1985b, 1987) also used a crossover design but employed an intervention period of six weeks. Subjects were also "blinded" to the level of alcohol intake by being given a low-alcohol lager with or without the addition of alcohol. The aims of blinding are to exclude placebo intervention effects and to remove potential observer bias. Both groups were able to demonstrate significant lowering of blood pressure with reduction of alcohol intake in heavy drinkers. This effect was seen both in normotensive and hypertensive subjects. Other reports confirm the blood pressure lowering effect of alcohol withdrawal using both crossover and parallel group designs (Howes and Reid 1986, Parker et al. 1990, Maheswaran et al. 1992). These studies have tended to show a greater fall in blood pressure in hypertensive subjects (see Table 2). In the only study to compare normotensive and hypertensive subjects directly, Malhotra et al. (1985) observed a substantially greater effect in hypertensive subjects. Unfortunately, this study is uncontrolled and some of the blood pressure fall reported may therefore be a placebo effect or result from regression to the mean. In particular, regression to the mean is more pronounced when blood pressure levels are higher, i.e., in the hypertensive range.

Table 2

Trials of changes in alcohol intake and impact on blood pressure (BP)

Study by first author	Subjects and alcohol intake by day (d) or week (wk)	n	Design	Initial Alcohol Intake	Final Alcohol Intake	Duration	Initial BP (mmHg)	Change BP (mmHg)	P-value
Potter 1984	H[a] (80 ml/d)	16	Crossover	80 ml/d 0 ml/d	0 ml/d 80 ml/d	3 days 4 days	174/104 156/100	−19/−5 +12/+5	< 0.05 < 0.01
Puddey 1985b	N[b] (366 ml/wk)	46	Crossover	426 ml/wk	85 ml/wk	6 weeks	130/73	−3.7/−1.4	< 0.001
Howes 1986	N[b] (40 ml/d)	10	Crossover	55 ml/d	0 ml/d	7 days	116/60	−3.0/−3.1	< 0.05 and < 0.01
Puddey 1987	H[a] (472 ml/wk)	44	Crossover	452 ml/wk	64 ml/wk	6 weeks	142/84	−5/−3	< 0.001
Parker 1990	H[a] (480 ml/wk)	59	Parallel group	537 ml/wk	57 ml/wk	4 weeks	138/85	−5.4/−3.2	< 0.01
Maheswaran 1992	H[a] (480 ml/wk)	41	Parallel group	480 ml/wk	240 ml/wk	8 weeks	149/101	−/−5.2 (Systolic blood pressure change n.s.)	< 0.05

[a]H = hypertensives.
[b]N = normotensives.

The intervention studies show a remarkable consistency in demonstrating a potentially valuable fall in blood pressure when heavy drinkers abstain or restrict their alcohol intake (see Table 2). The fall in blood pressure induced in these studies is similar in magnitude to that which would be predicted from the population associations if these represented a genuinely causal effect. Taken in conjunction, therefore, the observational and intervention studies create a powerful case for alcohol as an important life-style factor in elevated blood pressure.

From observational and intervention studies, a crude rule of thumb can be derived: above 30 g/day of alcohol intake, an increment of 10 g/day increases systolic blood pressure on average by 1–2 mmHg, and diastolic blood pressure by 1 mmHg.

Interpretation of the Findings

Measurement Problems

Methodological problems complicate interpretation of the data collected, especially those of nonexperimental observational studies. Measurement of alcohol intake is a fundamental issue in all population studies of the alcohol–blood pressure relationship (Colsher and Wallace 1989). As a rule, the alcohol intake in these studies is estimated on the basis of oral or written information provided by the subjects. Self reports may be obtained by having participants keep daily diaries of their alcohol consumption. Another way is to recall consumption over periods ranging from the most recent week to the entire lifetime (Colsher and Wallace 1989).

Such data are not always reliable. One issue is the exact amount of alcohol consumed over a period such as 1 day, week, month, or even longer periods. A second issue is the heterogeneity of the group that claims to consume no alcohol at all (Ference et al. 1986, Knupfer 1987). It has been reported that 50% of the patients of a clinic for hepatic diseases denied alcohol consumption, although alcohol could be demonstrated in the urine (Orrego et al. 1979).

The blood alcohol level provides a "gold standard" for the amount of alcohol recently consumed (Puddey et al. 1985a). Blood alcohol determination becomes impractical, however, when alcohol consumption in large numbers of people and over longer time periods must be assessed. Moreover, blood alcohol levels may not be elevated in moderate drinkers several hours after their last drink. A number of biochemical determinations are recommended in order to obtain more insight into alcohol consumption: γ GT, SGOT, SGPT, the mean cell volume (MCV), and high density lipoprotein (HDL) cholesterol (Ramsay 1977a,b, Chick et al. 1981). In general, studies relating biomarkers for alcohol intake to blood pressure levels have obtained results similar to studies relying on reported intake. However, none of these biochemical parameters appears sensitive or specific enough to replace or substantiate interview or questionnaire data.

Studies based on self-report measures of alcohol intake generally indicate that heavy drinkers tend to underreport or even deny alcohol consumption (Chick 1982, Poikolainen and Karkkainen 1983). In particular, the "no-alcohol-consumption group" is a problem group comprising lifelong abstainers, drinkers who deny their alcohol consumption, those who already suffer from health problems, and those who are too sick to drink alcohol (Barcha et al. 1968, Midanek et al. 1990, Wicklung et al. 1984). It has also been found that persons reporting to be teetotallers are often former heavy drinkers (Colsher and Wallace 1989). The effects of such misclassification on the alcohol–blood pressure relationship may be diverse. In this respect, it is important to note that a positive correlation between alcohol consumption and blood pressure was found, especially among those with more than an average alcohol intake. The findings for moderate and light alcohol consumption are less clear-cut. Some authors have described a "threshold phenomenon" whereby the mean blood pressure was only elevated if the alcohol intake exceeded approximately 3 glasses (30 g) per day (Klatsky et al. 1977, Dyer et al. 1977). Others have reported a J-shaped relationship between alcohol and blood pressure whereby moderate alcohol drinkers had a lower blood pressure than total abstainers (Gyntelberg and Meyer 1974, Harburg et al. 1980). Inadequate information on low- or no-alcohol consumption, so that the group of total abstainers becomes "contaminated" by subjects who do not admit their high alcohol consumption, may explain some of the inconsistency in findings. Such misclassification could cause an inverse relationship at the beginning of the curve, although the general view is that this phenomenon, if present, may not completely account for the absence of an association between light to moderate alcohol use and blood pressure.

Another problem is that people might underreport their alcohol intake. Such a general, nondifferential underreporting will probably result in an overestimate of the association at any specific level of actual alcohol intake, although the overall strength of the association will not be affected. Moreover, if a threshold really exists, its estimated level might be higher if there is a systematic underreporting of alcohol intake by subjects (MacMahon 1987, Colsher and Wallace 1989, Grobbee 1992).

Putative Confounders

Interpretation of the alcohol–blood pressure association is influenced not only by the quantification and potential misclassification of alcohol intake, but also by various putative confounding factors that may be associated with both blood pressure and alcohol intake and therefore might explain any eventual association. This applies in particular for age, sex, and body weight, and in most of the investigations adjustments have been made for these factors. Several other variables have often not been included in the analysis, however, because the relevant information was not available or assessment was too difficult. This applies, for example, to dietary factors such as electrolyte intake, notably sodium, potassium, and magnesium; medication; and physical activity. As it has also repeatedly been found that drinkers smoke more cigarettes (Gordon and Kannel 1983, Pincherle and Robinson 1974), it is not inconceivable that alcohol consumption is related to a life-style that could have an effect on blood pressure independent of alcohol intake (Calahan 1981). In addition, a generally poor nutritional condition could play a role, especially for heavy drinkers (West et al. 1984).

Perhaps even more difficult to assess is the potentially confounding effect of psychosocial stress. It is generally accepted that alcohol may serve a role in reduction of tension under stressful circumstances (Linsky et al. 1985, Pohorecki 1991). In view of the potential stress-buffering capacity of alcohol at a cognitive level, the blood pressure of subjects who do not drink may be more responsive to stressful conditions and life events.

A potential confounder that relates perhaps more closely to the mechanisms involved in alcohol-induced blood pressure elevation is the association between alcohol intake, alcohol withdrawal, and subsequent effects of withdrawal on blood pressure levels. It is well known that people decrease their alcohol intake in the period just before they visit their physician; this could similarly apply to participants in population surveys, which may lead to an increase in the serum catecholamine concentration. In addition, hypercorticism can develop. Both factors may well explain an increase in blood pressure, particularly systolic blood pressure. In two investigations of patients participating in a detoxification program, the level of blood pressure was correlated with the severity of the withdrawal symptoms (Saunders et al. 1979, 1981). Withdrawal symptoms occur not only as a result of the acute discontinuation of alcohol consumption, but also after a less pronounced decrease in the serum alcohol level (Mendelson and Mello 1979). It is conceivable that even the consumption of a few glasses of alcohol per day will already cause (subclinical) withdrawal symptoms. It is difficult, however, to estimate the importance of this phenomenon in the results of published observational studies. Clearly, alcohol withdrawal cannot explain the findings in several of the intervention studies discussed earlier.

Self-selection could cause the observed relationship due to the differences in risk of hypertension between individuals who choose to drink and those who prefer not to drink. The reverse also applies: specific personality characteristics of hypertensive individuals could give rise to the consumption of alcohol (Anonymous 1977). Finally, it is conceivable that genetic factors give rise to either elevated blood pressure or (excessive) alcohol consumption, but such a possibility remains rather remote and speculative, as there is still substantial discussion on the genetic basis and mechanisms of both high blood pressure and excessive alcohol use. The above explanations are not relevant to randomized trials. The question then arises, however, of the extent to which the acutely induced effects of alcohol can be extrapolated to the situation of chronic alcohol consumption. Another aspect that plays a role in both types of investigation is the fact that the researcher is never truly "blind" as far as alcohol consumption or the acute alcohol load is concerned, which could influence the findings. The importance of double blind studies is quite obvious, but the execution of such studies is exceedingly difficult.

Mechanisms (Pathogenesis)

Alcohol is widely distributed over body fluids and has important actions upon the physicochemical properties and biological function of cell membranes (Knochel 1983). In addition, its major active metabolite, acetaldehyde, has important cardiovascular actions with a slightly different pattern of activity (Altura et al. 1978). The tissue concentration of acetaldehyde is small, however, and it probably does not make a significant contribution to the haemodynamic actions of alcohol. Qualitatively different dose-dependent effects and divergence between acute and chronic actions make the interaction of alcohol and blood pressure a complex one, and it is extremely unlikely that a single mechanism accounts for the association between blood pressure and alcohol intake described in population studies.

The immediate pressor effect of alcoholic drinks probably reflects a reflex response to gastrointestinal irritation (Ireland et al. 1984) and concurrent administration of calorie-containing fluids (Stott et al. 1987). Later, a slight rise or no change in blood pressure has been reported with modest doses of alcohol or a fall in pressure with higher doses (Howes and Reid 1987). This fall is due to a reduction in total peripheral resistance with increased flow through some tissue beds, most notably the cutaneous bed. A reduction in venous return to the heart as a result of venous dilatation may also contribute and, after an interval, volume depletion as a result of diuresis. These effects are partly opposed by autonomic activation, which gives rise to a tachycardia and, in some studies, activation of the renin-angiotensin system (Ireland et al. 1984, Puddey et al. 1985b). In addition, there is evidence for decreased production of vasodilator prostanoids (Fostermann and Feuerstein 1987). Pharmacological blockade of the autonomic nervous system results in a consistent depressor effect (Child et al. 1979), suggesting that circulatory autonomic reflexes are important in limiting the alcohol-induced vasodepressor action. The acute withdrawal response in very heavy drinkers gives rise to biochemical evidence of sympathetic activation, together with increased plasma renin activity and plasma cortisol (Beevers et al. 1982, Bannan et al. 1984). While this phenomenon might contribute to the higher blood pressure reported among heavy drinkers in the population studies, it is unlikely to be a sufficient explanation in view of the consistent blood pressure lowering effect of sustained reduction of alcohol intake.

It is therefore likely that chronic alcohol administration directly or indirectly exerts a pressor effect upon the cardiovascular system that is not evident in acute studies where the predominant effect is blood pressure lowering. The pressor effect could be mediated by a neurogenic mechanism, a humoral mechanism, or directly through actions upon the vessels that maintain peripheral resistance. Plasma noradrenaline levels are not elevated by chronic alcohol administration (Arkwright et al. 1984, Ibsen et al. 1985), although heart rate is slightly elevated. Nevertheless, plasma catecholamines are an insensitive measure of sympathetic activity, and these findings are consistent with a modest increase in sympathetic tone. Chronic alcohol administration increases central and peripheral noradrenaline turnover in rats (Pohorecky 1974). However, noradrenaline spillover and release are uninfluenced by moderate alcohol intake in man, although noradrenaline clearance is reduced (Howes et al. 1986). Regular alcohol intake also reduces baroreceptor reflex sensitivity (Howes and Reid

1987). Whether this results from changes in central regulation of blood pressure or at the arterial level is uncertain. As a consequence, however, the circulatory mechanisms would not be as effective in opposing a rise in blood pressure.

There are reports of slightly elevated levels of plasma renin (Ibsen et al. 1985), cortisol (Potter and Beevers 1984, Arkwright et al. 1984), and vasopressin (Linkola 1979) in chronic drinkers. It is unlikely that the plasma concentration of any of those hormones is sufficient to account for elevated blood pressure, although plasma cortisol has been reported to correlate with blood pressure in both drinkers and non-drinkers (Arkwright et al. 1984). In some heavy drinkers, glucocorticoid levels are sufficiently elevated to give rise to the features of Cushing's syndrome. This may reflect a direct effect of alcohol on adrenocorticotrophic hormone (ACTH) release or potentiation of corticotrophin-releasing factor by vasopressin (Gilles et al. 1982). Under these circumstances, alcohol-induced glucocorticoid excess may be an important factor in hypertension.

It is possible that chronic alcohol intake has direct vascular actions that contribute to hypertension. Alcohol in concentrations observed in modest drinkers causes vasoconstriction in isolated arteries obtained from some vascular beds, such as the coronary tree or cerebral vasculature (Altura et al. 1983 a,b). This action is not associated with an overall increase in peripheral vascular resistance in vivo, however, and is therefore unlikely to contribute to blood pressure elevation. There is evidence that chronic exposure to alcohol produces more relevant distinct effects. Thus, while acute exposure of vascular smooth muscle to alcohol increases cell membrane fluidity, chronic exposure decreases it through increased incorporation of cholesterol (Knochel 1983). Decreased smooth muscle membrane fluidity has been implicated in some forms of genetic hypertension through vascular second-messenger systems that regulate contraction and structure (Bing et al. 1986). It has been suggested that alcohol-induced membrane changes (operating perhaps through depolarisation) increase inward leak of calcium (Knochel 1983). Alcohol may also inhibit active sodium pumping through an action upon sodium-potassium ATPase and thereby increase smooth muscle sodium through inhibition of sodium-potassium ATPase (Katz 1982). Some studies have reported a correlation between plasma calcium and blood pressure in drinkers and have suggested that vascular tone may become dependent on extracellular calcium concentrations (Arkwright et al. 1984). On the other hand, the thousand- to ten-thousand-fold differences in extra- and intracellular calcium concentrations imply that even very minor changes in extracellular calcium concentrations would produce disastrous effects upon intracellular calcium, if such a relationship were to develop as a result of impairment of transmembraneous ionic pathways. It seems unlikely, therefore, that extracellular calcium concentration is an important factor in alcohol-induced hypertension.

In summary, the acute and chronic physiological effects of alcohol on the cardiovascular system are quite distinct. The pressor effect of chronic ingestion is still poorly understood. At present, neural, humoral, and direct vascular mechanisms are thought to be possible mediators of the alcohol–blood pressure association. The role of each of these factors, if any, is still unclear.

Implications for Prevention and Treatment

In most epidemiological studies, blood pressure levels were greater at alcohol consumption levels of ≥ 40 g/day than they were at levels of 10–20 g/day (MacMahon 1987, Keil et al. 1989). About 25% of studies reported blood pressure elevations at alcohol consumption levels of < 30 g/day compared with blood pressure of nondrinkers. About 40% of studies reported blood pressure of nondrinkers to be greater than blood pressure of those consuming 10–20 g/day of alcohol. It is doubtful whether these findings actually reflect a blood pressure lowering effect of small amounts of alcohol. Thus, it is still unclear whether the alcohol–blood pressure relationship is linear or curvilinear. One possible explanation for the J-shaped relationship is the finding that nondrinkers are a heterogeneous group comprising extreme subgroups such as lifelong abstainers, heavy drinkers who deny their alcohol consumption, and those who are too ill to drink (Colsher and Wallace 1989). More research is needed to better understand the nondrinker group and its potential influence on the shape of the alcohol–blood pressure relationship.

If a threshold dose for hypertension risk exists, it is probably around 30–60 g/day of alcohol (lower for women than for men).

From the public health perspective, it is important to investigate what percentage of hypertension in the community might be caused by alcohol consumption and, more importantly, how much hypertension in the community could be eliminated if intake of, e.g. ≥ 40 g/day of alcohol were eliminated. Focusing on the population-attributable risk percent, it was calculated from LBS data that about 7% of hypertension in men in the community is due to alcohol consumption of ≥ 40 g/day (Keil et al. 1989). The respective calculations from U.S.

and Australian population studies revealed that alcohol consumption could account for as much as 11% of hypertension in men, but much less in women because of their much lower alcohol consumption (MacMahon et al. 1984, Friedman et al. 1982).

In spite of many unanswered questions (e.g., threshold level and shape of the association) concerning the alcohol–blood pressure relationship, it seems clear that a causal association exists between consumption of ≥ 30–60 g/day of alcohol and blood pressure elevation in men and women. The statement of a causal relationship is justified because chance and to a large degree bias and confounding have been ruled out as plausible explanations of the alcohol–blood pressure association in most observational studies. More importantly, the intervention studies support the observational studies and show a similar quantitative relationship. This indicates that confounding factors are not responsible for the observed relationship, even where these have not been specifically controlled for in observational studies. Furthermore, the consistency of the cross-sectional, prospective cohort, and intervention studies is high. In addition, a clear time sequence between cause and effect seems present. The underlying pathophysiology, however, must be clarified further. For example, the more recent techniques for studying vascular physiology and molecular mechanisms may shed more light on the mechanisms underlying the alcohol–blood pressure relationship.

Chronic alcohol consumption of ≥ 30–60 g/day can be viewed as the second most important nongenetic risk factor for hypertension, closely behind the well-established risk factor of being overweight.

From all epidemiological studies investigating the alcohol–blood pressure association, it has become clear that the accurate assessment of alcohol intake, including detailed information on lifetime specific use, is the paramount and crucial problem (Hennekens 1983).

It is conceivable that a major improvement in assessing the exposure variable alcohol will contribute to a more precise delineation of the alcohol–blood pressure association, and will transform the frequently found J-shaped curves to a more linear relationship with a more precise estimate of the threshold level in the range of a chronic intake of 30–60 g/day of alcohol for hypertension.

References

Altura BM, Carella A, Altura BT (1978) Acetaldehyde on vascular smooth muscle: possible role in vasodilator action of ethanol. Eur J Pharmacol 52:73–83

Altura BM, Altura BT, Gebrewold A (1983a) Alcohol-induced spasms of cerebral blood vessels: relation to cerebrovascular accidents and sudden death. Science 200:331–33

Altura BM, Altura BT, Carella A (1983b) Ethanol produces coronary vasospasm: evidence for a direct action of ethanol on vascular smooth muscle. Br J Pharmacol 78:260–62

Anonymous (1977) Alcohol and hypertension (leading article). Lancet 2:122–23

Arkwright PD, Beilin LJ, Rouse I, et al. (1981) Alcohol: effect on blood pressure and predisposition to hypertension. Clin Sci 61:373s–75s

Arkwright PD, Beilin LJ, Rouse I, et al. (1982) Effects of alcohol use and other aspects of lifestyle on blood pressure levels and the prevalence of hypertension in a working population. Circulation 66:60–66.

Arkwright P, Beilin L, Vandongen R, et al. (1984) Plasma calcium and cortisol as predisposing factors to alcohol-related blood pressure elevation. J Hypertens 2:387–92

Baghurst K, Dwyer T (1981) Alcohol consumption and blood pressure in a group of young Australian males. J Human Nutr 35:257–64

Bannan LT, Potter JF, Beevers DG, et al. (1984) Effect of alcohol withdrawal on blood pressure, plasma renin activity, aldosterone, cortisol and dopamine beta-hydroxylase. Clin Sci 66:659–63

Barcha A, Stewart MA, Guze MB (1968) The prevalence of alcoholism among general hospital ward patients. Am J Psychiat 125:30–41

Beevers G, Bannan L, Saunders J, et al. (1982) Alcohol and hypertension. Contrib Nephrol 30:92–97

Bing RF, Heagerty AM, Thurston H, Swales JD (1986) Ion transport in hypertension: are changes in the cell membrane responsible? Clin Sci 71:225–30

Bulpitt CJ, Shipley MJ, Semmence A (1987) The contribution of a moderate intake of alcohol to the presence of hypertension. J Hypertens 5:85–91

Cairns V, Keil U, Kleinbaum D, et al. (1984) Alcohol consumption as a risk factor for high blood pressure: Munich Blood Pressure Study. Hypertension 6:124–31

Calahan D (1981) Quantifying alcohol consumption: patterns and problems. Circulation 64:7–14

Chick J, Plant M, Kretiman N (1981) Mean cell-volume and gamma-glutamyltranspeptidase as markers of drinking in working man. Lancet 1:1249–51

Chick J (1982) Epidemiology of alcohol use and its hazards, with a note on screening methods. Br Med Bull 38:3–8

Child J, Kovick R, Levisman J, Pearce M (1979) Cardiac effects of acute ethanol ingestion unmasked by autonomic blockade. Circulation 59:120–25

Clark VA, Chapman JM, Coulson AH (1967) Effects of various factors on systolic and diastolic blood pressure in the Los Angeles Heart Study. J Chronic Dis 20:571–81

Coates RA, Corey PN, Ashley MJ, Steele CA (1985) Alcohol consumption and blood pressure: analysis of data from the Canada Health Survey. Prev Med 14:1–14

Colsher PL, Wallace RB (1989) Is modest alcohol consumption better than none at all? An epidemiologic assessment. Annu Rev Public Health 10:203–19

Cooke KM, Frost GW, Thornell IR, Stokes GS (1982) Alcohol consumption and blood pressure: survey of the relationship in a health screening clinic. Med J Aust 1:65–69

Cooke KM, Frost GW, Stokes GS (1983) Blood pressure and its relationship to low levels of alcohol consumption. Clin Exp Pharmacol Physiol 10:229–33

Criqui MH, Wallace RB, Mishkel M, et al. (1981) Alcohol consumption and blood pressure: the Lipid Research Clinics Prevalence Study. Hypertension 3:557–65

Dyer AR, Stamler J, Paul O, et al (1977) Alcohol consumption, cardiovascular risk factors, and mortality in two Chicago epidemiologic studies. Circulation 56:1067–74

Dyer AR, Stamler J, Paul O (1981) Alcohol, cardiovascular risk factors and mortality: the Chicago experience. Circulation 64 (suppl 3):20–27

Dyer AR, Cutter GR, Liu K, et al (1990) Alcohol intake and blood pressure in young adults: the Cardia Study. J Clin Epidemiol 43:1–13

Eisenhofer G, Whiteside EA, Johnson RH (1985) Plasma catecholamine responses to changes of posture in alcoholics during withdrawal and after continued absence from alcohol. Clin Sci 68:71–78

Elliott P, Fehily AM, Sweetnam PM, Yarnell JWG (1987) Diet, alcohol, body mass, and social factors in relation to blood pressure: the Caerphilly Heart Study. J Epidemiol Community Health 41:37–43

Ference RA, Truscott S, Whitehead PC (1986) Drinking and the prevention of coronary heart disease: findings, issues, and public health policy. J Stud Alcohol 47:394–408

Fortmann SP, Haskell WL, Vranizan K, et al (1983) The association of blood pressure and dietary alcohol: differences by age, sex and estrogen use. Am J Epidemiol 118:497–507

Fostermann U, Feuerstein TJ (1987) Decreased systemic formation of prostaglandin E and prostacyclin in alcoholics during withdrawal as estimated from metabolites in urine. Clin Sci 73:277–83

Friedman GD, Klatsky AL, Siegelaub AB (1982) Alcohol, tobacco and hypertension. Hypertension 4(suppl 3):143–50

Gilles GE, Linton EA, Lowri PJ (1982) Cortico-trophin releasing activity of the new CRF is potentiated several times by vasopressin. Nature 29:355–57

Gordon T, Kannel WB (1983) Drinking and its relation to smoking, blood pressure, blood lipids and uric acid. Arch Intern Med 143:1366–74

Gordon T, Doyle JT (1986) Alcohol consumption and its relationship to smoking, weight, blood pressure, and blood lipids: the Albany Study. Arch Intern Med 146:262–65

Grobbee DE (1992) Alcohol and blood pressure. In Veenstra J, van der Heij DG (eds), Alcohol and cardiovascular disease. Pudoc, Wageningen, pp 23–34

Gruchow HW, Sobocinski KA, Barboriak JJ (1985) Alcohol, nutrient intake, and hypertension in U.S. adults. JAMA 253:1567–70

Gyntelberg F, Meyer J (1974) Relationship between blood pressure and physical fitness, smoking and alcohol consumption in Copenhagen males aged 40–59. Acta Med Scand 195:375–80

Harburg E, Ozgoren F, Hawthorne VM, Schork MA (1980) Community norms of alcohol usage and blood pressure. Am J Public Health 70:813–20

Hennekens CH (1983) Alcohol. In Kaplan NM, Stamler J (eds), Prevention of coronary heart disease. Practical management of the risk factors. W.B. Saunders, Philadelphia, pp 130–38

Hofman A, Grobbee DE, Valkenburg HA (1985) Een epidemiologisch onderzoek naar het verband tussen alcohol en hoge bloeddruk. Ned Tijdschr Geneeskd 129:639–41

Howes LG, Reid JL (1985) Decreased vascular responsiveness to noradrenaline following regular ethanol consumption. Br J Clin Pharmacol 20:669–74

Howes LG, Reid JL (1986) Changes in blood pressure and autonomy reflexes following regular moderate alcohol consumption. J Hypertens 4:421–25

Howes LG, Reid JL (1987) The effects of alcohol on local neural and humoral cardiovascular regulation. Clin Sci 71:9–15

Howes LG, MacGilchrist A, Hawksby C, et al. (1986) Plasma (3H)-noradrenaline kinetics and blood pressure following regular moderate ethanol consumption. Br J Clin Pharmacol 22:521–26

Ibsen H, Christensen NJ, Rasmusen S, et al. (1985) Effect of high alcohol intake on blood pressure, adrenergic activity and the renin-angiotensin system. Scand J Clin Lab Invest 45(suppl):176:87–91

Ireland M, Vandongen R, Davidson L, et al. (1984) Acute effect of moderate alcohol consumption on blood pressure and plasma catecholamines. Clin Sci 66:643–48

Jackson R, Stewart A, Beaglehole R, Scragg R (1985) Alcohol consumption and blood pressure. Am J Epidemiol 122:1034–44

Kagan A, Yano K, Rhoads GG, McGee DL (1981) Alcohol and cardiovascular disease: the Hawaian experience. Circulation 64(suppl 3):27–31

Katz AM (1982) Effects of ethanol on ion transport in muscle membranes. Fed Proc 41:2456–59

Keil U, Chambless L, Remmers A (1989) Alcohol and blood pressure: results from the Lübeck Blood Pressure Study. Prev Med 18:1–10

Keil U, Chambless L, Filipiak B, Härtel U (1991) Alcohol and blood pressure and its interaction with smoking and other behavioural variables: results from the MONICA Augsburg Survey 1984/85. J Hypertens 9:491–98

Klag MJ, Moore RD, Whelton PK, et al. (1990) Alcohol consumption and blood pressure: a comparison of native Japanese to American men. J Clin Epidemiol 43:1407–14

Klatsky AL, Friedman GD, Siegeland AB, Gerard MJ (1977) Alcohol consumption and blood pressure. N Engl J Med 296:1194–1200

Klatsky AL, Friedman GD, Armstrong MA (1986) The relationships between alcoholic beverage use and other traits to blood pressure: a new Kaiser Permanente study. Circulation 73:628–36

Knochel JP (1983) Cardiovascular effects of alcohol. Ann Intern Med 98:849–54

Knupfer G (1987) Drinking for health: the daily light drinker myth. Br J Addict 82:547–55

Kondo K, Ebihara A (1984) Alcohol consumption and blood pressure in a rural community of Japan. In Lovenberg W, Yamori Y (eds), Nutritional prevention of cardiovascular disease. Academic Press, Orlando, FL, pp 217–24

Kornhuber HH, Lisson G, Suschka-Sauermann L (1985) Alcohol and obesity: a new look at high blood pressure and stroke; an epidemiological study in preventive neurology. Eur Arch Psychiatry Neurol Sci 234:357–62

Kozarevic DJ, Vojvodic N, Dawber T, et al. (1980) Frequency of alcohol consumption and morbidity and mortality: the Yugoslavia Cardiovascular Disease Study. Lancet 1:613–16

Kozarevic D, Racic Z, Gordon T, et al. (1982) Drinking habits and other characteristics: the Yugoslavia Cardiovascular Disease Study. Am J Epidemiol 116:287–301

Kromhout D, Bosschieter EB, de Lezenne Coulander C (1985) Potassium, calcium, alcohol intake and blood pressure: the Zutphen Study. Am J Clin Nutr 41:1299–1304

Lang T, Degoulet P, Aime F, et al. (1987) Relationship between alcohol consumption and hypertension prevalence and control in a French population. J Chronic Dis 40:713–20

Lian C (1915) L'alcoolisme, cause d'hypertension arterielle. Bull Acad Natl Med 74:525–28

Linkola J (1979) Alcohol and hypertension. N Engl J Med 98:849–54

Linsky A, Straus M, Colby J (1985) Stressful events, stressful conditions and alcohol problems in the United States: a partial test of Bayes' theory. J Stud Alcohol 46:47–80

MacMahon S (1987) Alcohol consumption and hypertension. Hypertension 9:111–21

MacMahon SW, Blacket RB, MacDonald GJ, Hall W (1984) Obesity, alcohol consumption and blood pressure in Australian men and women. The National Heart Foundation of Australia Risk Factor Prevalence Study. J Hypertens 2:85–91

Maheswaran R, Beevers M, Beevers DG (1992) Effectiveness of advice to reduce alcohol consumption in hypertensive patients. Hypertension 19:79–84

Malhotra H, Mathur D, Mehta SR, Khandewal PD (1985) Pressor effects of alcohol in normotensive and hypertensive subjects. Lancet 2:584–86

Marmot MG, Shipley MJ, Rose G, Thomas BJ (1981) Alcohol and mortality: a U-shaped curve. Lancet 2:580–83

Mendelson JH, Mello NK (1979) Biologic concomitants of alcoholism. N Engl J Med 301:912–21

Midanek LT, Klatsky AL, Armstrong MA (1990) Changes in drinking behaviour: demographic, psychosocial and biochemical factors. Int J Addict 25:599–619

Milon H, Froment A, Gaspard P, et al. (1982) Alcohol consumption and blood pressure in a French epidemiological study. Eur Heart J 3:59–64

Mitchell PI, Morgan MJ, Boadle DJ, et al. (1980) Role of alcohol in the etiology of hypertension. Med J Aust 2:198–200

Myrhed M (1974) Alcohol consumption in relation to factors associated with ischemic heart disease. Acta Med Scand 195(suppl I):567

Orrego H, Blake JE, Blendis LM, Kapur BM (1979) Reliability of assessment of alcohol intake based on personal interviews in a liver clinic. Lancet 2:1354–56

Parker M, Puddey IB, Beilin LJ, Vandongen R (1990) A 2-way factorial study of alcohol and salt restriction in treated hypertensive men. Hypertension 16:398–406

Paulin JM, Simpson FO, Waal-Manning HJ (1985) Alcohol consumption and blood pressure in a New Zealand community study. N Z Med J 98:425–28

Pincherle G, Robinson D (1974) Mean blood pressure and its relation to other factors determined at a routine executive health examination. J Chronic Dis 27:245–60

Pohorecky L (1974) Effects of ethanol on central and peripheral noradrenergic neurones. J Pharmacol Exp Ther 189:380–91

Pohorecky L (1991) Stress and alcohol interaction: an update on human research. Alcohol Clin Exp Res 15:438–59

Poikolainen K, Karkkainen P (1983) Diary gives more accurate information about alcohol consumption than questionnaire. Drug Alcohol Depend 11:209–16

Potter JF, Beevers DG (1984) Pressor effect of alcohol in hypertension. Lancet 1:119–22

Puddey IB, Vandongen R, Beilin LJ, Rouse IL (1985a) Alcohol stimulation of renin release in man—its relation to the hemodynamic, electrolyte and sympatho-adrenal responses to drinking. J Clin Endocrinol Metab 61:37–42

Puddey IB, Beilin LJ, Vandongen R, et al. (1985b) Evidence for a direct effect of alcohol consumption on blood pressure in normotensive men: a randomized controlled trial. Hypertension 7:707–13

Puddey IB, Beilin LJ, Vandongen R (1987) Regular alcohol use raises blood pressure in treated hypertensive subjects—a randomized controlled trial. Lancet 1:647–51

Ramsay LE (1977a) Liver dysfunction in hypertension. Lancet 1:111–14

Ramsay LE (1977b). Alcohol and hypertension. Lancet 2:300

Reed D, McGee D, Yano K (1982) Biological and social correlates of blood pressure among Japanese men in Hawaii. Hypertension 4:406–14

Salonen JT, Tuomilehto J, Tanskanen A (1983) Relation of blood pressure to reported intake of salt, saturated fats, and alcohol in a healthy middle aged population. J Epidemiol Community Health 37:32–37

Salvaggio A, Periti M, Miano L, et al. (1991) Analysis of the relation between blood pressure and both self-reported and biochemically inferred alcohol consumption. J Hypertens 9(suppl 6):S276–77

Saunders JB, Beevers DG, Paton A (1979) Factors influencing blood pressure in chronic alcoholics. Clin Sci 57:295s–98s

Saunders JB, Beevers DG, Paton A (1981) Alcohol-induced hypertension. Lancet 2:653–56

Savdie E, Grosslight GM, Adena MA (1984) Relation of alcohol and cigarette consumption to blood pressure and serum creatinine levels. J Chronic Dis 37:617–23

Schnall PL, Schwartz JP, et al. (1992) Relation between job strain, alcohol, and ambulatory blood pressure. Hypertension 19:488–94

Simon J, Filipovsky J, et al. (1988) Cross-sectional study of beer consumption and blood pressure in middle-aged men. J Human Hypertens 2:1–6

Stamler R, Stamler J, Grim MR, et al. (1987) Nutritional therapy for high blood pressure: final report of a four year randomised controlled trial—the Hypertension Control Program. JAMA 257:1484–91

Stott DJ, Ball SG, Inglis GC, et al. (1987) Effects of a single moderate dose of alcohol and blood pressure, heart rate and associated metabolic and endocrine changes. Clin Sci 73:411–16

Trevisan M, Krogh V, Farinaro E, et al. (1987) Alcohol consumption, drinking pattern and blood pressure: analysis of data from the Italian National Research Council Study. Int J Epidemiol 16:520–27

Ueshima H, Shimamoto T, Iada M, et al. (1984) Alcohol intake and hypertension among urban and rural Japanese populations. J Chronic Dis 37:585–92

Wannamethee G, Shaper AG (1991) Alcohol intake and variations in blood pressure by day of examination. J Human Hypertens 5:59–67

Weissfeld JL, Johnson EH, Brock BM, Hawthorne VM (1988) Sex and age interactions in the association between alcohol and blood pressure. Am J Epidemiol 128:559–69

West LJ, Maxwell DS, Noble EP, Solomon DH (1984) Alcoholism. Ann Intern Med 100:405–16

Wicklung RA, Sanne K, Vedin WJ, Wilhelmsen L (1984) Sick-role and attitude towards disease and working life two months after a myocardial infarction. Scand J Rehabil Med 16:57–84

Witteman JCM, Willett WC, Stampfer MJ, et al. (1989) A prospective study of nutritional factors and hypertension among U.S. women. Circulation 80:1320–27

Yamada Y, Ishizaki M, Kido T, et al. (1991) Alcohol, high blood pressure, and serum τ-glutamyl transpeptidase level. Hypertension 18:819–26

3

The Association Between Alcohol and Stroke

J. van Gijn
University of Utrecht, The Netherlands

M.J. Stampfer
Harvard Medical School, United States

C. Wolfe
St. Thomas's Hospital
London University, United Kingdom

A. Algra
University of Utrecht, The Netherlands

Abstract

Stroke can be either ischaemic (thromboembolism) or haemor-rhagic (intracerebral haemorrhage or subarachnoid haemorrhage). Theo-retically, alcohol may interact with a variety of intermediate factors that have been implicated in the pathogenesis of one or both types of stroke: increased blood pressure (ischaemic as well as haemorrhagic stroke), heart disease (ischaemic stroke), vasoconstriction (ischaemic stroke), total cholesterol (positively associated with ischaemic stroke, negatively with haemorrhagic stroke), and antiaggregant and fibri-nolytic effects (negative association with ischaemic stroke, positive as-sociation with haemorrhagic stroke). The relative importance of all these factors is unknown; epidemiological observations reflect the net effects.

From case-control studies, moderate drinkers (< 60 g/day) appear to have an equal or modestly elevated risk of total stroke com-pared with nondrinkers. There is some evidence of a J-shaped associa-tion between level of alcohol intake and total stroke in white popula-tions, with reduced risk for those reporting light drinking. All studies specifically addressing ischaemic stroke risk found no association with alcohol use. A nonlinear association cannot be ruled out in two of these studies but was not present in the third in a predominantly black population. For haemorrhagic stroke, a nonsignificant positive linear association was found between customary alcohol consumption and the relative risk of stroke in three nested case-control studies, but a high relative risk was estimated in a fourth study.

Some case-control studies suggest that stroke can be precipitated by the ingestion of large quantities of alcohol ("binge drinking"), but the association depends at least in part on confounding variables, and the precision of the odds ratio estimates is unclear.

At least 19 prospective studies, with an aggregate of nearly 2 mil-lion person-years of observation, have been reported to date. For total stroke, no strong evidence for any association is present, except for an apparently modest increase in risk in the highest level of alcohol intake. When the data are segregated according to the two broad cate-gories of stroke types, consistent patterns emerge. For haemorrhagic stroke, there is strong evidence for an association, with typically about a threefold excess risk for higher levels of alcohol consumption. In contrast, there is equally strong evidence against any material adverse association with ischaemic stroke.

Definitions of Stroke and Alcohol Consumption

Subtypes of Stroke

A stroke is a focal neurological deficit of sudden onset, presumably caused by a vascular lesion of the brain. These vascular lesions include occlusion of a vessel, usually an artery (brain infarction), as well as rupture of an intracerebral artery (brain haemorrhage). These two main categories of stroke can again be subdivided according to the site or the underlying cause (if known). Certain risk factors are common to both cerebral infarction and (intra)cerebral haemorrhage, hypertension being the most prominent example, but other factors act in an opposing fashion. For instance, inhibition of coagulation factors or of platelet aggregation decreases the risk of cerebral infarction but increases the risk of intracerebral haemorrhage. For this reason, the blanket term "stroke" shall, wherever possible, be subdivided in broad categories, according to the most important differences in pathophysiology.

The following three subtypes of stroke are distinguished in this report according to the different features that can be recognised morphologically:

(1) *Cerebral infarction* (approximately 85% of all strokes, according to Bamford et al. 1990 and Ricci et al. 1991): This consists of ischaemic necrosis of a part of the brain, most often in the territory of a large or small cerebral artery, more rarely in the border zone area between two such territories. The cause is an occlusion of the artery in question, usually by an embolus from an atherothrombotic lesion in an extracerebral artery or from the heart, less often by local thrombosis.

(2) *Intracerebral haemorrhage* (approximately 10% of all strokes): This is an extravasation of blood into the brain parenchyma, most often in the deep regions of the brain (basal ganglia, brain stem, or cerebellum). In older persons, the most common cause is rupture of a small perforating artery; in young adults, an arteriovenous malformation is the most frequent underlying anatomical abnormality.

(3) *Subarachnoid haemorrhage* (approximately 5% of all strokes): This condition is characterised by extravasation of blood primarily in the subarachnoid space at the base of the brain. The most common cause (90%) is a ruptured aneurysm of the circle of Willis.

It should be recognised that the clinical diagnosis is often less accurate than the pathological definition, depending on the clinical criteria and the use of ancillary investigations. As mentioned above, the term "stroke" is rather global, referring to a sudden, focal, and prolonged disturbance of cerebral function, presumably of vascular origin. In up to one-third of patients with a provisional diagnosis of stroke in the community, however, the final diagnosis is that of a non-vascular condition (Oxfordshire Community Stroke Project 1983). The most common errors are epilepsy, intoxications, psychogenic attacks, intracranial tumours, and traumatic haematomas, in that order (Norris and Hachinski 1982). In addition, the clinical distinction between intracerebral haemorrhage and cerebral infarction may be difficult. If a focal deficit is accompanied by headache or an impaired level of consciousness, an intracerebral haemorrhage is the most likely of the two, but the opposite is less often true: small haemorrhages may masquerade as infarcts. Subarachnoid haemorrhage differs clinically from the other two stroke types in that focal deficits are the exception rather than the rule, and that nonfocal symptoms such as headache or unconsciousness predominate.

The most important investigation is the computerised tomography (CT) scan. Cerebral haemorrhages are immediately recognisable as localised hyperdense lesions in the brain parenchyma (intracerebral haemorrhages) or in the subarachnoid cisterns (subarachnoid haemorrhage), whereas cerebral infarction is characterised by a hypodense area in the territory of a single artery (small or large), at least two or three days after onset; an additional advantage of CT scanning is that most other conditions in the differential diagnosis can be excluded.

Some but not all studies cited in this review have included CT scanning in the diagnostic criteria. Even if they have, CT scanning was often performed in only a minority. It is unavoidable that the accuracy with which these three subtypes of stroke have been separated from other conditions and from each other varies among the different studies cited in this report.

Alcohol Consumption

Camargo (1989) undertook an extensive search of the English-language literature and examined the relationship between moderate alcohol consumption (< 60 g/day ethanol) and the risk of stroke. To facilitate comparison between different studies, reported levels were converted to standard drinks per day, where the average drink is assumed to contain 12 g, 15 ml, or 0.5 fl oz of alcohol; 12 g is the appropriate content of 12 fl oz of beer, 4 fl oz of wine, or 1.5 fl oz of spirits. In this report, the same units have been adopted whenever possible.

Pathophysiological Background

Ethanol interacts with a variety of intermediate factors that are presumed to be involved in the pathogenesis of stroke (Gorelick 1987). The direction of this interaction is favourable in some respects and unfavourable in others. Current knowledge does not allow us to attribute the opposite trends for moderate and heavy use of alcohol, discussed in other sections of this report, to specific intermediate factors. Moreover, the effects on haemostasis may counteract infarction but promote haemorrhage, or vice versa.

The biochemical effects of ethanol can be subdivided into modification of established risk factors, influence on vessel diameter and blood flow, and effects on haemostasis (platelet aggregation and coagulation factors).

Modification of Risk Factors

Hypertension is by far the most important risk factor for stroke. The level of blood pressure is related to the incidence of stroke for severe, moderate, and even mild hypertensives (MacMahon et al. 1990). The presence of hypertension was found to be associated with the frequency of alcohol consumption in population studies in the United States (Klatsky et al. 1977, Witteman et al. 1990), and in former Yugoslavia (Kozarevic et al. 1980).

Cholesterol (total level) is significantly and independently related to the development of atherosclerosis in men and women. High density lipoprotein (HDL) cholesterol has an inverse association, and low density lipoprotein (LDL) cholesterol has a direct relationship to the incidence of coronary heart disease; but for total stroke or ischaemic stroke, the relationship with total serum cholesterol and cholesterol subfractions is less clear or consistent in different population-based studies (Wolf et al. 1992). The relationship to stroke in general may be obscured, because low levels of total cholesterol increase the risk of fatal intracerebral haemorrhage (Iso et al. 1989). Regular use of alcohol is associated with an increased total level of cholesterol (Kozarevic et al. 1980). On the other hand, data from five study populations indicated a consistently positive relationship between alcohol intake and HDL cholesterol, against an equally consistent though less strong negative relation with LDL cholesterol (Castelli et al. 1977).

Heart diseases such as atrial fibrillation, previous myocardial infarction, or congestive heart disease predispose to stroke, partly because thrombi that form in the heart can be dislodged to cause occlusion of cerebral arteries, and partly because of an indirect relationship, with atherosclerosis as a common cause. Heart disease may be related to alcohol consumption in different ways. Episodes of heavy drinking may induce disturbances of heart rhythm, particularly atrial fibrillation ("holiday heart"; Ettinger et al. 1978). In addition, alcoholic cardiomyopathy may lead to congestive heart failure, arrhythmias, and the formation of mural thrombi (Demakis et al. 1974). On the other hand, moderate intake of alcohol is known to reduce the risk of ischaemic heart disease.

Vessel Diameter and Blood Flow

Although most ischaemic strokes are caused by artery-to-artery embolism or by local thrombosis and not by haemodynamic factors, impairment of cerebral blood flow should be considered an adverse factor that may contribute to the pathogenesis of cerebral infarction.

Regional cerebral blood flow, measured by means of the ^{133}Xenon inhalation method, correlates inversely with the amount of alcohol consumed by healthy volunteers (Rogers et al. 1983), and is further reduced in patients with risk factors for stroke and in patients with Wernicke-Korsakow syndrome as a result of chronic alcoholism (Berglund 1981, Rogers et al. 1983). These effects may reflect a depression of cerebral metabolism by ethanol rather than a direct effect on cerebral blood flow and are not necessarily related to the risk of stroke.

On the other hand, in rats a direct vasoconstrictive effect has been demonstrated on the cerebral microvasculature in vivo as well as on large cerebral arteries in vitro (Altura et al. 1983). A further analysis of the influence of ethanol on cerebral arterioles in rats failed to demonstrate an alteration of the baseline diameter, but did demonstrate an impairment of the endothelium-dependent dilatation in response to acetylcholine, histamine, and adenosine diphosphate (Mayhan 1992).

Effects on Platelet Aggregation and Coagulation

An overview of placebo-controlled trials with antiplatelet agents in general (particularly aspirin), in a variety of patients at risk for arterial disease, demonstrated an overall reduction in the incidence of nonfatal stroke by approximately 30% and in the incidence of fatal vascular events of approximately 15% (Antiplatelet Trialists' Collaboration 1988). Agents that impair platelet aggregation are therefore potentially beneficial in the prevention of stroke.

An antiplatelet effect of ethanol is evident from a significant prolongation of the bleeding time in volunteers (Elmér et al. 1984). In another study with a smaller number of subjects, ethanol did not significantly prolong the bleeding times, but it had a powerful potentiating effect on the prolongation of the bleeding time induced by aspirin (Deykin et al. 1982). It is not quite clear how the effect of alcohol on platelets is mediated. Moderate doses of ethanol cause an increase in the level of prostacyclin, a powerful antiaggregant and vasodilator, when added to a culture of endothelial cells or measured in plasma of volunteers (Landolfi and Steiner 1984). Ethanol in vitro enhances the antiaggregating effects of prostacyclin as well as that of aspirin, independently and in a dose-dependent fashion (Jakubowski et al. 1988). Only one study found that ethanol caused, on average, a transient increase in the aggregatory response of platelets to adenoside diphosphate (Hillbom et al. 1985), but the variation among individuals was great; moreover, it is uncertain whether adenosine diphosphate is important as an aggregating agent in vivo.

Pharmacological interference with fibrinolysis can theoretically affect the risk of stroke. Increased fibrinolysis may promote intracerebral haemorrhage but lower the risk of cerebral infarction, and vice versa for impairment of fibrinolysis. That alcohol enhances fibrinolysis is suggested in vitro by augmented secretion of plasminogen activator by bovine endothelial cells (Laug 1983), and in a population study by the relation between reported alcohol consumption and increased fibrinolytic activity in plasma (Meade et al. 1979). Ethanol does not directly cause disorders of blood coagulation (Elmér et al. 1984). In chronic alcoholics with cirrhosis of the liver, the decreased capacity for protein synthesis results in a deficiency of clotting factors; in addition, these patients often have low platelet counts resulting from decreased survival and impaired thrombopoiesis (Cowan 1980). Coagulation disorders from liver damage and thrombocytopenia were reported in six consecutive alcoholic patients with intracerebral haemorrhage (Weisberg 1988).

Alcohol withdrawal after excessive consumption causes hyperaggregability in vitro after 1 week, as opposed to hypoaggregability on admission (Hutton et al. 1981). "Rebound thrombocytosis" was reported after alcohol withdrawal in five alcoholic patients, with peak values between 10 and 15 days after admission; two of these patients previously had recurrent episodes of venous thrombosis or pulmonary embolism (Haselager and Vreeken 1977). Thrombocytosis may predispose to arterial as well as venous thrombosis, and may well be a factor in the occurrence of ischaemic stroke in young adults after "binge drinking."

Habitual Intake of Alcohol and Stroke: Case-Control Studies

The case-control study is used primarily to assess risks, to study causes of disease in general, and involves observations of naturally occurring exposures and disease. Ideally, exposure-disease associations detected in an exploratory study should be considered tentative until more definitive evidence is obtained, fulfilling Bradford Hill's criteria of causality (Hill 1965). Two types of subject are sampled: persons with (cases) and without (controls) the disease of interest. The odds of having a particular risk factor in one group are compared to the odds in the other, providing an odds ratio of that risk factor for the disease. The advantages of case-control studies are that they are relatively cheap to undertake, compared to prospective studies, and do not depend on a long follow-up period to determine the results. Case-control studies can also be employed to assess the acute effects of high levels of alcohol consumption on the risk of stroke.

Potential Pitfalls of Case-Control Studies

Several methodological issues that should be addressed by those undertaking case-control studies are worth outlining before describing the literature on the association between stroke and alcohol. Cases should be representative of the disease under study, and a case definition that includes the World Health Organisation definition of stroke (Aho et al. 1980) and use of CT scan to confirm stroke and its subtype should be used. It is particularly relevant to the relationship between stroke and alcohol that the differentiation between cerebral ischaemia and haemorrhage be made. Also, imprecise ascertainment of stroke incidence and mortality will tend to weaken statistical associations with true risk factors.

Cases should be representative of the disease, and controls should be comparable with cases but without the disease under study. Much debate has surrounded the selection of cases and controls, the advantages and disadvantages of hospital- or community-based controls, and the generalisability of the results when different assessments are made of cases and controls in relation to alcohol and stroke. Of pivotal importance to alcohol studies is the recall of alcohol intake over the short and long term and how to record intake from patients who are either dead or unable to communicate. As no biological marker presently exists to accurately quantify the amount and frequency of chronic alcohol use, ascertainment of customary or typical alcohol consumption relies on direct enquiry and self-reported information, parameters that may be subject to recall bias. Recall bias is a systematic error due to differences of completeness of recall to memory of prior events or experiences that may occur between those that have had a stroke and those that have not. There is also a lack of a reference standard for validating self-reported drinking. For this reason, a relative risk calculated may achieve only rank-order validity. Another problem is that studies that fail to differentiate lifelong abstainers from former drinkers in the reference group may underestimate the relative risk at all levels of alcohol consumption. Finally, consensus on definition of light, moderate, and heavy alcohol consumption must be developed (Gorelick 1989). Causal inferences from observational studies should be made with caution, and it is important to adjust for the most likely confounders in the analysis, such as smoking, blood pressure, age, and sex, which may all have independent effects on the risk of stroke.

Although it is important to adjust for the confounding effect of such factors as cigarette smoking, age, and sex in order to assess the independent effect of alcohol on stroke, the biases introduced by controlling for hypertension, which itself may be caused by the moderate to high alcohol intake, need to be considered. Therefore, by controlling for hypertension in the analysis, one may be "over-controlling" for this effect, which may reduce the risk associated with alcohol. Control strategies initially should not include stroke risk factors that might serve as potential mediators of a causal association between alcohol intake and stroke. These mediators may include blood pressure, cardiac disease, atherosclerosis, lipoproteins, haematocrit and haemostasis parameters. Control of these factors should be reserved for final analysis aiming to assess to what extent measured variables explain the relationship between alcohol and stroke.

The choice of controls is a particular problem that has been discussed in relation to alcohol and stroke and is discussed in more detail below. It essentially revolves around how specific a group the controls are drawn from. For example, some studies have taken emergency surgical admissions as controls for the index stroke case. In that control group, alcohol-related disease is more prevalent, so the effect of high alcohol intake would be masked in the stroke group. The control group should be comparable with the stroke cases, and to use any group other than a random selection of cases from the community at large will introduce biases that need to be considered. Although it is virtually impossible to overcome these choice of control problems, more recent studies have addressed the effect of hospital and community controls on the estimated risk of alcohol on stroke.

Total Stroke

There is some evidence that chronic alcoholism and heavy drinking (> 60 g ethanol/day, or 4–6 drinks) are associated with increased risk of all types of stroke (Sundby 1967, Lindegard and Hillbom 1987, Calandre et al. 1986, Niizuma et al. 1988). It is the role of light or moderate alcohol intake, however, on which the present report is focused. This is important since the majority of the population reports light or moderate alcohol consumption, which, if associated with stroke, would have important implications for health promotion initiatives.

Seventeen case-control studies have been reviewed (see Table 1); these examined the relation between moderate alcohol intake and stroke. In the earliest study, Peacock (1972) described a modestly elevated odds ratio (1.5), but this was for total stroke, and no adjustment was made for confounding variables. However, 283 cases and 8519 controls were used. Further U.S. studies in the early 1980s (Taylor 1982, Taylor et al. 1984, Taylor and Combs-Orme 1985) estimated the risk of stroke generally, excluding subarachnoid haemorrhage, to be 2.2 after control for age, sex, and race. Further studies failed to demonstrate increased risk of stroke in drinkers (Oleckno 1986, 1988, Abu-Zeid et al. 1977, Herman et al. 1983). Oleckno compared young stroke patients from northern Illinois with both inpatient and community controls and in both analyses found comparable risk of total stroke in drinkers and nondrinkers. The first study to examine risk at different levels of alcohol intake (Herman et al. 1983) also failed to show any differences with nondrinkers.

More recently, von Arbin et al. (1985) studied a group of patients in which the case definition included first stroke, repeat stroke, and transient ischaemic attack; controls were admitted for acute surgical disorders, thereby representing a potentially biased group. The authors observed a J-shaped association, cases being more likely to report

Table 1
Case-control studies of moderate drinking and stroke

Reference	Population	Cases	Control	Alcohol (drinks/days)	Odds ratios[a]	Controlled for
Peacock 1972	Birmingham, Alabama M+W, age 50–69 years 283 cases, 8519 controls	Community, with history of stroke	Community	Nondrinkers Drinkers	Total stroke 1.0 1.5 (1.2–1.9)	No adjustment
Taylor 1985	St. Louis, Missouri M+W, aged 24–87 years 64 cases, 64 controls	Hospitalized (excludes SAH)	Inpatient	Nondrinkers Drinkers	Total stroke[b] 1.0 2.2 (1.1–4.4)	Age, sex, race
Oleckno 1986	Northern Illinois M+W, age 15–40 years 80 cases, 321 controls	Hospitalized with first stroke (excludes SAH)	Inpatient	Nondrinkers Drinkers	Total Stroke 1.0 0.6	Age, sex, diabetes, HTN, CVD
Oleckno 1988	Northern Illinois M+W, age 15–40 years 50 cases, 864 controls	Hospitalized with first stroke (excludes SAH)	Community	Nondrinkers Drinkers	Total Stroke 1.0 1.5	Age, sex, race, diabetes, smoking, HTN, CVD
Abu-Zeid 1977	Winnipeg, Canada M+W, mean age 67 years 606 cases, 606 controls	Hospitalized with first stroke	Inpatient	Nondrinkers Drinkers	HS IS 1.0 1.0 1.4 1.5	Age, sex, residence

M men; W women; IS ischemic stroke; HS hemorrhagic stroke; ICH intracerebral hemorrhage; SAH subarachnoid hemorrhage; TIA transient ischemic attack; HTN hypertension; CVD cardiovascular disease. Alcohol in standard drinks per day (12 g ethanol/drink); see text.
[a]95% confidence interval in parentheses.
[b]Unmatched analysis of matched data.

Table 1. *Continued*

Reference	Population	Cases	Control	Alcohol (drinks/days)	Odds ratios[a]		Controlled for
Herman 1983	Tilburg, The Netherlands M+W, age 40–74 years 132 cases, 239 controls	Hospitalized with first stroke	Inpatient	Nondrinkers < 2 ≥ 2	Total stroke 1.0 0.9 1.3		Age, sex
Von Arbin 1985	Stockholm, Sweden M+W, age ≥ 50 years 209 cases, 209 controls	Hospitalized (includes TIA)	Inpatient	Nondrinkers < 0.4 0.4–1.9 > 1.9	Total stroke (%, case vs. control) 22 vs. 12 ($p < 0.01$) 53 vs. 64 ($p < 0.05$) 29 vs. 23 18 vs. 14		Age, sex
Gill 1988	Birmingham, England M+W, age 20–70 years 230 cases, 577 controls	Hospitalized	Community	Nondrinkers ≤ 1.3 1.4–4.1 ≥ 4.2	Total stroke (M) 1.0 0.5 (0.2–1.2) 1.0 1.8 (0.8–4.5)	Total stroke (F) 1.0 0.4 (0.2–1.1) 0.4	Age, sex, race, smoking, medication, social stratum
Gorelick 1989	Chicago, Illinois M+W, age > 44 years 205 cases, 410 controls	Hospitalized with first IS	Outpatient	Nondrinkers < 1.2 1.2–3.5 ≥ 3.6	IS 1.0 1.9 (0.9–3.9) 2.0 (1.0–3.7) 1.7 (0.8–3.4)		Age, sex, race, smoking, method of hospital payment, HTN

Study	Population	Outcome	Design	Exposure / Results	Adjusted for
Stemmermann 1984	Honolulu, Hawaii M, age 45–68 years 79 cases, 191 controls	Stroke on autopsy, 16 yr follow-up	Autopsied cohort	Average drinks/day (case vs. control) IS: 1.1 vs. 1.7 HS: 2.4 vs. 1.7	Age, sex
	79 cases, 6753 controls	Stroke on autopsy, 16 yr follow-up	Living cohort	Average drinks/day (case vs. control) IS: 1.2 vs. 1.1 HS: 2.5 vs. 1.1 ($p < 0.01$)	Age, sex (see text)
Sacco 1984	Framingham, Mass. M+W, age 30–62 years 36 cases, 144 controls	First SAH during 26-yr follow-up	Cohort	"No significant differences" in average daily intake of SAH cases vs. controls[c]	Age, sex
Petitti 1979	Walnut Creek, California W, age 18–54 years 34 cases, ? controls	First stroke during 6.5 yr follow-up (includes TIA)	Cohort	Other Stroke / SAH Nondrinkers 1.0 / 1.0 Drinkers 1.3 / 2.5	Age, sex
Monforte 1990	Spain M+W, 33–63 years 24 cases, 48 controls	Hospitalized, CT scan proven (includes intracerebral hemorrhage)	Medical admissions	>100g Univariate 15.82 (2–124) Multivariate 13.31 (1.5–119)	Alcohol, HTN, sex, age, smoking
Ben-Shlomo 1991	Birmingham, England M+W, 15–69 years 164 cases, 165 general controls, 115 select controls, 752 community controls	Hospitalized with first stroke	General medical, selected admissions, community	>300 g General 0.73 (0.54–3.49) Select 1.53 (0.42–4.05) Community 1.93 (0.87–4.28) No significant difference	HTN, cigarettes, CVD, race

M men; W women; IS ischemic stroke; HS hemorrhagic stroke; ICH intracerebral hemorrhage; SAH subarachnoid hemorrhage; TIA transient ischemic attack; HTN hypertension; CVD cardiovascular disease. Alcohol in standard drinks per day (12 g ethanol/drink); see text.
[a] 95% confidence interval in parentheses.
[b] Details of odds ratio not given in this study; p value in parentheses.
[c] "No significant differences" in average daily intake of SAH cases vs. controls.

nondrinking, less likely to report light drinking (< 0.4 drinks/day), and yet having a higher average daily alcohol intake than controls (1.6 vs. 1 drink; $p < 0.05$), but because of the methodological inadequacies of the study these findings should be considered with caution.

The studies from Gill et al. in Birmingham, England (1985, 1986, 1988) demonstrate the J-shaped association of total stroke more strongly. This group addressed in detail the methodological problems with the selection of controls from general hospital, select hospital, and community, although the latter are actually drawn from industry rather than electoral registers. In the first report, cases were compared with matched inpatient controls. Controls were admitted for routine surgical procedures and were excluded if there was a history of previous stroke, conditions related to excessive alcohol use, or diseases that alter liver function. There was criticism of the choice of criteria for selecting cases and controls, the criteria being applied only to controls (Kiefe et al. 1987). Reanalysis of the data for first strokes only did not affect the results, and the authors indicated that only one case would have been excluded had the criteria been applied to cases. Recent alcohol consumption and haematological alcohol markers were assessed. A lower risk was observed in light drinkers than in nondrinkers, which was the same as the trend seen in the biochemical markers. Multivariate analysis revealed the J-shaped association among men ($p < 0.01$) but not among women.

The second study using the industrial workers as community controls came up with the same J-shaped association, but the odds ratio in the heavier drinkers was reduced from 4.2 to 1.8. The reduced relative risk of female light drinkers almost reached statistical significance. The validation of a structured alcohol intake questionnaire with liver enzymes lends support to the associations observed in these studies. These studies employed the Allen score to differentiate type of stroke, only 20% having a CT scan.

The final study from this group (Ben-Shlomo et al. 1992) illustrated how the relative risk associated with alcohol varied depending on whether community, general medical admissions, or selected (excluding possible alcohol-related admissions) controls were used. The relative risks for alcohol intake of more than 300 g/week ranged from 0.73 (with confidence intervals of 0.54–3.49) for general medical controls to 1.93 (with confidence intervals of 0.87–4.28) for community-based controls. None of these associations was significant, and no dose-response effect was observed. There was also a poor (37%) response rate from community controls, potentially biasing the results. It was also only possible to obtain an alcohol history from 29 out of 49 cases. The authors considered that their study, like previous studies, had insufficient power to significantly detect a modest increase in risk of total stroke associated with moderate alcohol consumption. Because of the biases involved in choosing control groups, the true risk may be underestimated by hospital controls and overestimated by community controls.

Ischaemic Stroke

From the data presented it is not possible to determine whether the J-shaped association is related to ischaemic or haemorrhagic stroke, but since 70–85% of strokes are ischaemic, one might assume that the J-shaped association resulted from a similar relation with ischaemic stroke. Gorelick et al. (1989) compared predominantly black ischaemic stroke patients with matched medical outpatients in whom the diagnosis was not reported. Drinking was found to have a modest positive association with ischaemic stroke at all levels of alcohol intake. This association was lost after controlling for smoking and hypertension, indicating that moderate drinking was not independently associated with ischaemic stroke in middle-aged and elderly blacks. A nonlinear association cannot be excluded in studies by von Arbin et al. (1985) and Stemmermann et al. (1984).

Haemorrhagic Stroke (Intracerebral or Subarachnoid Haemorrhage)

Monforte et al. (1990) reported an increased risk of stroke in chronic high ethanol drinkers in young and middle-aged intracerebral haemorrhage cases that was independent of chronic hypertension. Although the selection criteria differed from previous studies, the authors considered that this provided strong evidence of a pathogenic link between chronic high ethanol intake and haemorrhagic stroke.

There have been three "nested" case-control studies that assessed alcohol exposure and then followed subjects for the occurrence of fatal and nonfatal strokes. Stemmermann et al. (1984) showed that autopsy-proven haemorrhagic stroke patients tended to have drunk more than controls showing no cerebrovascular disease at autopsy and more than living members of the original cohort, but these associations were lost after adjustment for various confounding factors. Similar nonsignificant associations were found in the other two nested studies (Sacco et al. 1984, Petitti et al. 1979).

Binge Drinking and Stroke

Case reports suggest a direct relationship between the drinking of large quantities of alcohol ("binge drinking") and the subsequent occurrence of stroke (Wilkens and Kendall 1985). Though promising with regard to causality because of the time order of the events—first binge then stroke—evidence on a causal relationship between the two entities is sparse. All epidemiological evidence is from case-control studies.

No standardized definition of "binge drinking" exists. In Finnish studies, the definition was the consumption of ≥ 80 g of ethanol over a few hours within 24 hours before the onset of symptoms (Hillbom and Kaste 1990). A binge has also been defined as 100 g of ethanol above the subject's normal average daily intake during the 24 hours before the stroke (Gill 1986). In yet another study, attempts were made to detect a threshold dose of alcoholic ingestion for the precipitation of stroke (Gorelick 1987). Whatever the definition, binge drinking may be rather frequent, because almost one-third of U.S. drinkers acknowledge that they "sometimes drink more than they should" (Gallup 1988); however, considerable differences among countries may exist.

Biological plausibility for an association between binge drinking and stroke may be inferred from several factors: vasoconstriction, interference with haemostasis, and blood pressure (Anonymous 1983; see also "Pathophysiological Background," above).

At least five case-control studies on the relation between binge drinking and stroke have been published; three studies originate from Finland (Hillbom and Kaste 1982, 1983, Syrjänen et al. 1986), and two originate from the United States (Taylor et al. 1984, Gorelick 1987). All Finnish studies used the prevalence of drinking habits in the Finnish population from an earlier time period as "control," and report odds ratios of binge drinking ranging from 6–35 for ischaemic stroke and 2.4–6.7 for subarachnoid haemorrhage; however, the precision of the odds ratio estimates was not given, no control for incomparability of other stroke risk factors between cases and controls was attempted apart from age, and ascertainment of alcohol ingestion was different between the cases and the "control" population. The two U.S. studies are true case-control studies. In the study by Taylor et al. (1984), alcohol use in ≤ 24 hours was compared between 64 hospitalized stroke cases and 64 hospital controls, resulting in an odds ratio of 5.1 after adjustment for age, sex, and race. Gorelick et al. (1987) performed a study in 205 elderly predominantly black patients with ischaemic stroke (cases) and 410 controls matched for age, sex, race, and method of hospital payment. The crude unmatched odds ratio was 1.6; however, if smoking behaviour was taken into account, the apparent association was completely lost.

The conclusion reached by Camargo (1989) that "the results of epidemiologic studies provide meagre evidence that recent alcohol use affects risk of stroke" still holds true in 1992. Future studies should be carefully designed and address at least the following issues: (1) confounding by other recreational drugs, including cigarette smoking; (2) the distinction between binge drinking and the usual level of alcohol ingestion; and (3) the use of laboratory measures of recent alcohol use (Camargo 1989). Moreover, the use of hospital controls in a case-control study on binge drinking and stroke is problematic if not improper, because it is very hard to identify diseases not associated with alcohol intake one way or the other. Most hospitalized patients have been sick for a while before admission; this would decrease their likelihood for recent binge drinking. On the other hand, patients admitted for trauma would be at increased risk for recent binge drinking. Population-based case-control studies should therefore be encouraged. Finally, diagnosis of the subtype of stroke proven by CT scan may unravel different pathophysiological factors in the causation of the repository of "alcohol-related-stroke."

Habitual Intake of Alcohol and Stroke: Prospective Cohort Studies

Methodological Issues

Prospective cohort studies have several important strengths for studying the relation between alcohol intake and risk of stroke. Chief among these is that this design avoids the problem of selecting and enroling appropriate controls, and avoids recall bias. The major potential source of bias associated with cohort studies is differential follow-up of the population under observation, i.e., if strokes among drinkers are more (or less) likely to be ascertained than those among nondrinkers. This problem can be minimized by maintaining a high rate of overall follow-up. Operationally, the main disadvantages of cohort studies are that considerable resources are required to establish the cohort and to collect information, and one must wait until a sufficient number of endpoints has accrued to perform the analysis.

Usually, habitual alcohol intake is ascertained at baseline from the population, which is then followed for the occurrence of stroke and other endpoints of interest. If alcohol intake is not repeatedly ascertained, then changes in intake in the population over time will not be captured. Thus, with an increasing interval following a single assessment of alcohol intake, the data will be increasingly flawed in terms of representing true long-term intake. Another difficulty with the prospective design is that it generally is not useful to assess the acute effects of high levels of alcohol consumption. During the course of follow-up, improvements in diagnostic tools could alter the ascertainment of stroke. This should not alter estimates of the association between risk of stroke and alcohol unless the changes in diagnosis were selective for alcohol-related stroke.

The prospective study design shares with case-control studies the potential problems of inaccurate assessment of alcohol intake and possible confounding. Some individuals, particularly heavy drinkers, may not tell the truth about their alcohol consumption. Also, some past heavy drinkers may report only on current consumption; if their past alcohol abuse has an adverse impact, this could bias the findings by making it appear that having no alcohol intake carries a greater risk than is real. Perhaps somewhat mitigating this problem in some cohorts is the finding that problem drinkers are less likely to enrol in health surveys (Alanko 1984). This of course would lead to underrepresentation of this important segment of the population. The main area of public health interest, however, is in the effect of moderate alcohol consumption, since the ill effects of excess alcohol are well-known. A high degree of validity of self-reported alcohol intake has been established for two large cohorts (Giovannucci et al. 1991).

Individuals who drink alcohol differ in other important respects from nondrinkers, and these differences may be manifest across different amounts of usual alcohol consumption. Drinkers typically smoke more than nondrinkers, and because smoking is an independent risk factor both for ischaemic and haemorrhagic stroke (Colditz et al. 1988, U.S. Department of Health and Human Services 1990), it is critical to adjust for smoking in the analysis to assess the independent effect of alcohol. Hypertension presents a more difficult problem because excessive alcohol intake increases blood pressure, and this may be one mechanism whereby alcohol acts to increase risk of stroke (see "Pathophysiological Background," above). Hence, adjustment for hypertension may represent "overcontrol" in the analysis and could artifactually reduce an elevated relative risk.

Total Stroke

At least 19 reports from prospective studies have been published. Many of these have reported only on total stroke, without distinguishing the type. As noted earlier, different types of stroke have different causes, and it seems unlikely a priori that the effect of alcohol would be the same for all types. By combining all types, one addresses an important public health issue of the overall association between alcohol and stroke, but it is easy to obscure differences in associations by specific type. Fifteen studies reported results for total stroke (see Table 2). The studies range widely in geographic location, coming from Europe, North America, Australia, and Japan. The cohorts also vary in size, from 359 (Tofler 1985) to 123,840 (Klatsky et al. 1990), and in the range and categories of alcohol intake. Overall, there is little evidence for an association between alcohol and risk of total stroke except in the highest category of intake, for which the evidence suggests a modest excess risk. The findings are reasonably consistent for the largest studies (more than 100 cases) and the ones with the best control of confounding factors (Boysen et al. 1988, Wolf et al. 1988, Klatsky et al. 1990, Stampfer et al. 1988, Kono et al. 1986, Donahue et al. 1986). In each of those studies, individuals in the highest alcohol consumption category had an elevated relative risk. The definition of the highest category, which was open-ended in each study, varied from 2+ (Wolf et al. 1988) to 6+ drinks per day (Klatsky et al. 1990), so it is possible that the apparent modest excess risk is attributable entirely to a high excess risk among heavy drinkers.

Haemorrhagic Stroke (Intracerebral or Subarachnoid Haemorrhage)

The reports with data on individual type of stroke are more informative. Table 3 summarizes the results from studies of haemorrhagic stroke, classified where possible as total haemorrhagic stroke, intracerebral haemorrhage, and subarachnoid haemorrhage. For total haemorrhagic stroke, a more consistent finding emerges. In each of the eight studies that reported data either on total haemorrhagic stroke or the specific subtypes, individuals in the highest category of alcohol intake had an elevated risk. Moreover, this excess risk was quite substantial, ranging from 1.6 (Kono et al. 1986) to 4.7 (Klatsky et al. 1990); in the majority of studies, the elevated risk in the top category was statistically significant. The data suggesting a dose-response effect were not impressive, however.

Table 2
Prospective studies of alcohol and total stroke

References	City/state country	Number followed	Sex, age range (yrs)	Follow-up (yrs)	Number of strokes	Categories of alcohol	Relative risk (95% CI)
Cullen 1982	Busselton, Australia	2209	M,F 40+	13	72 fatal	Nondrinker Drinker	1.0 0.94
Boysen 1988	Copenhagen, Denmark	13,088	M,F 35+	5	295	Not daily drinker Daily drinker	1.0 1.3
Semenciw 1988	Canada	7117	M,F 35–79	10	58 fatal	< 3 drinks/day ≥ 3 drinks/day	1.0 3.2 (1.3–8.0)
Peacock 1972	Birmingham, Alabama	10,876	M,F 50–69	4	87	Nondrinkers Drinkers	1.0 1.7 (1.1–2.7)
Wolf 1988	Framingham, Massachusetts	4722	M,F 50–79	32	523	Men—nondrinkers ≤ 2 drinks/day > 2 Women—nondrinkers ≤ 1 drink/day > 1	(p = 0.03) compared to nondrinkers and heavy drinkers n.s.
Khaw 1987	Rancho Bernardo, California	859	M,F 50–79	12	24 fatal	Alcohol per 10 g	0.92 (0.72–1.16)

Study	Location	N	Sex/Age	Years	Events	Category	stroke (%)
Klatsky 1990	California	123,840	M,F mean age 40.5	average 5.3	138 fatal	Nondrinkers	1.0
						Ex-drinkers	1.0
						<1 drink/month	0.8
						<1 drink/day	0.8
						1–2	0.8
						3–5	0.7
						≥6	1.4
Paganini-Hill 1988	Laguna Hills, California	8841	F median age 73	17	63 fatal	Nondrinkers	1.0
						≤1 drink/day	0.81
						≥2 drinks/day	0.75
Tofler 1985	Perth, Australia	359	M mean age 45	17	11 fatal	nondrinkers	4.2
						<2.9	0
						≥2.9	2.6
Gordon 1987	Albany, New York	1762	M 38–55	18	33 fatal	Nondrinkers	1.0
						<2 drinks/day	0.29
						≥2	0.92
Kozarevic 1983	Yugoslavia	11,121	M 35–62	7	49 fatal	<1 drink/month	1.0
						≥1/month to 1/week	0.4
						≥1/week to 1/day	0.3
						≥1/day (not inebriated)	0.8
						≥1/day (inebriated)	1.0

Table 2. *Continued*

References	City/state country	Number followed	Sex, age range (yrs)	Follow-up (yrs)	Number of strokes	Categories of alcohol	Relative risk (95% CI)
Stampfer 1988	United States	87,526	F 34–59	4	120	Nondrinkers	1.0
						< 1.5 g/day	0.9 (0.5–1.6)
						1.5–4.9	0.6 (0.3–1.0)
						5.0–14.9	0.6 (0.3–1.0)
						15.0–24.9	0.5 (0.2–1.2)
						25.0+	1.2 (0.7–2.2)
Kono 1986	Japan	5135	M 25+	19	230	Nondrinkers	1.0
						Ex-drinkers	2.3 (1.5–3.5)
						Occasional drinkers	1.1 (0.7–1.6)
						< 3.6 drinks/day	1.2 (0.8–1.8)
						≥ 3.6	1.7 (1.1–2.6)
Donahue 1986	Honolulu, Hawaii	7878	M 45–68	12	290	Nondrinkers	1.0
						< drink/day	1.2 (0.9–1.6)
						1–2.7	1.3 (0.9–1.9)
						2.7+	1.5 (1.1–2.2)
Shaper 1991	Great Britain	6422	M 40–59	8	63	< 1 drink/week	1.0 ⎫ Relative risks
						< 3 drinks/day	1.3 ⎪ estimated from
						3–6	1.3 ⎬ Figure 2
						> 6	1.5 ⎭ (Shaper 1991)

Table 3
Prospective studies of alcohol and hemorrhagic stroke classified by total, intracerebral, and subarachnoid hemorrhage

References	City/state country	Number followed	Sex, age range (yrs)	Follow-up (yrs)	Number of strokes	Categories of alcohol	Relative risk (95% CI)
					Total Hemorrhagic		
Kono 1986	Japan	5135	M 25+	19	89	Nondrinkers Ex-drinkers Occasional drinkers < 3.6 drinks/day ≥ 3.6	1.0 1.0 (0.4–2.4) 1.2 (0.7–2.2) 0.9 (0.5–1.8) 1.6 (0.8–3.1)
Donahue 1986	Honolulu, Hawaii	7895	M 45–68	12	76	Nondrinkers < 1 drink/day 1–2.7 2.8+	1.0 2.3 (1.2–4.3) 2.5 (1.2–4.2) 2.9 (1.4–6.0)
Omae 1982	Hisayama, Japan	1621	M,F 40+	18	41	Nondrinkers ≤ 2.8 drinks/day > 2.8	% stroke 2 4.5 5.5
Klatsky 1989	California	10,751	M,F 70% < 50	3.5 average	43	Nondrinkers Former drinkers < 1 drink/day 1–2 ≥ 3	1.0 1.47 (0.28–7.83) 1.02 (0.39–2.65) 0.94 (0.28–3.17) 3.85 (1.19–12.41)

Table 3. *Continued*

References	City/state country	Number followed	Sex, age range (yrs)	Follow-up (yrs)	Number of strokes	Categories of alcohol	Relative risk (95% CI)
Klatsky 1990	California	123,840	M,F 40.5 average	5.3 average	41 fatal	Nondrinkers	1.0
						Former drinkers	1.4
						<1 drink/month	1.5
						<1 drink/day	1.6
						1–2	1.8
						3–5	1.3
						6+	4.7
					Intracerebral Hemorrhage		
Peacock 1972	Birmingham, Alabama	10,876	M,F 50–69	4	22	Nondrinkers	1.0
						Drinkers	3.1 (1.4–7.2)
Tanaka 1982	Taisho, Japan	1673	M,F 40+	10	30	<1.9 drinks/day	1.0
						≥1.9	3.0 ($p < 0.05$)
Okada 1976	Akabane and Asahi, Japan	4186	M,F 40–79	7	143	Nondrinker	1.0
						Occasional	4.4 ($p < 0.001$)
						Regular	4.5 ($p < 0.001$)
Donahue 1986	Honolulu, Hawaii	7895	M 45–68	12	44	Nondrinkers	1.0
						<1 drink/day	2.0 (0.9–4.5)
						1–2.7	2.0 (0.8–5.2)
						2.8+	2.4 (0.9–6.2)

Subarachnoid Hemorrhage

Stampfer 1988	United States	87,526	F 34–59	4	28	Nondrinkers	1.0
						< 1.5 g/day	2.4 (0.5–12.1)
						1.5–4.9	2.9 (0.7–11.5)
						5.0–14.9	3.7 (1.0–13.8)
						15.0+	2.6 (0.7–10.3)
Donahue 1986	Honolulu, Hawaii	7895	M 45–68	12	32	Nondrinkers	1.0
						< 1 drink/day	2.8 (0.9–8.6)
						1–2.7	3.5 (1.1–12.0)
						2.8+	3.8 (1.1–13.3)

In most populations, haemorrhagic stroke makes up a minority of total stroke, but clinically these tend to be the most severe and usually predominate among fatal strokes. For this reason, the number of cases in most studies of haemorrhagic stroke is sparse, and when attention is limited to the highest level of alcohol intake, the estimates of the relative risk are imprecise and have wide confidence intervals. For example, in the large study by Klatsky et al. (1990), with 123,840 men and women, only 41 fatal haemorrhagic strokes were recorded. In Stampfer's report based on 87,526 women, just 28 cases of subarachnoid haemorrhage were documented; the relative risk for those drinking 25+ g/day of alcohol (one drink containing 10–15g) was 3.9, with 95% confidence intervals of 0.9–17.4 (Stampfer et al. 1988). Although the number of cases in each individual study is small (the largest has 143 cases [Okada et al. 1976]), the findings are remarkably consistent. Elevated risks for high alcohol intake were also observed in studies with good control of potential confounding variables. Overall, the prospective studies provide strong evidence to support the view that higher levels of alcohol intake are associated with an increased risk of haemorrhagic stroke. Data are more limited for the specific forms of haemorrhagic stroke but suggest an increase in risk both for subarachnoid haemorrhage as well as intracerebral haemorrhage.

Ischaemic Stroke

Table 4 summarizes the results from nine prospective studies that reported on the association between alcohol consumption and risk of ischaemic stroke. A reasonably consistent pattern emerges from this summary. In no case is there a statistically significantly elevated relative risk of ischaemic stroke for any category of alcohol intake. For the highest category of intake, relative risks are null in three studies (Stampfer et al. 1988, Tanaka et al. 1982, Donahue et al. 1986), somewhat but not significantly reduced in two (Klatsky et al. 1989, 1990), and slightly but not significantly elevated in the remaining four studies. Studies that distinguished moderate levels of alcohol intake tended to observe an inverse association (Stampfer et al. 1988, Klatsky et al. 1989, 1990), with a borderline significant protective effect for under one drink per day. Donahue et al. (1986), however, reported a relative risk of 1.0 for men drinking less than one drink per day.

Overall, the weight of evidence from the prospective studies of alcohol and ischaemic stroke does not support a direct association. The data provide strong evidence against even a modest increase in risk, and indeed there is some suggestion of a possible decrease in

Table 4

Prospective studies of alcohol and ischemic stroke

Reference	City/state country	Number followed	Sex, age range (yrs)	Follow-up (yrs)	Number of strokes	Categories of alcohol	Relative risk (95% CI)
Peacock 1972	Birmingham, Alabama	10,876	M,F 50–69	4	55	Nondrinkers Drinkers	1.0 1.5 (0.9–2.7)
Stampfer 1988	United States	87,526	F 34–59	4	66	Nondrinkers <1.5 g/day 1.5–4.9 5.0–14.9 15.0+	1.0 0.7 (0.4–1.6) 0.4 (0.2–0.9) 0.3 (0.1–0.7) 0.5 (0.2–1.1)
Omae 1982	Hisayama, Japan	1621	M,F 40+	18	171	Nondrinkers ≤2.8 drinks/day >2.8	% stroke 13% 9.5% 16%
Tanaka 1982	Taisho, Japan	1673	M,F 40+	10	81	<1.9 drinks/day ≥1.9	1.0 1.19 (n.s.)
Okada 1976	Akabane and Asahi, Japan	4186	M,F 40–79	7	58	Nondrinker Occasional Regular	1.0 1.0 1.6 (n.s.)
Tanaka 1985	Shibata, Japan	960	M,F 40+	6.5	16	g/ethanol/kg weight	1.46 (n.s.)

Table 4. *Continued*

References	City/state country	Number followed	Sex, age range (yrs)	Follow-up (yrs)	Number of strokes	Categories of alcohol	Relative risk (95% CI)
Donahue 1986	Honolulu, Hawaii	7895	M 45–68	12	190	Nondrinkers < 1 drink/day 1–2.7 2.8+	1.0 1.0 (0.7–1.4) 1.2 (0.8–1.8) 1.1 (0.7–1.7)
Klatsky 1989	California	10,751	M,F 70% < 50	3.5 average	143	Nondrinkers Former drinkers < 1 drink/day 1–2 ≥ 3	1.0 1.05 (0.49–2.24) 0.61 (0.37–1.00) 0.73 (0.41–1.28) 0.62 (0.29–1.31)
Klatsky 1990	California	123,840	M,F 40.5 average	5.3 average	34 fatal	Nondrinkers Former drinkers < 1 drink/month < 1 drink/day 1–2 3+	1.0 0.9 0.5 0.5 0.3 0.4

risk associated with low levels of alcohol consumption. The protective effect of alcohol on coronary disease is reasonably well-established (Rimm et al. 1991, Stampfer et al. 1988). To the extent that ischaemic stroke and coronary disease share atherosclerosis and related thrombosis as common aetiologies, a modest level of protection among moderate drinkers is plausible.

Conclusions and Review of the Evidence

The possible specific associations between alcohol consumption and stroke are:

(1) Does habitual alcohol consumption increase the risk of stroke overall?

(2) Does habitual alcohol consumption increase the risk of haemorrhagic stroke?

(3) Does habitual alcohol consumption increase the risk of ischaemic stroke?

(4) Does moderate habitual alcohol consumption decrease the risk of ischaemic stroke?

(5) Does binge drinking of alcohol increase the risk of stroke overall, and the major subtypes specifically?

The consensus for each of these possible associations can be summarised as:

(1) No. Substantial evidence suggests little association between habitual alcohol consumption and risk of stroke, except for a modest increase in risk at high levels of intake. Very high levels of alcohol consumption increase risk of stroke by a variety of biochemical changes. The content of the consensus and the body of evidence is summarized in the report. The dose range where some adverse effect may be present for stroke overall is unclear but appears to be at several drinks per day. No further research on "unspecified stroke" would be useful because of the need to distinguish between stroke types in studying the effects of alcohol.

(2) Yes. Substantial evidence suggests an association between habitual alcohol consumption and risk of haemorrhagic stroke at high levels of intake. The content of the consensus and the body of evidence is summarized in the report. The dose range where the adverse effect begins is unclear but appears to be at several drinks per day. A two-to threefold

increase in risk is present at high levels of consumption. It is unclear whether this association reflects habitual or short-term intake of alcohol. Further research efforts should concentrate on establishing the dose range for the apparent adverse effect, identifying susceptible individuals, and distinguishing between habitual and short-term effects ("binge drinking"; see question 5, above).

(3) No. Substantial evidence suggests no association between habitual alcohol consumption and risk of ischaemic stroke, even at high levels of intake. The content of the consensus and the body of evidence is summarized in the report. The evidence regarding this association is fairly persuasive, and it is unlikely that further research of this specific question will alter the general consensus.

(4) No consensus exists regarding the possible decreased risk of ischaemic stroke with low to moderate levels of alcohol intake. Studies are divided on this point. Many of the methodological problems and potential pitfalls of the epidemiologic studies are discussed in the report. Further epidemiologic studies that take account of these problems and specifically assess low levels of intake would be useful to help resolve this issue.

(5) No consensus exists for this question, though the data are suggestive of a positive relation between binge drinking and stroke overall. The data are sparse and difficult to interpret because of methodological problems. Methodologically sound studies of this association would be quite useful to resolve the issue and to explore the effects on different stroke subtypes. Moreover, such data would also be important to resolve whether the association between habitual intake and haemorrhagic stroke may be explained wholly or in part by binge drinking.

Sound biological evidence is available to support the observations from the epidemiologic studies, but further investigation, particularly into the mechanisms for the apparent effect of alcohol on haemorrhagic stroke, would be quite useful. In general, the findings are not overly dependent on any single study, and we do not recommend that increased attention be paid to contrary evidence for any of the hypotheses we have listed. We do not see evidence for biases of investigators influencing the degree to which any hypothesis has received attention.

References

Abu-Zeid HAH, Choi NW, Maini KK, et al. (1977) Relative role of factors associated with cerebral infarction and cerebral hemorrhage: a matched pair case-control study. Stroke 8:106–12

Aho K, Harmsen P, Hatono S, et al. (1980) Cerebrovascular disease in the community: results of the WHO collaborative study. Bull World Health Organ 58:113–30

Alanko T (1984) An overview of techniques and problems in the measurement of alcohol consumption. In Smart RG, Glaser FB, Cappell HD, et al. (eds), Research advances in alcohol and drug problems. Plenum Press, New York, vol 8, pp 209–26

Altura BM, Altura BT, Gebrewold A (1983) Alcohol-induced spasms of cerebral blood vessels: relation to cerebrovascular accidents and sudden death. Science 220:331–33

Anonymous (1983) "Binge" drinking and stroke. Lancet 2:660–61

Antiplatelet Trialists' Collaboration (1988) Secondary prevention of vascular disease by prolonged antiplatelet treatment. Br Med J 296:320–31

Bamford J, Sandercock P, Dennis M, et al. (1990) A prospective study of acute cerebrovascular disease in the community: the Oxfordshire Community Stroke Project 1981–86. 2. Incidence, case fatality rates and overall outcome at one year of cerebral infarction, primary intracerebral and subarachnoid haemorrhage. J Neurol Neurosurg Psychiatry 53:16–22

Ben-Shlomo Y, Markowe H, Shipley M, Marmot M (1991) Stroke risk from alcohol consumption using different control groups. Stroke 23:1093–98

Berglund M (1981) Cerebral blood flow in chronic alcoholics. Alcohol Clin Exp Res 5:295–303

Blackwelder WC, Yano K, Rhoads GG, et al. (1980) Alcohol and mortality. The Honolulu Heart Study. Am J Med 68:164–69

Boysen G, Nyboe J, Appleyard M, et al. (1988) Stroke incidence and risk factors for stroke in Copenhagen, Denmark. Stroke 19:1345–53

Calandre L, Arnal C, Ortega JF, et al. (1986) Risk factors for spontaneous cerebral hematomas: case-control study. Stroke 17:1126–28

Camargo CA (1989) Moderate alcohol consumption and stroke. The epidemiological evidence. Stroke 20:1611–26

Castelli WP, Doyle JT, Gordon T, et al. (1977) Alcohol and blood lipids—the Cooperative Lipoprotein Phenotyping Study. Lancet 2:153–55

Colditz GA, Bonita R, Stampfer MJ, et al. (1988) Cigarette smoking and elevated risk of stroke in a cohort of middle-aged women. N Engl J Med 318:937–41

Cowan DH (1980) Effect of alcoholism on hemostasis. Semin Hematol 17:137–47

Cullen K, Stenhouse NS, Wearne KL (1982) Alcohol and mortality in the Busselton Study. Int J Epidemiol 11:67–70

Demakis JG, Proskey A, Rahimtoola S, et al. (1974) The natural course of alcoholic cardiomyopathy. Ann Intern Med 80:293–97

Deykin D, Janson P, McMahon L (1982) Ethanol potentiation of aspirin-induced prolongation of the bleeding time. N Engl J Med 306:852–54

Donahue RP, Abbott RD, Reed DM, Yano K (1986) Alcohol and hemorrhagic stroke. The Honolulu Heart Study. JAMA 255:2311–14

Elmér O, Göransson G, Zoucas E (1984) Impairment of primary hemostasis and platelet function after alcohol ingestion in man. Hemostasis 14:223–28

Ettinger PO, Wu CF, De La Cruz C, et al. (1978) Arrhythmias and the "holiday heart": alcohol-associated cardiac rhythm disorders. Am Heart J 95:555–62

Gallup G Jr (1988) The Gallup poll: public opinion 1987. Scholarly Resources, Wilmington, DE

Gill JS, Shipley MJ, Hornby RH, et al. (1988) A community case-control study of alcohol consumption in stroke. Int J Epidemiol 17:542–47

Gill JS, Zezulka AV, Beevers DG (1985) Stroke affecting young men after alcoholic binges (letter). Br Med J 291:1645

Gill JS, Zezulka AV, Shipley MJ, et al. (1986) Stroke and alcohol consumption. N Engl J Med 315:1041–46

Giovannucci E, Colditz GA, Stampfer MJ, et al. (1991) The assessment of alcohol consumption by a simple self-administered questionnaire. Am J Epidemiol 133:810–17

Gordon T, Doyle JT (1987) Drinking and mortality. The Albany Study. Am J Epidemiol 125:263–70

Gordon T, Kannel WB (1983) Drinking habits and cardiovascular disease. The Framingham Study. Am Heart J 105:667–73

Gorelick P (1989) The status of alcohol as a risk factor for stroke. Stroke 20:1607–10

Gorelick PB (1987) Alcohol and stroke. Stroke 18:268–71

Gorelick PB, Rodin MB, Langenberg P, et al (1987) Is acute alcohol ingestion a risk factor for ischemic stroke? Results of a controlled study in middle-aged and elderly stroke patients at three urban medical centers. Stroke 18:359–64

Gorelick PB, Rodin MB, Langenberg P, et al. (1989) Weekly alcohol consumption, cigarette smoking and the risk of ischemic stroke: results of a case-control study at three urban medical centers in Chicago, Illinois. Neurology 39:339–43

Haselager EM, Vreeken J (1977) Rebound thrombocytosis after alcohol abuse: a possible factor in the pathogenesis of thromboembolic disease. Lancet 1:774–75

Herman B, Schmitz PIM, Leyten ACM, et al. (1983) Multivariate logistic analysis of risk factors for stroke in Tilburg, The Netherlands. Am J Epidemiol 118:514–25

Hill AB (1965) The environment and disease: association or causation? Proc R Soc Med 58:295–300

Hillbom M, Kangasaho M, Kaste M, et al. (1985) Acute ethanol ingestion increases platelet reactivity: is there a relationship to stroke? Stroke 16:19–23

Hillbom M, Kaste M (1978) Does ethanol intoxication promote brain infarction in young adults? Lancet 2:1181–83

Hillbom M, Kaste M (1981a) Ethanol intoxication: a risk factor for ischemic brain infarction in adolescents and young adults. Stroke 12:422–25

Hillbom M, Kaste M (1981b) Does alcohol intoxication precipitate aneurysmal subarachnoid haemorrhage? J Neurol Neurosurg Psychiatry 44:523–26

Hillbom M, Kaste M (1982) Alcohol intoxication: a risk factor for primary subarachnoid hemorrhage. Neurology 32:706–11

Hillbom M, Kaste M (1983) Ethanol intoxication: a risk factor for ischemic brain infarction. Stroke 14:694–99

Hillbom M, Kaste M (1990) Alcohol abuse and brain infarction. Ann Med 22:347–52

Hutton RA, Fink FR, Wilson DT, Marjot DH (1981) Platelet hyperaggregability during alcohol withdrawal. Clin Lab Haematol 3:19–23

Iso H, Jacobs DR, Wentworth D, et al. for the MRFIT Research Group (1989) Serum cholesterol levels and six-year mortality from stroke in 350,977 men screened for the multiple risk factor intervention trial. N Engl J Med 320:904–10

Jakubowski JA, Vaillancourt R, Deykin D (1988) Interaction of ethanol, prostacyclin, and aspirin in determining human platelet reactivity in vitro. Arteriosclerosis 8:436–41

Kagan A, Popper JS, Rhoads GG (1980) Factors related to stroke incidence in Hawaiian Japanese men: the Honolulu Heart Study. Stroke 11:14–21

Kagan A, Popper JS, Rhoads GG, Yano K (1985) Dietary and other risk factors for stroke in Hawaiian Japanese men. Stroke 16:390–96

Kagan A, Yano K, Rhoads GG, McGee DL (1981) Alcohol and cardiovascular disease. The Hawaiian experience. Circulation 64(suppl III):III-27–III-31

Kannel WB (1971) Current status of the epidemiology of brain infarction associated with occlusive arterial disease. Stroke 2:295–318

Kannel WB, Wolf PA, Dawber TR (1975) An evaluation of the epidemiology of atherothrombotic brain infarction. Milbank Mem Fund Q 53:405–48

Kannel WB, Woosley P (1975) Alcohol and cardiovascular risk (abstract). Circulation 52(suppl II):II-200

Katsuki S (1971) Hisayama Study. Jpn J Med 10:167–75

Khaw KT, Barrett-Connor E (1987) Dietary potassium and stroke-associated mortality. A 12-year prospective study. N Engl J Med 316:235–40

Kiefe C, Freiman J, Corman LC, et al. (1987) Stroke and alcohol consumption. N Engl J Med 319:1214–15

Kiyohara Y, Ueda K, Hasuo Y, et al. (1986) Hematocrit as a risk factor of cerebral infarction. Long-term prospective population survey in a Japanese rural community. Stroke 17:687–92

Klatsky AL, Armstrong MA, Friedman GD (1989) Alcohol use and subsequent cerebrovascular disease hospitalizations. Stroke 20:741–46

Klatsky AL, Armstrong MA, Friedman GD (1990) Risk of cardiovascular mortality in alcohol drinkers, ex-drinkers and nondrinkers. Am J Cardiol 66:1237–42

Klatsky AL, Friedman GD, Siegelaub AB (1981) Alcohol use and cardiovascular disease. The Kaiser-Permanente experience. Circulation 64(suppl III):III-32–III-41

Klatsky AL, Friedman GD, Siegelaub AB (1981) Alcohol and mortality. A ten-year Kaiser-Permanente experience. Ann Intern Med 95:139–45

Klatsky AL, Friedman GD, Siegelaub AB, Gérard MJ (1977) Alcohol consumption and blood pressure—Kaiser Permanente multiphasic health examination data. N Engl J Med 296:1194–1200

Kono S, Ikeda M, Ogata M, et al. (1983) The relationship between alcohol and mortality among Japanese physicians. Int J Epidemiol 12:437–41

Kono S, Ikeda M, Tokudome S, et al. (1986) Alcohol and mortality: a cohort study of male Japanese physicians. Int J Epidemiol 15:527–32

Kozarevic D, McGee D, Vojvodic N, et al. (1980) Frequency of alcohol consumption and morbidity and mortality. The Yugoslavia Cardiovascular Disease Study. Lancet 1:613–16

Kozarevic DJ, Vojvodic N, Gordon T, et al. (1983) Drinking habits and death. The Yugoslavia Cardiovascular Disease Study. Int J Epidemiol 12:145–50

Landolfi R, Steiner M (1984) Ethanol raises prostacyclin in vivo and in vitro. Blood 64:679–82

Laug WE (1983) Ethyl alcohol enhances plasminogen activator secretion by endothelial cells. JAMA 250:772–76

Lindegard B, Hillbom M (1987) Associations between brain infarction, diabetes and alcoholism: observations from the Gothenburg population cohort study. Acta Neurol Scand 75:195–200

MacMahon S, Peto R, Cutler J, et al. (1990) Blood pressure, stroke, and coronary heart disease. Part 1. Prolonged differences in blood pressure: prospective observational studies corrected for the regression dilution bias. Lancet 335:765–74

Mayhan WG (1992) Responses of cerebral arterioles during chronic ethanol exposure. Am J Physiol 262:H787–91

Meade TW, Chakrabarti R, Haines AP, et al. (1979) Characteristics affecting fibrinolytic activity and plasma fibrinogen concentrations. Br Med J 1:153–56

Monforte E, Estruch R, Graus F, et al. (1990) High ethanol consumption as risk factor for intracerebral hemorrhage in young and middle-aged people. Stroke 21:1529–32

Niizuma H, Suzuki J, Yonemitsu T, Otsuki T (1988) Spontaneous intracerebral hemorrhage and liver dysfunction. Stroke 19:852–56

Norris JW, Hachinski VC (1982) Misdiagnosis of stroke. Lancet 1:328–32

Okada H, Horibe H, Ohno Y, et al. (1976) A prospective study of cerebrovascular disease in Japanese rural communities, Akabane and Asahi. Part 1: evaluation of risk factors in the occurrence of cerebral hemmorrhage and thrombosis. Stroke 7:599–607

Oleckno WA (1986) Selected factors and stroke in young adults, 15–40 years of age. J R Soc Health 106:102–07

Oleckno WA (1988) The risk of stroke in young adults: an analysis of the contribution of cigarette smoking and alcohol consumption. Public Health 102:45–55

Omae T, Ueda K (1982) Risk-factors of cerebral stroke in Japan. prospective epidemiological study in Hisayama community. In Katsuki S, Tsubaki T, Toyokura Y (eds), Proceedings of the 12th World Congress of Neurology, Kyoto, Japan. Excerpta Medica, Amsterdam, pp 119–35

Oxfordshire Community Stroke Project (1983) Incidence of stroke in Oxfordshire: first year's experience of a community stroke register. Br Med J 287:713–17

Paganini-Hill A, Ross RK, Henderson BE (1988) Postmenopausal oestrogen treatment and stroke. A prospective study. Br Med J 297:519–22

Peacock PB, Riley CP, Lampton TD, et al. (1972) The Birmingham stroke, epidemiology and rehabilitation study. In Stewart G (ed), Trends in epidemiology: applications to health service research and training. Charles C. Thomas, Springfield, IL, 1972, pp 231–345

Petitti DB, Wingerd J, Pellegrin F, Ramcharan S (1979) Risk of vascular disease in women: smoking, oral contraceptives, noncontraceptive estrogens, and other factors. JAMA 242:1150–54

Ricci S, Celani MG, La Rosa F, et al. (1991) SEPIVAC: a community-based study of stroke-incidence in Umbria, Italy. J Neurol Neurosurg Psychiatry 54:695–98

Rimm EB, Giovannucci E, Stampfer MJ, et al. (1991) A prospective study of alcohol consumption and the risk of coronary disease in men. Lancet 338:464–68

Rogers RL, Meyer JS, Shaw TG, Mortel KF (1983) Reductions in regional cerebral blood flow associated with chronic consumption of alcohol. J Am Geriatr Soc 31:540–43

Sacco RL, Wolf PA, Bharucha NE, et al. (1984) Subarachnoid and intracerebral hemorrhage: natural history, prognosis, and precursive factors in the Framingham Study. Neurology 34:847–54

Semenciw RM, Morrison MI, Mao Y, et al. (1988) Major risk factors for cardiovascular disease mortality in adults. Results from the Nutrition Canada Survey Study. Int J Epidemiol 17:317–24

Shaper AG, Phillips AN, Pocock SJ, et al. (1991) Risk factors for stroke in middle age British men. Brit Med J 302:1111–15

Stampfer MJ, Colditz GA, Willett WC, et al. (1988) A prospective study of moderate alcohol consumption and the risk of coronary disease and stroke in women. N Engl J Med 319:267–73

Stemmermann GN, Hayashi T, Resch JA, et al. (1984) Risk factors related to ischemic and hemorrhagic cerebrovascular disease at autopsy: the Honolulu Heart Study. Stroke 15:23–8

Sundby P (1967) Alcoholism and Mortality. Publ No 6, National Institute for Alcohol Research, Universitetsforlaget, Oslo

Syrjänen J, Valtonen VV, Iivavainen M, et al. (1986) Association between cerebral infarction and increased serum bacterial antibody levels in young adults. Acta Neurol Scand 73:273–78

Takeya Y, Popper JS, Shimizu Y, et al. (1984) Epidemiologic studies of coronary heart disease and stroke in Japanese men living in Japan, Hawaii and California. Incidence of stroke in Japan and Hawaii. Stroke 15:15–23

Tanaka H, Hayashi M, Date C, et al. (1985) Epidemiologic studies of stroke in Shibata, a Japanese provincial city. Preliminary report on risk factors for cerebral infarction. Stroke 16:773–80

Tanaka H, Ueda Y, Hayashi M, et al. (1982) Risk factors for cerebral hemorrhage and cerebral infarction in a Japanese rural community. Stroke 13:62–73

Taylor JR (1982) Alcohol and strokes (letter). N Engl J Med 306:1111

Taylor JR, Combs-Orme T (1985) Alcohol and strokes in young adults. Am J Psychiatry 142:116–68

Taylor JR, Combs-Orme T, Anderson D, et al. (1984) Alcohol, hypertension, and stroke. Alcoholism 8:283–86

Tofler OB (1985) The Heart of the Social Drinker. Lloyd-Luke, London

Ueda K, Hasuo Y, Kiyohara Y, et al. (1988) Incidence, changing pattern during long-term follow-up, and related factors. Stroke 19:48–52

U.S. Department of Health and Human Services (DHHS) (1990) The Health Benefits of Smoking Cessation. DHHS Publ No (CDC)90-8416, U.S. DHHS Public Health Service, Centers for Disease Control, Center for Chronic Disease Prevention and Health Promotion, Office on Smoking and Health

von Arbin M, Britton M, De Faire U, Tisell A (1985) Circulatory manifestations and risk factors in patients with acute cerebrovascular disease and in matched controls. Acta Med Scand 218:373–80

Weisberg LA (1988) Alcoholic intracerebral hemorrhage. Stroke 19:1565–69

Wilkens MR, Kendall MJ (1985) Stroke affecting young men after alcoholic binges. Br Med J 291:1342

Witteman JCM, Willett WC, Stampfer MJ, et al. (1990) The relation of moderate alcohol consumption and increased risk of hypertension in women. Am J Cardiol 65:633–37

Wolf PA, Belanger AJ, D'Agostino RB (1992) Management of risk factors. In Barnett HJM, Hachinski VC (eds), Cerebral ischemia: treatment and prevention. Neuro Clin 10:177–91

Wolf PA, D'Agostino RB, Odell P, et al. (1988) Alcohol consumption as a risk factor for stroke. The Framingham Study (abstract). Ann Neurol 24:177

Wolf PA, Kannel WB, Verter J (1983) Current status of risk-factors for stroke. Neurol Clin 1:317–43

4

Alcohol Drinking and Coronary Heart Disease

S. Renaud
INSERM, France

M.H. Criqui
San Diego Medical School
University of California, United States

G. Farchi
Istituto Superiore di Sanita, Italy

J. Veenstra
TNO Institute, The Netherlands

Abstract

Results of ecologic, case-control, and prospective studies are concordant in that a moderate intake of alcohol in the form of beer, wine, or spirits apparently protects by 10–70%, according to studies of both morbidity and mortality resulting from coronary heart disease (CHD). Particular confidence can be given to the very large cohort studies published in the last 3 years and involving more than 500,000 subjects (more subjects than in all the studies published before) with results totally unanimous. At dosages of 10–20 g/day in the United States, even mortality from all causes was significantly decreased. It is generally agreed that there is a J-shaped relationship between alcohol intake and total mortality with an increase in heavier drinkers in deaths from different causes, including total cardiovascular disease. The protective effect of alcohol seems to be present at all ages, in women as in men, whatever the length of follow-up (2–22 years), with other risk factors taken into consideration in addition to alcohol. It is not due to the inclusion in the nondrinkers of ex-drinkers with prevalent CHD.

This protection afforded by alcohol seems to be due only partly to less anterosclerosis. In most of the autopsy studies, when alcohol drinkers were compared to adequate controls, significant differences in the atherosclerotic lesions were not observed between the two groups. In clinical (angiography) and experimental studies, a significant protective effect of alcohol on atherosclerosis was observed, but at a higher dosage than that optimally beneficial for CHD and total mortality. This partial inhibitory effect of alcohol on atherosclerosis seems to be due to an increase in the reverse transport of cholesterol through the level of high density lipoprotein (HDL) consistently enhanced, in a dose-related manner, by alcohol drinking, even binge drinking (which does not protect from CHD). As a confirmation of the only partial protective effect of the raised level of HDL, multivariate analysis of epidemiologic data indicates that HDL could explain only 50% of the preventive effect of alcohol on CHD.

The additional effect of alcohol, especially at low dosage, could be to protect from myocardial infarction, i.e., from coronary thrombosis. Since alcohol may predispose to cerebral hemorrhage, part of the mechanism could be through hemostatic functions. Blood platelets, the primary factor involved in thrombosis, have been consistently shown to have their aggregability decreased by alcohol, in vitro and ex vivo, after acute and long-term ingestion in man and animals.

In epidemiologic studies, platelet aggregability to ADP was decreased to the same extent as CHD, by different intakes of alcohol, in a dose-related manner. In the explanation of the protective effect of alcohol on thrombosis, this does not exclude further contribution of fibrinogen, its level being consistently decreased by alcohol drinking, and fibrinolytic activity that is apparently increased.

The epidemiological literature consistently shows that light to moderate alcohol consumption is associated with a reduced risk of CHD and even of total mortality in middle-age and elderly people. A number of alternative explanations for the findings have been suggested but do not appear to explain the observed prospective association. These findings are backed up by numerous animal, clinical, and biochemical studies. Despite the absence of randomized intervention trial probably impossible to complete, the likelihood that the protective association is high.

From a public health point of view, out of fear of stimulating drinking and giving comfort to heavy drinking that is harmful to health and predisposing to violence and accidents, it is difficult for this panel to encourage any level of alcohol consumption.

Introduction

Alcohol drinking, especially in the form of wine, held a prominent place in many ancient cultures. Plato, the Greek philosopher who lived to the age of 80, wrote, "No thing more excellent nor more valuable than wine was ever granted mankind by God." This concept still prevailed in Mediterranean countries in the 19th century, the French microbiologist L. Pasteur writing that "wine is the most healthful and hygienic of beverages."

Beneficial effects of alcohol on the cardiovascular system have been recognized since Heberden (1786), who was the first to describe angina pectoris, and who recommended wine or spirits for its treatment.

Paul D. White, in his famous textbook on heart disease (1951), noted that "the most effective drug after the nitrites is alcohol" for rapid relief from angina pectoris. Only in the second part of this century, however, has sound, indisputable scientific evidence been accumulating on the beneficial cardiovascular effects of moderate alcohol drinking.

Public Beliefs on the Relationship Between Alcohol Drinking and Health

It is difficult to find information on public beliefs about alcohol and health in the international literature. These beliefs differ from country to country, but it can be assumed that in any country it is strongly believed that binge drinking is harmful for health, predisposes to violence and accidents, and should be strictly avoided.

In Mediterranean countries, moderate drinking can be considered good for health, or at least nondamaging, while in the United States, for fear of stimulating drinking and giving comfort to heavy drinking, even moderate drinking is probably not considered as healthy. Nevertheless, some evolution can be observed in recent years.

For millenaries, drinking wine at meals was considered a good or necessary habit, even in Christian religions. Nowadays it is still considered a good habit in Mediterranean countries. Surprisingly, by 1985 in the United States, 53% of the hospitals in 65 of the largest metropolitan areas offered wine service to their patients, and others were looking into serving wine with food. One-third of the hospitals reported that they used wine as soporific instead of tranquilizers. In addition, wine boosted patient morale and satisfaction. In geriatric hospitals, a small amount of wine or beer every day seems to increase the number of ambulatory patients, and they socialize more actively and attend chapel more often (Mansson 1989).

In Italy, and probably other Mediterranean countries, it is believed that drinking moderately between meals is a "sinful" habit and that taking some spirit during a heart attack is protective. As mentioned in the introduction, the apparently correct concept of protection by wine and spirits against heart attack was spread throughout the world for the last two centuries. Finally, in Italy, a recent opinion poll (Osservatorio Permanente 1992) on young men and women aged 15–24 years reports that 15% thought that one glass of wine per day is not dangerous for health, 44% answered two glasses, 20% answered three glasses, and 17% answered more than three glasses. The mean value is 2.4 glasses per day.

The Association Between Alcohol and CHD

In almost all epidemiological studies, an inverse correlation between moderate alcohol use and CHD incidence has been found. These studies can be classified as ecological studies, case-control studies, and cohort studies.

In recent years, Moore and Pearson (1986), Kannel (1988), Veenstra (1991), Marmot and Brummer (1991), Poikolainen (1991), and Jackson and Beaglehole (1993) have produced extensive reviews and discussed the scientific evidence available.

Ecological Studies

A number of ecological studies (Brummer 1969, St Leger et al. 1979, La Porte et al. 1980, Hegsted and Ausman 1988, Renaud et al. 1992) have investigated the relationship between average alcohol consumption and CHD in various countries. A clear inverse relation between average alcohol consumption and CHD mortality was found. Ecological studies are very suggestive but are no real proof of a favourable effect of alcohol consumption on CHD development. Results just indicate a relationship on a population level, and differences among countries with regard to culture, living and working conditions, and other potential confounders are not taken into account. A second drawback of these studies is that alcohol consumption is derived from alcohol sales data, uncorrected for sales to visitors from abroad or for self-produced alcoholic beverages.

Case-Control Studies

Several case-control studies have shown that moderate drinkers of alcohol have a lower risk of CHD when compared with nondrinkers. Among the 11 studies listed in Table 1 with their confidence limits or p-values, only Kaufman et al. (1985) found no effect of moderate alcohol consumption. The majority of studies showed statistically significant lower CHD risk among drinkers: none showed a significant higher risk. Studies include populations of men and of women and of young and old adults; they were undertaken mainly in the United States, but also in the United Kingdom, New Zealand, and Japan. The most recent published study (Jackson et al. 1991), which separately analyzed men and women and nonfatal and fatal myocardial infarction (MI), confirms the previous findings for drinkers but found different relative risks for fatal and nonfatal MI between former drinkers and "never" drinkers. Former drinkers were somewhat preserved from nonfatal but not from fatal MI.

Longitudinal Studies

In longitudinal studies, i.e., cohort or prospective studies, large study populations are classified into categories with different alcohol consumption levels. After a number of years, the association between

Table 1
Case-control studies of alcohol consumption and coronary artery disease

First author/year	Population	Cases	Controls	Alcohol measure	Relative risk	Adjusted for
Stason 1976	M, W age 40–69 United States	Hospitalized nonfatal MI	Hospitalized	< 6 drinks/day ≥ 6 drinks/day	1.0 0.6 (0.3–1.1)	Age, sex, cigarette use
Klatsky 1974	M, W United States	Hospitalized first MI	Hospitalized	< 3 drinks/day 3–5 drinks/day 6 drinks/day	1.0 0.7 ($p < 0.05$) 0.4 ($p < 0.01$)	Cigarette use, age, sex, weight, BP, cholesterol
Hennekens 1978	M age 30–70 United States	Death from CHD	Living community	None ≤ 2 ounces/day > 2 ounces/day	1.0 0.4 (0.3–0.6) 0.7 (0.4–1.1)	Cigarette use, weight, religion
Petitti 1979	W age 18–54 United States	AMI	Non-MI, same year of birth	Nondrinker Drinker	3.1 (1.6–6.0) 1.0	Cigarette use, hypertension, hypercholesterolemia, obesity, gallbladder disease
Ramsay 1979	M age 50–59 United Kingdom	Past history MI	No history of MI	Nil or occasional Frequent or heavy	3.4 (1.2–9.9) 1.0	
Rosenberg 1981	W age 30–49 United States	Hospitalized ml	Hospitalized	Never drinker Current drinker	1.0 0.7 (0.5–1.0)	Age hospital, cigarette use, lipid levels, hypertension, obesity, oral contraceptive use

Study	Population	Outcome	Setting	Alcohol category	Relative risk	Adjustments
Ross 1981	W ≤ age 80 United States	Fatal CAD	Community	No alcohol < 2 drinks/day	1.0 0.4 (p < 0.01)	
Kaufman 1985	M age 30-54 United States	Hospitalized nonfatal first MI	Hospitalized	Never drinkers 1-7 drinks/week	1.0 1.2 (0.8-1.8)	
Siscovick 1986	M age 25-75 United States	Primary cardiac arrest	Community	< 1 drink/month < 1 drink/day 1-3 drinks/day	1.0 0.7 (0.5-1.0) 0.5 (0.3-1.0)	Cigarette use, hypertension, habitual vigorous activity
Kono 1991	M age 40-69 Japan	Nonfatal AMI	Community	Never drinkers Past drinkers < 30 ml/day 30-59 ml/day ≥ 60 ml/day	1.0 0.5 (0.14-1.86) 1.11 0.31 (0.11-0.83) 0.13 (0.05-0.36)	Age, smoking, exercise BMI, hypertension, diabetes, heart disease in parent, job class
Jackson 1991	M age 25-64 New Zealand	Nonfatal MI	Community	Never drinkers Former drinkers ≤ 4 drinks/week 5-14 drinks/week 15-35 drinks/week 36-56 drinks/week > 56 drinks/week	1.0 0.4 (0.2-0.9) 0.6 (0.3-1.0) 0.6 (0.3-1.0) 0.5 (0.3-0.9) 0.6 (0.3-1.3) 1.2 (0.4-1.8)	Age, smoking, hypertension, social class, exercise, recent change in drinking

Table 1. *Continued*

First author/year	Population	Cases	Controls	Alcohol measure	Relative risk	Adjusted for
Jackson 1991 *Continued*	W age 25–64 New Zealand	Nonfatal MI	Community	Never drinkers Former drinkers ≤ 4 drinks/week 5–14 drinks/week 15–35 drinks/week 36–56 drinks/week	1.0 0.1 (0.2–0.9) 0.5 (0.2–0.1) 0.2 (0.1–0.5) 0.2 (0.0–0.5) 0.4 (0.0–4.4)	Age, smoking, hypertension, social class, exercise, recent change in drinking
	M age 25–64 New Zealand	Fatal CHD	Community	Never drinkers Former drinkers ≤ 4 drinks/week 5–14 drinks/week 15–35 drinks/week 36–56 drinks/week > 56 drinks/week	1.0 1.1 (0.3–3.3) 0.4 (0.2–0.8) 0.4 (0.2–0.8) 0.4 (0.2–0.8) 0.2 (0.1–0.6) 0.5 (0.2–1.5)	Age, smoking, hypertension, social class, exercise, recent change in drinking
	W age 25–64 New Zealand	Fatal CHD	Community	Never drinkers Former drinkers ≤ 4 drinks/week 5–14 drinks/week 15–35 drinks/week 36–56 drinks/week	1.0 1.1 (0.2–4.2) 0.0 (0.0–0.2) 0.0 (0.0–0.3) 0.5 (0.0–0.7) 0.9 (0.0–32.3)	Age, smoking, hypertension, social class, exercise, recent change in drinking

alcohol consumption and CHD incidence is analyzed. In the last 40 years, the effect of alcohol drinking on CHD incidence has been investigated in more than 30 cohorts all over the world.

Table 2 shows the results of 16 studies where alcohol consumption was measured in a quantitative or semiquantitative way (for example, the number of drinks per day) in such a way that the consumption in grams of alcohol per unit of time could be evaluated with some degree of precision. Some of the results observed in man are summarized in Figure 1. In contrast to all other studies, a recent study in Finland (Suhonen et al. 1987) showed a positive association between consumption of alcohol, especially spirit, and CHD mortality. In another study (Camacho et al. 1987), the protective effects of small amounts of alcohol on CHD mortality was not confirmed, but an excess of risk was not found either. In all other studies listed in Table 2, relative risks of CHD are less than 1 in moderate drinkers compared to nondrinkers.

Particular confidence can be given to the results of the most recent studies, which considered very large cohorts. The studies of Stampfer et al. (1988) (87,526 women followed for 4 years), Boffetta and Garfinkel (1990) (276,802 men followed for 12 years), Klatsky et al. (1986, 1990) (123,840 men followed for 8 years), and Rimm et al. (1991) (51,529 men followed for 2 years), all significantly confirm that the CHD risk is lower in moderate drinkers.

Figure 1
Alcohol and CAD, longitudinal studies, men

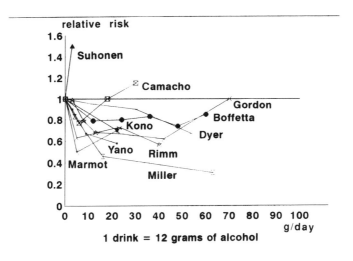

Table 2

Cohort studies of alcohol consumption and coronary artery disease

First author/ year	Population	Follow-up	Alcohol meaure	Relative risk	Adjusted for
Yano 1977	7705 M age 45–66 United States	6 years	0 ml/day 1–6 ml/day 7–15 ml/day 16–39 ml/day 40+ ml/day	**CHD incidence** 1.00 0.90 0.67 0.58 0.46	Age
Dyer 1980	1832 M age 40–55 United States	17 years	< 1 drink/day 1 drink/day 2–3 drinks/day 4–5 drinks/day 6+ drinks/day	**CHD mortality** 1.00 0.95 0.90 0.67 1.83	Age, smoking, diastolic BP, cholesterol, pulse rate
Marmot 1981	1422 M age 40–64 United Kingdom	10 years	0 g/day 0.1–9.0 g/day 9.1–34 g/day 34+ g/day	**CAD mortality** 2.1 1.0 1.5 0.9	Age, BP, smoking, cholesterol, grade of employment
Klatsky 1981	8060 M, W United States	10 years	0 drinks/day ≤ 2 drinks/day 3–5 drinks/day 6+ drinks/day	**CAD mortality** 1.0 0.61 0.70 0.82	
Gordon 1983	2026 M age 31–64 United States	22 years	0 oz/month 1–9 oz/month 10–19 oz/month 20–29 oz/month 30–59 oz/month 60+ oz/month	**CHD incidence** 1 0.90 0.88 0.75 0.58 0.72	Age, systolic BP, relative weight, lipoprotein level
Gordon 1983	2599 W age 31–64 United States		0 oz/month 1–9 oz/month 10–19 oz/month 20–29 oz/month 30–59 oz/month 60+ oz/month	**CHD incidence** 1 1.05 0.68 0.72 0.75 0.76	Age, systolic BP, relative weight, lipoprotein level
Colditz 1985	1184 M, W age 63+ United States	4.75 years	0 g/day 0.1–8.9 g/day 9–34 g/day 34+ g/day	**CHD mortality** 1 0.3 (0.1–0.7) 0.5 (0.2–1.1) 0.8 (0.2–3.4)	Age, sex, smoking, cholesterol

Table 2. *Continued*

First author/ year	Population	Follow-up	Alcohol meaure	Relative risk	Adjusted for
Gordon 1987	1910 M age 38–55 United States	18 years after 1953–1954	0 oz/month 1–9 oz/month 10–19 oz/month 20–29 oz/month 30–59 oz/month 60–89 oz/month 90+ oz/month	**CHD incidence** 1 0.63 0.68 0.67 0.62 1.0 1.4	
Gordon 1987	823 M age 56–73 United States	10 years after 1971–72	0 oz/month 1–9 oz/month 10–19 oz/month 20–29 oz/month 30–59 oz/month 60–89 oz/month 90+ oz/month	**CHD incidence** 1 1.1 0.93 0.55 1.0 0.74 0.62	
Kono 1986	5477 M Japan	19 years	Nondrinkers Ex-drinkers Occasional drinker < 2 go (54 ml) $\geq$ 2 go (54 ml)	**CHD mortality** 1.0 1.5 (1.0–2.4) 0.6 (0.4–0.9) 0.7 (0.5–1.1) 0.7 (0.4–1.1)	Age, smoking
Camacho 1987	4590 M, W age 35+ United States	15 years M	0 drink/month 1–30 drinks/month 31–60 drinks/month 61–90 drinks/month 91+	**CHD mortality** 1.3 (0.8–2.0) 1.0 1.3 (0.8–2.1) 1.5 (0.8–2.9) 1.5 (0.6–2.4)	Age
		W	0 drink/month 1–30 drinks/month 31–60 drinks/month 61–90 drinks/month	1.1 (0.8–1.6) 1.0 1.0 (0.5–2.2) 1.0 (0.2–4.5)	
Suhonen 1987	4532 M age 40–64 Finland	5 years	0 g/month < 200 g/month $\geq$ 200 g/month	**CHD mortality** 1 1.5 1.5	
Stampfer 1988	87,526 W age 34–59 United States	4 years	0 g/day < 1.5 g/day 1.5–4.9 g/day 5.0–14.9 g/day 15–24.9 g/day $\geq$ 25 g/day	**CHD incidence** 1.0 0.7 (0.5–1.1) 0.5 (0.4–0.8) 0.5 (0.4–0.8) 0.6 (0.3–1.1) 0.6 (0.3–1.1)	Age

Table 2. *Continued*

First author/ year	Population	Follow-up	Alcohol meaure	Relative risk	Adjusted for
Miller 1990	1341 M age 35–69 Trinidad	7.5 years	**CHD incidence** Never drinkers 1–4 drinks/week 5–14 drinks/week 15–59 drinks/week	**CHD incidence** 1.0 0.83 (0.4–1.7) 0.46 (0.2–1.0) 0.31 (0.1–0.8)	Age, ethnic group, smoking, systolic BP, cholesterol
Boffetta 1990	276,802 M age 40–59 United States	12 years	Nondrinkers Occasional drinkers 1 drink/day 2 drinks/day 3 drinks/day 4 drinks/day 5 drinks/day 6+ drinks/day Irregular drinkers	**CHD mortality** 1 0.86 (0.81–0.92) 0.79 (0.76–0.83) 0.80 (0.76–0.85) 0.83 (0.77–0.89) 0.74 (0.68–0.82) 0.85 (0.75–0.98) 0.92 (0.85–1.01) 0.96 (0.91–1.02)	Age, smoking
Klatsky 1990	123,840 M, W mean age 40.5 United States	8 years	Never drinkers Ex-drinkers < 1 drink/month < 1 drink/day 1–2 drinks/day 3–5 drinks/day 6+ drinks/day	**CAD mortality** 1 1.0 0.9 0.8 0.7 (p≤ 0.001) 0.6 (p≤ 0.05) 0.8	Age, gender, race, smoking, BMI, marital status, education
Rimm 1991	51,529 M age 40–75 United States	2 years	0 g/day 0.1–5.0 g/day 5.1–10.0 g/day 10.1–15.0 g/day 15.1–30.0 g/day 30.1–50.0 g/day > 50 g/day	**CAD mortality** 1 0.99 (0.74–1.33) 0.79 (0.55–1.14) 0.68 (0.45–1.01) 0.73 (0.51–1.05) 0.57 (0.35–0.79) 0.41 (0.20–0.84)	
Farchi 1992	1563 M age 45–64 Italy	15 years	**Mean Value of Quintiles** 22.7 g/day 56.4 g/day 77.8 g/day 108.2 g/day 164.7 g/day	**CHD mortality** 1.0 0.84 (0.46–1.54) 0.61 (0.31–1.18) 0.90 (0.50–1.61) 1.02 (0.57–1.81)	Age, smoking, occupation

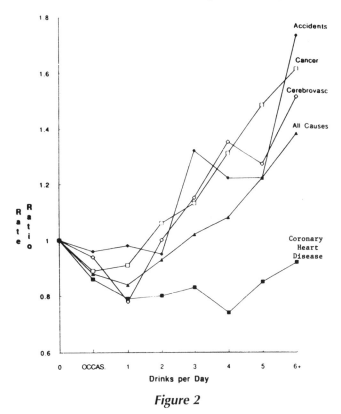

Figure 2

R. Curtis Ellison, Epidemiology, September 1990, Volume 1

Is There a U-Shaped Curve for Alcohol and CHD?

It is generally agreed that there is a J-shaped rather than a U-shaped relationship between alcohol intake and total mortality, with increases in death from cirrhosis, accidents, violence, and cancer in heavier drinkers (Boffetta and Garfinkel 1990) (see Figure 2). In addition, there is a general concurrence that there is a U-shaped curve for the association between alcohol and total cardiovascular disease (CVD) mortality, which includes stroke and noncoronary heart disease deaths (Kagan 1981, Klatsky et al. 1981a, Criqui et al. 1987a, Shaper et al. 1988). However, the Whitehall Study found protection for CVD at 9 g/day of alcohol intake and above (Marmot et al. 1981), with little evidence for a U-shaped relationship. Much of the U-shape for total CVD mortality is presumably due to the association of heavier alcohol consumption with stroke (Gill et al. 1986), and particularly with hemorrhagic stroke (Kagan et al. 1981, Stampfer et al. 1988).

Some studies of the alcohol-CHD association address only mortality data, while others have reported both morbidity and mortality.

The Lipid Research Clinics (LRC) Follow-up Study evaluated mortality only and showed a benefit limited to < 3 drinks per day, beyond which CHD began to increase (Criqui et al. 1987a). Similarly, the American Cancer Society prospective study of 276,802 men revealed a benefit up to 4 drinks per day for CHD mortality, but less benefit at higher intakes (Boffetta and Garfinkel 1990). The MRFIT Study also evaluated CHD mortality only and found that the alcohol benefit reached a maximum at 2–3 drinks per day (Suh et al. 1992).

Studies that have evaluated both CHD morbidity and mortality include a Swedish prospective study (Petersson 1988). After 9 years of follow-up, middle-aged men who had been at some time in their life registered with the Temperance Board, a rough index of alcohol intemperance, had a significantly increased risk of CHD independent of other risk factors. Nonfatal and fatal CHD events were not separately analyzed in this study. In the Honolulu Heart Study there was a similar benefit for both CHD morbidity and mortality up to alcohol intake levels of 3 drinks per day (Yano et al. 1977). However, a later publication showed some loss of benefit for mortality at 4 or more drinks per day (Kagan et al. 1981). In a New Zealand case-control study, the effect for nonfatal MI and fatal CHD was similar, with a plateau of benefit at about 1 drink per day and a beginning reversal of benefit at very high drinking levels of > 56 drinks/week (Jackson et al. 1991).

By contrast, data from the Yugoslavia Cardiovascular Disease Study did not suggest a plateau of benefit at low levels of intake, but did indicate a stronger benefit for nonfatal MI than for CHD death (Kozarevic et al. 1980). Similarly, in the Health Professionals Follow-Up Study, the benefit for nonfatal MI and for coronary artery bypass graft or percutaneous transluminal coronary angioplasty was somewhat greater than for fatal CHD, due to a slightly smaller protective effect of alcohol for fatal CHD at > 3 drinks/day compared to 1–2 drinks/day (Rimm et al. 1991). The Kaiser Study data show the biggest discrepancy between morbidity and mortality data. Both acute MI and all coronary disease are lower in the highest drinking category of 6+ drinks/day (Klatsky et al. 1981b), whereas the lowest coronary mortality was in the group consuming 1–2 drinks/day (Klatsky et al. 1981a).

In summary, the evidence suggests that, similar to total mortality and all CVD, there is a U-shaped relationship between alcohol and CHD as well. The threshold at which the right side of the U begins to increase for all CVD and total mortality is about 2 drinks/day.

However, the threshold for the right side of the U for CHD is somewhat less clear, and could be as few as 2 or as many as 6 drinks/day. In addition, the maximal protective effect for fatal CHD appears to occur at a lower dose (< 2 drinks/day), while the maximal protective effect for nonfatal CHD may be at higher levels of consumption.

The above discussion is consistent with the known continued increase in HDL at high levels of alcohol consumption (Castelli et al. 1977), the reported reduced atherosclerosis in alcoholics (La Porte et al. 1980), but also the known direct toxic effect of high levels of alcohol on blood pressure and on the heart, including arrhythmias, cardiomyopathy, and left ventricular hypertrophy (Criqui 1990). This could logically lead to an increase of sudden CHD death but not necessarily nonfatal CHD at higher levels of alcohol intake (Kittner et al. 1983).

Consensus

It seems important to examine the independence of the observed association with regard to possible confounding or effect-modifying variables.

Age

Almost all findings are age-adjusted. Moreover, the studies cover a large range of age intervals, including young adults of 18 years (Petitti et al. 1979), adults 25 years and older (Jackson et al. 1991), or, as in the study of Colditz et al. (1985), men and women aged 63 and over. The association between alcohol consumption and 15-year total mortality was studied in a cohort of 49,464 Swedish conscripts (Andreasson et al. 1988) mostly aged 18–19. In this study, a strong direct association with alcohol was found for total mortality, but the highest mortality from CVD was found in the abstinent group. As CVD accounted for only 3.9% of total deaths, the benefit was outweighed other risks.

Gender

The majority of studies concern men, but there are studies of women only or of women and men considered together, as above in Tables 1 and 2. The lower risk in drinkers seems to be similar for both sexes. Nevertheless, women drink lower quantities than men, get a protective effect at a lower dosage, but also experience noxious effects at a smaller dosage than men.

Fatal and Nonfatal Events

Many studies considering as endpoints fatal CHD, nonfatal only, or fatal and nonfatal incidence at the same time did not give clear evidence that alcohol could be more protective for a particular kind of event. Nevertheless, in certain studies mentioned above (Kozarevic et al. 1980, Rimm et al. 1991, Klatsky et al. 1981), the benefit for nonfatal MI is somewhat greater than for fatal CHD.

Length of Follow-Up

The study of Rimm et al. (1991) considered a follow-up of only 2 years and observed a relative risk of 0.57 for 30–50 g of alcohol per day. The follow-up of Gordon and Kannel (1983) was 22 years and obtained for a similar intake of alcohol a relative risk of 0.58. In longitudinal studies, whatever the length of follow-up, the results are surprisingly similar. Very seldom papers on these longitudinal studies include life tables showing the survival of people by alcohol consumption. It would be interesting to know if and how differences in survival change along time. Farchi et al. (1992) observed that maximum differences in survival were reached 10 years after entry screening and then remained almost constant thereafter up to 20 years.

Countries

There is also a remarkable consistency of the findings in diverse populations in different states of the United States; in different regions of the United Kingdom; and in Yugoslavs, Italians, Puerto Ricans, Japanese Americans in Hawaii, Australians, New Zealanders, and others; except in Finland (Suhonen et al. 1987), as already indicated. The difference in Finland can probably be attributed to the type of alcohol (mostly spirit) and type of drinking (weekend only) or other confounding factors.

Other Possible Confounders

Almost all studies adjusted the relative risks by age and smoking habits. Many of them also adjusted the results for other possible confounders such as blood pressure, serum cholesterol, pulse rate, education, marital status, occupation, and others. The relative risks are generally weakly affected by these adjustments. In the study of Rimm et al. (1991a), after adjustment for coronary risk factors including dietary intake of cholesterol, fat, dietary fibre, and aspirin use (Rimm et al. 1991b), the alcohol intake was still inversely related to coronary disease incidence.

Problems related to adjustment have been raised by Smith and Shipley (1991). If there is a direct effect of alcohol on the value of a biological variable included in the model, the risk associated with alcohol is under- or overestimated if the effect is positive or negative. This has been shown by Criqui et al. (1987a). The inclusion of HDL cholesterol in Criqui's model reduced the apparent protective effect of alcohol by about half for both cardiovascular and coronary heart disease, and the p-value for cardiovascular disease was no longer close to significance.

Type of Alcoholic Beverage

Several studies (Hennekens et al. 1978, Rosenberg et al. 1981, Yano et al. 1977, Stampfer et al. 1988, Klatsky et al. 1986, 1990, Rimm et al. 1991a, Frideman and Kimball 1986) separately measured the consumption of wine, beer, and spirit and estimated the relative risks for each type of alcoholic beverage. From these studies it can be inferred that there is no clear evidence that one type of beverage is more protective than another, although there is a hint that wine might offer some more protection, at least in certain studies. In the comparison between countries, the inverse association between alcohol and CHD mortality was observed only for wine; beer and spirits showed no significant relationship (St Leger et al. 1979). In the recent report from the Kaiser Permanente Medical Center on 129,000 persons (Klatsky et al. 1992), wine preference was associated with significantly lower relative risk for cardiovascular death (0.7, $p = 0.01$). Finally, in the only study in which wine was the main alcoholic beverage (Farchi et al. 1992), the lower mortality rate from both CVD and cancer (see Figure 3) was observed with an intake of 56 g of alcohol per day. This is a substantially higher amount than the most beneficial in the Boffetta study (1990) (1 drink/day or approximately 12 g alcohol). This suggests that wine drinking could be a safer way of drinking alcohol, at least under Italian conditions. Nevertheless, even if wine, through its regular moderate consumption at meals, could fit best with the idea of a protective effect, especially in Mediterranean countries, its superiority over other alcoholic beverages has not yet been satisfactorily established.

Drinking Pattern

Only a few studies addressed the question of drinking pattern directly. Rimm et al. (1991) found that the average number of days

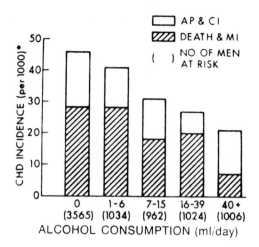

Figure 3
**Six-year incidence of coronary heart disease according
to alcohol consumption**

*Age-adjusted in five-year groups by the direct method according to the age structure of the entire population at risk. CHD denotes coronary heart disease, AP angina pectoris, CI acute coronary insufficiency, and MI myocardial infarction.

per week on which alcohol was consumed was also inversely associated with risk of coronary artery disease (CAD). Men who reported drinking, on average, on 3–4 days per week had a relative risk of 0.66 (0.46–0.96) compared with men who drank on less than 1 day a week. Because total alcohol intake and average number of days per week on which alcohol was consumed were so highly correlated (r = 0.89), the two predictors were not modelled simultaneously.

Kannel (1988) states that a small amount of alcohol taken weekly is beneficial only if it is spread out over the week. "Binge drinking" of the entire week's allocation is harmful. The only study showing an increased risk of CHD with any alcohol intake (Suhonen et al. 1987) was the result of the weekend consumption of spirits.

Quantity of Alcohol

Several case-control studies (see Table 1) and longitudinal studies (see Table 2) estimated the relative risks by different amounts of alcohol consumption. If the very few studies unable to find any protective role of alcohol are excluded, it appears that the estimated lower relative risk in alcohol drinkers is very similar for consumptions ranging from a few grams per day to about 40 g/day (see Figure 1).

Continuing Controversies

Each of the studies relating alcohol to CVD has its flaws. Although consistency of the finding is often cited as one of the criteria making an observed association more likely to be causal than artefactual, studies can be wrong consistently. Two main arguments concerning non-drinkers are questioned in the international literature and deal with "sick quitters" and "ill health in abstainers." These possible biases were first raised by Shaper et al. (1988). They found an inverse relationship between alcohol consumption and CVD mortality in their whole cohort, but the inverse relationship could no longer be found in the subcohort initially free from heart disorders.

The argument suggests that it is the inclusion of "sick quitters" with the nondrinkers that accounts for the high incidence of CHD in nondrinkers compared with moderate drinkers. Several studies (Jackson et al. 1991, Kono et al. 1991, Yano et al. 1977, Kono et al. 1986, Stampfer et al. 1988, Miller et al. 1990, Klatsky et al. 1990, Lazarus et al. 1991) have been able to separate lifetime abstainers from people who stopped drinking. Stampfer et al. (1988) stated that separate analyses that excluded women who had reported a great decrease in intake of alcohol during the past 10 years yielded the same results. Other studies estimated quantitatively the risks of "never" drinkers and former drinkers. The risk of CHD in former drinkers was generally equal or greater than that of never drinkers, and the latter was greater than that of drinkers. Jackson et al. (1991) observed a lower risk for nonfatal but not for fatal CHD in former drinkers as compared to never drinkers. Kono et al. (1991) also observed a lower risk in past drinkers.

In addition, in the report from Klatsky et al. (1990), moderate alcohol consumption was associated with lower CHD mortality, even in the population left after exclusion of anyone who had one of 17 indicators of cardiovascular illness or risk factors. In the study by Boffetta and Garfinkel (1990), 33% of the cohort was classified as sick at the enrolment. Among the healthy remainder, the higher incidence of CHD in nondrinkers compared with moderate drinkers was clear.

Thus, it seems that the inclusion of former drinkers in the non-drinking group did not account for the higher incidence of CHD in nondrinkers in the studies that have the data to address this question directly.

The Association Between Alcohol and Atherosclerosis in Relation to Coronary Heart Disease

Autopsy and Relevant Studies

It has been frequently reported, especially when cirrhosis of the liver was used as a marker of excessive alcohol consumption, that chronic alcoholism is associated with a lesser degree of atherosclerosis and lower incidence of MI (Hall et al. 1953, Howell and Manion 1960, Ruebner et al. 1961). Nevertheless, in these studies controls were frequently patients dying from CVD with severe atherosclerosis. Thus, any group compared to these subjects would exhibit some protective effect. By contrast, in the autopsy studies performed by Parrish and Eberly (1961) in people dying from car accidents, there was not a lower severity of coronary atherosclerosis in patients with liver cirrhosis.

In autopsy studies reported by Moore and Pearson (1986) in which alcohol consumption was estimated by interview instead of relying on cirrhosis as a marker, five (Hirst et al. 1965, Viel et al. 1966, Sackett et al. 1968, Rissanen 1974, Rhoads et al. 1978) out of seven studies did not observe any significant lowering of atherosclerotic lesions in alcohol consumers, especially after adjusting for age, smoking, cholesterol, and blood pressure. The main difficulty of these studies is in the selection of adequate controls. They should not be patients dying from CHD, or even from wasting diseases such as cancer, which are known to be associated with a lesser degree of atherosclerosis. It seems that the controls should ideally be violent deaths as in the studies of Parrish and Eberly (1961), Viel et al. (1966), Rissanen (1974), and others. Under these conditions, significantly less atherosclerosis in alcohol consumers has not been found. Nevertheless, it can be argued that, since alcohol drinking is frequently associated with violent death, reliable information on alcohol consumption of these people could be difficult to obtain.

In the study of Rhoads et al. (1978), alcohol consumption was lower in men with infarcts. Concordant with these studies is the observation in the cohort of Japanese men living in Hawaii that the negative association of alcohol consumption with the risk of CHD was particularly strong with hard endpoints (death and MI), but not with angina pectoris (see Figure 4) (Yano et al. 1977). In addition, this protection was observed in the range of moderate consumption rather than with heavy drinking.

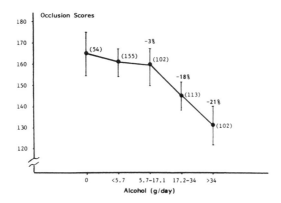

Figure 4

By contrast, in the Puerto Rico Heart Health program (Kittner et al. 1983), opposite results were found since the most significant inhibitory effects on CHD was on angina pectoris ($p < 0$–0.5). But it was not clear whether the group of angina pectoris comprised unstable angina, which is rather a thrombotic phenomenon, stable angina being primarily dependent on the severity of atherosclerotic lesions per se.

In conclusion, it does not seem that the inhibitory effect of alcohol on atherosclerotic lesions has been clearly demonstrated in man by autopsy and clinical observations, especially for a moderate intake of alcohol; the data do not exclude such a possibility, however.

Clinical Studies

In a series of studies, Barboriak et al. (1982) observed, in more than 2500 patients undergoing diagnostic coronary arteriographyn, an inverse relationship between the extent of coronary occlusion and the amount of alcohol consumed, for both males and females. The coronary obstruction–limiting effect of alcohol was apparent in spite of the higher prevalence of hypertension, heavier smoking, and higher levels of plasma triglycerides. In further studies (Gruchow et al. 1982) it was found that a consumption of 5.7 to 17.1 g of alcohol per day decreased the occlusion score by 3% (see Figure 4). To be emphasized is that a similar intake of alcohol was associated, in prospective studies, with a 10–50% lower incidence of CHD (see Figure 1). It was only

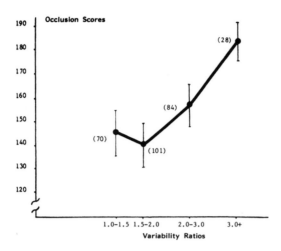

Figure 5

with an intake higher than 17.2 ml of alcohol, and mostly higher than 34 g, that a decrease of approximately 20% in the score could be observed. The more consistent the intake of alcohol, the more significant was the lower level of occlusions. By contrast, drinkers with variable drinking patterns had higher occlusion scores, regardless of amounts consumed (see Figure 5). They also suggested that the retarding effect of alcohol on CHD may be at least partially explained by the alcohol-induced rise of plasma-HDL cholesterol (Barboriak et al. 1979). However, drinkers with a variable pattern of drinking, thus with a high occlusion score, had a similar high level of HDL cholesterol as the regular drinkers (Gruchow et al. 1982).

By contrast, in a study of 1000 patients who underwent coronary angiography, the inverse association between coronary occlusion and alcohol consumption was found only in white females 50 years of age or older (Pearson et al. 1979).

The results with angiography suggest a different pattern compared to epidemiologic studies concerning the inverse relationship between alcohol intake and CHD. At moderate intake, there is little or no protective effect, while high consistent intake of alcohol is associated with substantial lessening of coronary lesions.

Experimental Atherosclerosis in Animals

Very few studies have been done in this field. The most classical experiment has been done by Eberhard (1936) in rabbits fed a high cholesterol diet for approximately 5 months. The inclusion of 25% ethanol in the drinking water, although it increased the level of cholesterol in plasma and liver, decreased the extent of atherosclerotic lesions in the aorta and its content in cholesterol. More recently, these studies have been reproduced by Goto et al. (1974), also in rabbits, this time with a more physiologic level of alcohol in the drinking water (5–10%) and 0.5% cholesterol in the diet. Again, most of the plasma lipid fractions were significantly higher in the alcohol-fed animals, although the severity of lesions in the aorta was significantly decreased, especially with 10% alcohol in the drinking water. Renaud et al. (1979), in preliminary studies, confirmed these results in rabbits fed for 20 weeks a purified diet containing 45% of calories from butter, 0.05g/100g cholesterol, and drinking 6% alcohol. The content of cholesterol in the aorta was significantly decreased ($p < 0.01$) in the group with alcohol drinking, although plasma cholesterol was similar to the group fed the same diet without alcohol. By contrast, platelet aggregation to thrombin was significantly decreased in the group with alcohol drinking, suggesting a possible effect of platelet reactivity in the formation of atherosclerotic lesions. Thus, the effect on platelet reactivity could also be a possible mechanism involved in the protective effect of alcohol on experimental atherosclerosis, under conditions where plasma lipids are increased by alcohol drinking.

Nevertheless, the protective effect of alcohol was not reproduced in rabbits by Feller and Huff (1955) over a much shorter period of time and a much higher level of dietary cholesterol. They confirmed the hypercholesterolemic effect of alcohol observed by previous investigators under conditions of a high intake of dietary cholesterol and alcohol. In other animal species, such as cockerels (Nichols et al. 1956) and rat (Gottlieb et al. 1959), a protective effect of alcohol on atherosclerosis was not confirmed.

More recently, Rudel et al. (1981) investigated the effect of alcohol (36% of calories) included in a liquid diet rich in cholesterol on atherosclerotic lesions in primates (*Macaca memestrima*). Alcohol induced a significant increase in the plasma level of cholesterol and triglycerides, especially at the highest level of dietary cholesterol. Nevertheless, ethanol appeared to prevent much of the cholesterol–induced coronary atherosclerosis, and to some extent that of the aorta. The severity of lesions was significantly related to the fatty acid composition of the LDL fraction in blood. They concluded that their work was consistent with a protective effect of alcohol, especially on coronary atherosclerosis, but that the need for further work was readily apparent.

In conclusion, further work is certainly needed, but under more physiologic conditions with diets more comparable to that of humans and alcohol intake not higher than 10–15% of calories.

Lipid Metabolism

Ethanol is oxidized almost exclusively in the liver. Since the liver also plays a central role in the metabolism of lipids, there are several interactions of ethanol with lipid metabolism. The main interest in the present review is the effect of alcohol in human studies on lipids and lipoprotein particles known to be associated with CHD.

In numerous epidemiological studies, a positive association has been observed between alcohol consumption and the level of HDL cholesterol (Moore and Pearson 1986, Veenstra 1991). In addition, in a number of experimental studies in man, even moderate amounts of alcohol were shown to increase HDL cholesterol within a few weeks. There is some evidence that HDL3-cholesterol is more sensitive to the alcohol-induced increase than HDL2-cholesterol subfraction (Valimaki et al. 1988). In epidemiological studies, however, both subfractions of HDL cholesterol are associated with a reduced risk of CHD (Miller et al. 1988, Stampfer et al. 1991). Epidemiological and experimental studies that have included measurements of the HDL associated apolipoproteins A1 and A2 confirm the positive association between alcohol consumption and HDL.

There is little doubt that alcohol, even at moderate consumption, increases HDL cholesterol. Before definite conclusions can be drawn as to whether the increased level of HDL cholesterol contributes to a reduction in CHD risk, it seems necessary to have a better understanding of the mechanism underlying this increase. Also, definite evidence of an increase in the excretion of cholesterol and bile acid with moderate alcohol consumption seems to be needed to support the reverse cholesterol transport hypothesis, as well as definite evidence that reverse cholesterol transport inhibits atherosclerosis.

The relationship between moderate alcohol consumption and HDL cholesterol as observed in epidemiological studies has been confirmed by many clinical studies, which proves the causality of the relationship. The mechanism, however, is still unclear.

It should be realised that it may not be the HDL cholesterol that causes the decrease in CHD risk, but a factor that is closely associated with HDL cholesterol. The fact that not more than 50% of the reduced risk can be explained by HDL cholesterol (Criqui et al. 1987a) already points to the fact that other factors play a significant role. Other lipid mechanisms as well as nonlipid mechanisms could be involved.

In general, especially in the case of moderate alcohol consumption, clinical research in humans has to be preferred to studies in animals, for which moderate alcohol consumption is not a normal habit.

Finally, this area is dominated by studies in which only HDL cholesterol or apolipoproteins are measured without further investigation of the mechanisms. More studies showing simply an increase in HDL will not give stronger evidence for a beneficial effect or moderate alcohol consumption. As an example, it has been reported that alcohol decreases the antiatherogenic fraction Lp Al instead of increasing it (Puchois et al. 1990). These authors found it unlikely that the antiatherogenic effect of alcohol consumption would be based on its action on HDL.

Does the Effect of Alcohol on Lipoproteins Explain the Effect of Alcohol on Coronary Heart Disease?

Given the multiplicity of effects of alcohol on the cardiovascular system, it would appear that much of the benefit on the left side of the U-shaped curve should be attributable to the increase in HDL cholesterol and related apolipoproteins (Criqui et al. 1990). This question has been explored in the LRC Follow-Up Study. If modest alcohol consumption had a protective effect on CHD incidence via an increase in HDL cholesterol, adding HDL cholesterol to a multivariate model predicting CHD incidence as a function of alcohol (and other variables) would show a lesser benefit for alcohol than a model without HDL, since the benefit of moderate alcohol through an HDL cholesterol pathway would be statistically controlled. This was exactly the result obtained in both men and women (Criqui et al. 1987a). The 50% reduction of the protective strength of the alcohol coefficient after addition of HDL cholesterol to the model suggested that about half of the alcohol's effect was mediated by HDL cholesterol. There was not a pathway via low density lipoprotein (LDL) cholesterol in these analyses. However, alcohol consumption in men was not associated with lower LDL cholesterol in the LRC Study (Criqui et al. 1986a).

The probable validity of these findings has increased with similar findings in two subsequent publications. In the Honolulu Heart Study, cross-sectional analyses at baseline had shown that alcohol was associated both with decreased LDL cholesterol and increased HDL cholesterol (Castelli et al. 1977). Controlling for LDL cholesterol reduced the alcohol coefficient by about 18%, indicating a small contribution of alcohol to decreased CHD risk through this mechanism (Langer et al. 1992). Further addition of term for HDL cholesterol to the model reduced the alcohol coefficient by 45%, indicating striking agreement with the LRC Study that about half of alcohol's effect is mediated by HDL cholesterol.

Data from 11,688 men participating in the MRFIT Study have recently been published on the association of alcohol with CHD mortality (Suh et al. 1992). Using a statistical methodology essentially the same as used in the LRC and Honolulu studies, the authors showed that the protective effect of alcohol was reduced by 45% after inclusion of HDL cholesterol in the multivariate model. Thus, the findings from this third publication are strikingly concordant with the earlier two studies indicating that about half of moderate alcohol consumption's protective effect appears to be mediated by increases in HDL cholesterol. Nevertheless, the effect attributable to HDL cholesterol may actually be somewhat larger than estimated in these three studies, since misclassification due to measurement error will attenuate the degree to which HDL appears to mediate the effects of alcohol in these regression models.

The results in each of the three studies were controlled for other major cardiovascular risk factors. However, these studies were not controlled for potential dietary differences in drinkers. Although such dietary differences have been reported (Jones et al. 1982, Rimm et al. 1991), this is not always the case (Fisher 1985). In addition, in the study by Rimm et al., despite dietary differences in drinkers, adjustment for these differences produced little change in the risk estimates for alcohol.

Since the results of the above three studies suggest only half the protective effect of moderate alcohol consumption appears to be mediated by an HDL cholesterol pathway, or by a variable very highly correlated with HDL, alcohol, and CHD, what are other possible mechanisms for moderate alcohol's protective effect? One likely additional pathway is the coagulation system. Alcohol can lower fibrinogen (Meade et al. 1979) and inhibit platelet aggregation (Mikhailidis et al. 1983; Renaud et al. 1992). Thus, it is tempting to speculate that moderate alcohol consumption can inhibit CHD incidence both by inhibiting atherosclerosis (the HDL cholesterol pathway) and thrombotic occlusion of the coronary arteries (the coagulation pathway).

Interestingly, similar statistical models in both the LRC Study (Criqui 1987b) and the Honolulu Study (Langer et al. 1992) suggested that blood pressure elevations accompanying higher levels of alcohol con-

Table 3
**Relative risk (RR) of CHD, ischemic stroke and subarachnoid hemorrhage
according to alcohol intake after adjustment for risk factors
in proportional-hazards model**

Alcohol (g/day)	Coronary heart disease (No. of cases = 200)	Ischemic stroke (No. of cases = 66)	Subarachnoid hemorrhage (No. of cases = 28)
		RR (95% CI)	
0	1.0 (referent)	1.0 (referent)	1.0 (referent)
< 1.5	0.8 (0.5–1.2)	0.7 (0.4–1.6)	2.4 (0.5–12.1)
1.5–4.9	0.6 (0.4–1.0)	0.4 (0.2–0.9)	2.9 (0.7–11.5)
5.0–14.9	0.6 (0.4–0.9)	0.3 (0.1–0.7)	3.7 (1.0–13.8)
> 15	0.6 (0.3–1.1)	0.5 (0.2–1.1)	2.6 (0.7–10.3)

Adapted from Stampfer et al. 1988.

sumption do promote CVD incidence. The evidence that such a blood pressure increase may be due to withdrawal has been reviewed (Criqui 1987b). The effect of moderate alcohol consumption (< 2 drinks/day) on blood pressure is uncertain, with studies variously showing a decrease, no change, or an increase in blood pressure. (For an extensive review of alcohol's effect on blood pressure, see the chapter entitled "Alcohol Intake and its Relation to Hypertension.")

The Association Between Alcohol and Hemostasis in Relation to Coronary Heart Disease

Alcohol and Cerebral Hemorrhage

A high rate of stroke has been reported among populations with low CHD (Kuller and Reisler 1971), especially in Japanese in Japan compared to Japanese in California (Gordon 1957). In the Japanese cohort living in Hawaii, it seems that the high risk of hemorrhagic stroke can be at least partly attributed to alcohol drinking (Reed 1990). The relationship between alcohol intake and cerebral hemorrhage was also noted in other prospective studies in Japan (Tanaka et al. 1982) as well as in American women (Stampfer et al. 1988), but was already observed through many case reports (Hilbom 1987), especially after alcohol intoxication. Alcohol seems to protect from ischemic stroke to the same extent it protects from CHD (Stampfer et al. 1988) (see Table 3), but at the same time increases the risk of subarachnoid hemorrhage. This strongly suggests a marked effect of alcohol on hemostasis, probably through several factors as reviewed by Gorelick (1989) and Hillbom (1987). Therefore, any studies on the mechanism involved in the effect of alcohol on the cardiovascular system should consider the possible effect on hemostasis.

Platelet Function

Since moderate alcohol drinking seems to mostly prevent MI, a parameter of special interest is platelet function. It is now accepted that coronary thrombosis is the main factor responsible for MI, and that platelet aggregates are the primary events in its formation. Antiplatelet drugs such as aspirin reduce coronary events by about half in unstable angina (Fuster et al. 1989) and even in primary prevention (Steering Committee 1989). The main effect of aspirin on platelets is to decrease secondary platelet aggregation to ADP (Zucker 1968) as evaluated by the ex vivo classical tests of platelet aggregation.

In animals, these tests have been closely associated with the tendency to develop thrombosis (Renaud and Godu 1969; Renaud et al. 1970).

In man, the platelet aggregation tests have been shown to predict coronary events (Thaulow et al. 1991, Trip et al. 1990) and to be significantly correlated with prevalent cases of MI (Elwood et al. 1991), independent of serum lipids, in 1800 subjects in the Caerphilly Study.

Influence of Alcohol

In Vitro and Animal Studies

Following the demonstration of Haut and Cowan (1974) that alcohol added in vitro at physiologic dosage to human platelets markedly reduces the aggregation to thrombin, epinephrine, and ADP (mostly secondary wave), several studies have confirmed that ethanol inhibits platelet aggregation and secretion (Fenn and Littleton 1982, Benistant and Rubin 1990, Mikhailidis et al. 1990, Renaud et al. 1988, Rubin 1989).

Adding 6% ethanol to the drinking fluid in rats significantly decreased platelet aggregation to thrombin and ADP, but only in animals fed a saturated fat diet (McGregor and Renaud 1981). Further studies with this model (Renaud et al. 1984) indicated that the inhibitory effect of alcohol was lost rapidly with rebound effects. For platelet thrombi formed in stenosed dog coronary arteries, Folts et al. (1983) have shown their inhibition by ethanol, even under the influence of the prothrombotic effect of cigarette smoke (Keller and Folts 1988).

Acute Effects Ex Vivo in Man

Collagen-induced platelet aggregation, ex vivo, was inhibited 30 minutes following the ingestion in man of 1 ml ethanol/kg body weight (Mikhaïldis et al. 1983). This effect was lost in 60 minutes. In preliminary studies (Renaud et al, 1984), similar results were obtained on collagen and ADP aggregation, with rebound effects in some subjects.

These studies indicate that the acute effect of alcohol on platelets is transient in man, as also observed in rats (Renaud et al. 1984). Thus, it can be expected that any acute study failing to take a blood sample within 30 minutes of alcohol ingestion will not observe inhibitory effects on platelets. That was the case for the study by Dunn et al. (1981) and Veenstra et al. (1990). In the study of Hillbom et al. (1985), blood samples were obtained 4 hours later. As a result, they observed a significant increase in the response of platelets to ADP-induced aggregation, after ingestion of 1.5 g alcohol/kg body weight, which lasted for an additional 8 hours. This rebound effect, observed in alcoholics after alcohol withdrawal (Fink and Hutton 1983), could constitute an explanation for sudden CHD deaths after drunkenness episodes (Kozarevic et al. 1988). By contrast, as shown recently (Jackson et al. 1992), the risks of nonfatal MI and coronary death were consistently lower in people who drank alcohol in the previous 24 hours.

Long-Term Effects Ex Vivo in Man

More importantly for the usual relationship with CHD is the effect of long-term alcohol drinking on platelet reactivity. Pikaar et al. (1987) studied over a period of 5 weeks the effect of a standard consumption of wine. A significant decrease in collagen-induced platelet aggregation was observed, even when alcohol was not present in the circulation. Already after 2 weeks of alcoholic beverage administration, other investigators (Seigneur et al. 1990) found that red wine, but not diluted alcohol or white wine, would decrease platelet aggregability to ADP. A conclusion of Veenstra et al. (1990b) was that on the long run, the acute effect of alcohol results in a permanent decrease of aggregation tendency. This has been confirmed by epidemiological studies. In fasted British farmers, Renaud et al. (1981) found that platelet aggregation to ADP, collagen, and epinephrine was significantly inversely related to the intake of alcohol. In further

Table 4
Comparison between the effect of alcohol on platelets in Caerphilly and risk of CHD in the Harvard Health Professionals Study

Alcohol intake (g/day) 1	0	0.10–5.00	5.10–30.00	> 30.0	Trend P
Odds ratio for high ADP-S 95% CI (36)	1.0	0.40–1.13	0.19–0.80	0.08–0.54	< 0.001
RR for CHD 95% CI (12)	1.0	0.74–1.33	0.56–0.97	0.35–0.79	< 0.0001

Caerphilly, 1600 subjects (Amer J Clin Nutr 55:1012–17, 1992).
Harvard, 51,529 subjects (Lancet 338:464, 1991).

analyses (Renaud et al. 1984), the intake of alcohol was most significantly inversely related to secondary aggregation to ADP and epinephrine. That was subsequently observed for epinephrine and collagen in a multivariate analysis on 250 French and British farmers (Renaud et al. 1986). The inverse relationship to ADP-induced aggregation was also observed by Meade et al. (1985) in a prospective study. Finally, in 1600 subjects in Caerphilly (Renaud et al. 1992), the intake of alcohol, in a dose-related manner, was inversely related to the response of platelets to collagen, ADP, and, most significantly, secondary aggregation to ADP. As shown in Table 4, for each category of alcohol intake, the odds ratio of a high response to ADP in this study was quite comparable to the relative risk of CHD in the study of Rimm et al. (1991), suggesting a close relationship between the effect of alcohol on ADP-induced aggregation and on CHD.

Consensus

There is a consensus that part of the effect of alcohol on CHD seems to be through an effect on hemostasis. There is also a consensus that in vitro, alcohol inhibits platelet aggregation induced by several agonists, especially secondary aggregation to ADP. An acute inhibitory effect of alcohol drinking has been observed, but only in the reports having removed blood within 30 minutes of alcohol drinking. Although there are only a few studies on the long-term, these indicate inhibitory effects of moderate alcohol drinking on the tests of platelet aggregation, especially aggregation to ADP, the test the most closely associated with MI (Elwood et al. 1991).

Although ex vivo tests of platelet aggregation have been criticized as not necessarily reflecting what occurs in vivo, there is increasing evidence that these tests are good indicators of CHD risk. Nevertheless, further studies are certainly required to definitely prove the role of platelet reactivity in CHD in relation to alcohol. In vivo indicators of platelet reactivity are currently developed and should be used in addition to previous tests in the evaluation of the effect of alcohol drinking on platelets.

Fibrinogen and Fibrinolytic Function

In several epidemiologic studies (Broadhurst et al. 1990), the level of fibrinogen has been found to be independently significantly associated with the risk of CHD. In about 10 epidemiologic studies, the relationship between fibrinogen and alcohol consumption has been reported (Kluft et al. 1992). In half of them an inverse association was observed. The effect, however, was not very large, which may be the reason why it was not significantly present in the other half of the studies.

The relationship between alcohol consumption and fibrinolytic activity has been reviewed recently by Veenstra (1990c) and Kluft et al. (1992). In only one epidemiologic study has fibrinolytic activity been evaluated (Meade et al. 1979) in relation to alcohol consumption. The positive association found suggests that an increase in fibrinolytic activity also may contribute to the reduced CHD risk of moderate drinkers.

On the other hand, several studies have shown a decrease in fibrinolytic activity after acute alcohol consumption. Owing to technical difficulties, the global assays of fibrinolytic activities do not necessarily reflect the in vivo situation. Through recent improvements in methodology, the fibrinolytic system can be now studied more accurately.

Recent results show large effects of moderate alcohol consumption on the specific fibrinolytic factors t-PA and PA1, which play a crucial role in the ability to prevent unnecessary clot formation and to dissolve already existing ones (Veenstra 1992, Veenstra et al. 1992). The activity of t-PA was significantly decreased in the hours after consumption of beer, wine, or spirits, whereas t-PA activity was significantly increased the next morning. No longer-term experimental or epidemiologic studies using the improved blood sampling techniques are currently available. Since both t-PA and PA1 display a strong circadian pattern, the effect of alcohol consumption will strongly depend on the time of drinking.

Another new and promising development in this area is the possibility of measuring activation and degradation of fibrin. Turnover of fibrin in vivo continuously happens at a very low level, and changes in this situation can now be recorded by measuring fibrin degradation products and plasmin-alpha-2 antiplasmin complexes.

Studies in which these newly developed procedures are applied will lead to a better understanding of the effects of alcohol on the fibrinolytic system, the underlying mechanisms, and to what extent these effects contribute to a reduced CHD risk in moderate drinkers.

Future Research

In almost every aspect of the inverse association between the intake of alcohol and CHD, further research seems to be needed.

Epidemiology

There are now a large number of both case-control and prospective cohort studies addressing the question of alcohol and CHD, and these reveal quite consistent findings (Marmot and Brummer 1991). In only the last 3 years, prospective studies on more than 500,000 subjects have been reported, more than all the studies published before 1989. Additional observational studies may help to refine certain questions.

Reanalysis of Existing Studies

- Meta-analysis of the association between alcohol and CHD is needed.
- Analysis of the results using the same unit of measure and with the same methodology (survival curves and proportional hazards model) are also needed.
- A few studies suggest that wine could have more beneficial effects than other alcoholic beverages (see Figure 6). This problem should be further investigated in countries such as France and Italy, where wine is consumed mostly at meals, to determine whether wine is really more protective than other alcoholic beverages:
  (1) through its drinking at meals or
  (2) through substances other than alcohol present in red

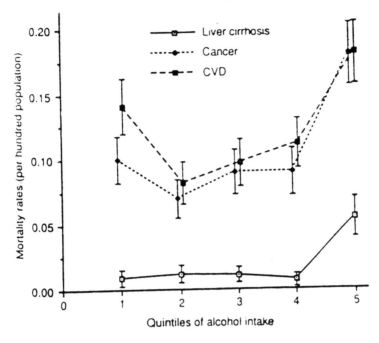

Figure 6
Italian rural cohorts of the Seven Countries Study

15 year cancer, cardiovascular and liver cirrhosis mortality rates in quintile classes of alcohol (as percentage of total energy intake) almost exclusively under the form of wine. The mean value of daily alcohol consumption in each quintile is 22.7, 56.4, 77.8, 108.2, 164.7 g.

In these cohorts, there were very few people not drinking wine. Therefore the mortality rates could not be assessed for 0 intake of alcohol. Nevertheless, it seems that the same U shape curve as in other studies on alcohol can be expected. The conclusion of the authors was that in a rural population drinking wine at mealtime, a relatively wide range of consumption had no measurable effect on mortality. (Farchi et al. 1992, by permission.)

wine as emphasized recently (Sharp 1993). These substances have oxygen free radical scavenger capacity (Ricardo da Silva et al. 1991), prevent LDL oxidation more effectively than α-tocopherol (Frankel et al. 1993), increase the production of HDL cholesterol, and modify the eicosanoid metabolism of leucocytes (Kimura et al. 1985).

• Several studies on smoking habit tried to estimate (1) the risk of diseases versus the number of smoked cigarettes; (2) the risk versus the number of years of smoking; and (3) for people who stopped smoking, the risk versus the number of years since cessation. In the field of drinking habit, almost nothing is known on points (2) and (3).

- Only a few studies measured alcohol consumption and other nutrient intake at the same time. It seems that a strong interaction exists between alcohol and other nutrients, like, for example, a negative association between the intake of alcohol and that of carbohydrates found in several studies. Therefore, it would be useful to separate the alcohol by adjusting for other nutrient intake.
- Drinking pattern such as binges cannot be detected. Persons who take one drink per day over a 7-day period are treated as identical to those who take seven drinks in one day.

Randomized Controlled Trials

- The dose-response U-shape of the alcohol-CHD curve needs further evaluation. Where data are available, cohort studies should evaluate the timing of alcohol consumption during the course of the day, the association for ex-drinkers, possible differences in other dietary factors as potential confounding variables, and should utilize measures of change in alcohol consumption over time. Prospective observational studies with repeated noninvasive vascular measures, or invasive measures such as angiography, would be helpful.
- The value of ecological studies could be improved by a standardized measure of alcohol consumption across populations, as well as data on change in alcohol consumption over time. Nevertheless, it will be only an intervention trial that will be able to address causality.
- A randomized double blind trial of alcohol consumption and CHD events could give a definitive answer, but it seems unlikely that such a trial will be ever done. Methodological problems include the difficulty of maintaining controls on a zero-alcohol regimen over several years, and the obvious difficulty with providing an appropriate placebo for the control group and maintaining blinding. Other approaches will be required.

Clinical Studies

Since large intervention trials by alcohol drinking on CHD morbidity and mortality cannot be undertaken, limited intervention studies in healthy human volunteers to evaluate the specificity of alcohol's effects on CVD risk factors would be useful, since risk factors such as blood pressure; lipids and lipoproteins; as well as fibrinogen, platelets, fibrinolysis, and other coagulation factors are likely mediating variables for alcohol's effect (Criqui et al. 1987a, Renaud, 1992). Experimental studies to date reveal some inconsistency concerning platelets and fibrinolysis (Veenstra 1991), which could be solved by using recently developed techniques and procedures. If we could determine dose-response relationships, including some probable nonlinear relationships between alcohol and such mediating variables, we could begin to investigate whether such effects could be produced by specific dietary or other behavioral regimens not including alcohol.

These studies should be completed by the difficult evaluation of stress reduction induced by alcohol. This factor could also play a role in the decreased risk for CHD associated with moderate alcohol drinking.

Animal Studies

There are only a few studies in animals on the effect of alcohol on atherosclerosis and thrombosis, especially under physiologic conditions. Such experimental studies in animals could add significantly to our knowledge in the field. Studies should be done to see whether (1) alcohol stimulates reverse cholesterol transport as well as raising HDL, (2) reverse cholesterol transport interferes with the development of atherosclerosis, and (3) alcohol has other effects on the development of atherosclerosis through either other lipid or nonlipid mechanisms.

Acknowledgments: Prof. R. Jackson, University of Auckland (NZ) is gratefully acknowledged for his contribution in critically reviewing the manuscript.

References

Andreasson S, Allebeck P, Romelsjo A (1988) Alcohol and mortality among young men: longitudinal study of Swedish conscripts. Brit Med J 296:1021–25

Barboriak JJ, Anderson AJ, Hoffmann RG (1979) Interrelationship between coronary artery occlusion, high-density lipoprotein cholesterol, and alcohol intake. J Lab Clin Med 94:348–53.

Barboriak JJ, Anderson AJ, Hoffmann RG (1982) Smoking, alcohol and coronary artery occlusion. Atherosclerosis 43:277–82.

Benistant C, Rubin R (1990) Ethanol inhibits thrombin-induced secretion by human platelets at a site distinct from phospholipase C or protein kinase C. Biochem J 269:489

Boffetta P, Garfinkel L (1990) Alcohol drinking and mortality among men enrolled in an American Cancer Society prospective study. Epidemiol 1:342–48

Broadhurst P, Kelleher C, Hughes L, et al. (1990) Fibrinogen, factor VII clotting activity and coronary disease severity. Atherosclerosis 85:169–73

Brummer P (1969) Coronary mortality and living standard II. Coffee, tea, cacao, alcohol and tobacco. Acta Med Scand 186:61–63

Camacho TC, Kaplan GA, Richard D (1987) Alcohol consumption and mortality in Almeda County. J Chronic Dis 40:229–36

Castelli WP, Doyle JT, Gordon T, et al. (1977) Alcohol and blood lipids. The Cooperative Lipoprotein Phenotyping Study. Lancet 2:153–55

Colditz GA, Branch LG, Lipnick RJ, et al. (1985) Moderate alcohol and decreased cardiovascular mortality in an elderly cohort. Am Heart J 109:886–89

Criqui MH (1985) Alcohol and Cardiovascular Mortality. In Kaplan RM, Criqui MH (eds), Behavioral Epidemiology and Disease Prevention. Plenum, New York

Criqui MH (1986b) Alcohol consumption, blood pressure, lipids, and cardiovascular mortality. Alcoholism: Clinical and Experimental Research 10:564–69

Criqui MH (1987b) Alcohol and hypertension: new insights from population studies. Eur Heart J 8(suppl B):19–26

Criqui MH (1987c) The roles of alcohol in the epidemiology of cardiovascular disease. Acta Med Scand 717(suppl):73–85

Criqui MH (1990) The reduction of coronary heart disease with light to moderate alcohol consumption: effect or artifact? Br J Addict 85:854–57

Criqui MH, Cowan LD, Heiss G, et al (1986a) Frequency and clustering of non-lipid coronary risk factors in dyslipoproteinemia. The Lipid Research Clinics Program Prevalence Study. Circulation 73(suppl 1):40–50

Criqui MH, Cowan LD, Tyroler HA, et al. (1987a) Lipoproteins as mediators for the effects of alcohol consumption and cigarette smoking on cardiovascular mortality. Results from the Lipid Research Clinics Follow-up Study. Am J Epidemiol 126:629–37

Dunn EL, Cohen RG, Moore EE, Hamstra RD (1981) Acute alcohol ingestion and platelet function. Arch Surg 116:1082–83

Dyer AR, Stamler J, Paul O, et al. (1980) Alcohol consumption and 17-year mortality in the Chicago Western Electric Company Study. J Prev Med 9:78–90

Eberhard TP (1936) Effect of alcohol on cholesterol-induced atherosclerosis in rabbits. Arch Pathol 21:616–22

Elwood PC, Renaud S, Sharp DS, et al. (1991) Ischaemic heart disease and platelet aggregation. The Caerphilly collaborative heart disease study. Circulation 83:38–44

Ernst E (1992) Fibrinogen: the plot thickens. J Clin Epidemiol 45:561–62

Farchi G, Fidanza F, Mariotti S, Menotti A (1992) Alcohol and mortality in the Italian rural cohorts of the Seven Countries Study. Int J Epidemiol 21:74–82

Feller DD, Huff RL (1955) Lipid synthesis by arterial and liver tissue obtained from cholesterol-fed and cholesterol-alcohol-fed rabbits. Am J Physiol 182:237–42

Fenn CG, Littleton JM (1982) Inhibition of platelet aggregation by ethanol in vitro shows specificity for aggregating agent used and is influenced by platelet lipid composition. Thromb Haemost 48:49–53

Fink R, Hutton RA (1983) Changes in the blood platelets of alcoholics during alcohol withdrawal. J Clin Pathol 36:337–40

Fisher M, Gordon T (1985) The relation of drinking and smoking habits to diet: the Lipid Research Clinics Prevalence Study. Am J Clin Nutr 41:623–30

Folts J, Bertha B, Ballantyne F (1983) Inhibition of platelet thrombus formation in stenosed dog coronary arteries with ethanol. Thromb Haemost 50:379

Frankel EN, Kanner J, German JB, et al. (1993) Inhibition of oxidation of human low-density lipoprotein by phenolic substances in red wine. Lancet 341:454–57

Friedman LA, Kimball AW (1986) Coronary heart disease mortality and alcohol consumption in Framingham. Am J Epidemiol 124:481–89

Fuster V, Cohen M, Halpern J (1989) Aspirin in the prevention of coronary disease (editorial). N Engl J Med 321:183–85

Gill JS, Zezulka AV, Shipley MJ, et al. (1986) Stroke and alcohol consumption. N Engl J Med 315:1041–46

Goodwin DW (1978) Hereditary factors in alcoholism. Hosp Pract 13:121–24, 127–30

Gordon T (1957) Mortality experience among the Japanese in the United States, Hawaii and Japan. Public Health Rep 72:543–53

Gordon T, Doyle J (1987) Drinking and mortality. Am J Epidemiol 125:263–70

Gordon T, Kannel WB (1983) Drinking habits and cardiovascular disease. The Framingham Study. Am Heart J 105:667–73

Gorelick PB (1989) The status of alcohol as a risk factor for stroke. Stroke 20:1607–10

Goto Y, Kikuchi H, Abe K, et al. (1974) The effect of ethanol on the onset of experimental atherosclerosis. Tohoku J Exp Med 114:35–43

Gottlieb LS, Broitman SA, Vitale JJ, Zamcheck N (1959) The influence of alcohol and dietary magnesium upon hypercholesterolemia and atherogenesis in the rat. J Lab Clin Med 53:433–41

Gruchow HW, Hoffmann RG, Anderson AJ, Barbosiak JJ (1982) Effects of drinking patterns on the relationship between alcohol and coronary occlusion. Atherosclerosis 43:393–404

Hall EM, Olsen AY, Davies FE (1953) Clinical and pathologic review of 782 cases from 16,600 necropsies. Am J Pathol 29:993–1027

Haut MJ, Cowan DH (1974) The effect of ethanol on hemostatic properties of human blood platelets. Amer J Med 56:22–33

Hegsted DM, Ausman LM (1988) Diet, alcohol and coronary heart disease in men. J Nutr 118:1184–89

Hennekens CH, Rosner B, Cole DS (1978) Daily alcohol consumption and fatal coronary heart disease. Am J Epidemiol 107:196–200

Hennekens CH, Willet W, Rosner B, et al. (1979) Effects of beer, wine, and liquor in coronary death. JAMA 242:1973–74

Hillbom ME (1987) What supports the role of alcohol as a risk factor for stroke? Acta Med Scand 717(suppl):93–106

Hirst AE, Hadley GG, Gore I (1965) The effect of chronic alcoholism and cirrhosis of the liver on atherosclerosis. Am J Med Sci 46:143–49

Howell WL, Manion WC (1960) The low incidence of myocardial infarction in patients with portal cirrhosis of the liver: a review of 639 cases of cirrhosis of the liver from 17,731 autopsies. Am Heart J 60:341–44

Jackson R, Beaglehole R (1993) The relationship between alcohol and coronary heart disease: is there a protective effect? Curr Opin Lipidology 4:21–26

Jackson R, Scragg R, Beaglehole R (1991) Alcohol consumption and risk of coronary heart disease. Brit Med J 303:211–16

Jackson R, Scragg R, Beaglehole R (1992) Does recent alcohol consumption reduce the risk of acute myocardial infarction and coronary death in regular drinkers? Am J Epidemiol 136:819–824

Jones BR, Barrett-Connor E, Criqui MH, et al. (1982) A community study of calorie and nutrient intake in drinkers and non-drinkers of alcohol. Am J Clin Nutr 35:135–39

Kagan A, Katsuhiko Y, Rhoads GG, et al. (1981) Alcohol and cardiovascular disease: the Hawaiian experience. Circulation 64(suppl III):27–31

Kannel WB (1988) Alcohol and cardiovascular disease. Proc Nutr Soc 47:99–110

Kaufman DW, Rosemberg L, Hemrich SP, Shapiro S (1985) Alcoholic beverages and myocardial infarction in young men. Am J Epidemiol 121:548–54

Keller JW, Folts JD (1988) Relative effects of cigarette smoke and ethanol on acute platelet thrombus formation in stenosed canine coronary arteries. Cardiovasc Res 22:73–78

Kimura Y, Okuda H, Arichi S (1985) Effects of stilbenes on arachidonate metabolism in leukocytes. Biochim Biophys Acta 834:275–78

Kittner SJ, Garcia-Palmieri MR, Costas R, et al. (1983) Alcohol and coronary heart disease in Puerto Rico. Am J Epidemiol 117:538–50

Klatsky AL, Friedman GD, Siegelaub AB (1974) Alcohol consumption before myocardial infarction. results from the Kaiser-Permanente epidemiologic study of myocardial infarction. Ann Intern Med 81:294–301

Klatsky AL, Friedman GD, Siegelaub AB (1981a) Alcohol use and cardiovascular disease: the Kaiser-Permanente experience. Circulation 64(suppl III):32–41

Klatsky AL, Friedman GD, Siegelaub MS (1981b) Alcohol and mortality. a ten year Kaiser-Permanente experience. Ann Intern Med 95:139–45

Klatsky AL, Armstrong MA, Friedman GD (1986) Relation of alcoholic beverage use to subsequent coronary artery disease hospitalization. Am J Cardiol 58:710–14

Klatsky AL, Armstrong MA, Friedman GD (1990) Risk of cardiovascular mortality in alcohol drinkers, ex drinkers and non-drinkers. Am J Cardiol 66:1237–42

Kluft C, Jie AFH, Kooistra T, et al. (1992) Alcohol and fibrinolysis. In Veenstra J, van der Heij DG (eds), Alcohol and cardiovascular diseases. Pudoc, Wageningen

Kono S, Ikeda M, Tokudome S, et al. (1986) Alcohol and mortality: a cohort study of male Japanese physicians. Int J Epidemiol 15:527–31

Kono S, Handa K, Kawano J, et al. (1991) Alcohol intake and nonfatal acute myocardial infarction in Japan. Am J Cardiol 68:1011–14

Kozarevic DJ, McGee D, Vojvodic N, et al. (1980) Frequency of alcohol consumption and morbidity and mortality: the Yugoslavia Cardiovascular Disease Study. Lancet 1:613–16

Kozarevic DJ, Vojvodic N, Gordon T, et al. (1988) Drinking habits and death. the Yugoslavia cardiovascular disease study. In J Epidemiol 12:145–50

Kuller L, Reisler DM (1971) An explanation for variations in distribution of stroke and arteriosclerotic heart disease among populations and racial groups. Am J Epidemiol 63:1–9

La Porte RE, Cresanta JL, Kuller LH (1980) The relationship of alcohol consumption to atherosclerotic heart disease. Prev Med 9:22–40

Langer RD, Criqui MH, Reed DM (1992) Lipoproteins and blood pressure as biologic pathways for the effect of moderate alcohol consumption on coronary heart disease. Circulation 85:910–15

Lazarus NB, Kaplan GA, Cohen RD, Len DJ (1991) Change in alcohol consumption and risk of death from all causes and ischaemic heart disease. Brit Med J 303:553–56

Lifsic AM (1976) Alcohol consumption and atherosclerosis. Bull World Health Organ 53:3482–83

Mansson PH (1989) Wine and good health. Wine Spectator, Feb 28, pp 21–27

Marmot M, Brummer E (1991) Alcohol and cardiovascular disease: the status of the U-shaped curve. Brit Med J 303:565–68

Marmot MG, Rose G, Shipley MJ, Thomas BS (1981) Alcohol and mortality: a U-shaped curve. Lancet 1:580–83

McGregor L, Renaud S (1981) Inhibitory effect of alcohol on platelet functions of rats fed saturated fats. Thromb Res 22:221–25

Meade TW, Chakrabarti R, Haines A, et al. (1979) Characteristics effecting fibrinolytic activity and plasma fibrinogen concentrations. Brit Med J 1:153–56

Meade TW, Vickers MV, Thompson SG, et al. (1985) Epidemiological characteristics of platelet aggregability. Br Med J 290:428–32

Mikhailidis DP, Barradas MA, Jeremy JY (1990) The effect of ethanol on platelet function and vascular prostanoids. Alcohol 7:171–80

Mikhailidis DP, Jeremy JY, Barradas A, et al. (1983) Effect of ethanol on vascular prostacyclin (prostaglan oodin I$_2$) synthesis, platelet aggregation, and platelet thromboxane release. Br Med J 287:1495–98

Miller GJ, Beckles GLA, Maude GH, Carson DC (1990) Alcohol consumption: protection against coronary heart disease and risks to health. Int J Epidemiol 19:923–30

Miller NE, Bolton CH, Hayes TM, et al. (1988) Associations of alcohol consumption with plasma high-density lipoprotein cholesterol and its major subfractions: the Caerphilly and Speedwell Collaborative Heart Disease studies. J Epidemiol Community Health 42:220–25

Moore MC, Guzman MA, Schilling PE, Strong JP (1975) Dietary-atherosclerosis study on deceased persons. J Am Diet Assoc 67:22–28

Moore RD, Pearson TA (1986) Moderate alcohol consumption and coronary artery disease. a review. Medicine 65:242–67

Nichols CW, Siperstein MD, Gaffey W, et al. (1956) Does the ingestion of alcohol influence the development of arteriosclerosis in fowls? J Exp Med 103:465–75

Osservartorio Permanente su Giovani e l'Alcool (1992) Indagine Doxa. I giovani a l'alcool. Quademi dell'Osservatorio n.2. OTET 132

Parrish HM, Eberly AL, Jr (1961) Negative association of coronary atherosclerosis with liver cirrhosis and chronic alcoholism. a statistical fallacy. J Indiana Med Assoc 54:341–47

Pearson TA, Bulkley BH, Achuff SC, et al. (1979) The association of low levels of HDL cholesterol and arteriographically defined coronary artery disease. Am J Epidemiol 109:285–95

Peterson B (1988) Analysis of the role of alcohol in mortality, particularly sudden unwitnessed death, in middle-aged men in Malmö, Sweden. Alcohol Alcohol 23:259–63

Petitti DB, Wingerd J, Pellegrin F, Ramcharan S (1979) Risk of vascular disease in woman. smoking, oral contraceptives, noncontraceptive estrogens, and other factors. JAMA 242:1150–54

Pikaar NA, Wedel M, van der Beek E, et al. (1987) Effects of moderate alcohol consumption on platelet aggregation, fibrinolysis, and blood lipids. Metabolism 36:538–47

Poikolainen K (1991) Epidemiologic assessment of population risks and benefits of alcohol use. Alcohol Alcohol 1(suppl):27–34

Puchois P, Chalim N, Zylberger G, et al. (1990) Effect of alcohol intake on human apolipoprotein A-I-containing lipoprotein subfractions. Arch Intern Med 150:1638–41

Ramsay LE (1979) Alcohol and myocardial infarction in hypertensive men. Am Heart J 98:402–3

Rand ML, Groves HM, Packham MA, et al. (1990) Acute administration of ethanol to rabbits inhibits thrombus formation induced by indwelling aortic catheters. Lab Invest 63:742

Rand ML, Packham MA, Kinlough-Rathbone RL, Mustard JF (1988) Effects of ethanol on pathways of platelet aggregation in vitro. Thromb Haemost 59:383

Reed DM (1990) The paradox of high risk of stroke in populations with low risk of coronary heart disease. Am J Epidemiol 131:579–88

Renaud S, Beswick AD, Fehily AM, et al. (1992) Alcohol and platelet aggregation: the Caerphilly prospective heart disease study. Am J Clin Nutr 55:1012–17

Renaud S, de Lorgeril M (1992) Wine, alcohol, platelets and the French paradox for coronary heart disease. Lancet 339:1523–26

Renaud S, Godu J (1969) Induction of large thrombi in hyperlipemic rats by epinephrine and endotoxin. Lab Invest 21:512–18

Renaud S, Kuba K, Goulet C, et al. (1970) Relationship between platelet fatty-acid composition of platelets and platelet aggregation in rat and man. relation to thrombosis. Circ Res 26:553–64

Renaud S, McGregor L, Martin JL (1984) Influence of alcohol on platelet functions in relation to atherosclerosis. In Pozza G, et al. (eds), Diet, diabetes and atherosclerosis. Raven Press, New York, pp 177–87

Renaud S, Morazain R, Godsey F, et al. (1981) Platelet function in relation to diet and serum lipids in British farmers. Br Heart J 46:562–70

Renaud S, Morazain R, McGregor L, Baudier F (1979) Dietary fats and platelet functions in relation to atherosclerosis and coronary heart disease. Hemostatis 8:234–51

Rhoads GG, Blackwelder WC, Stemmermann GN, et al. (1978) Coronary risk factors and autopsy findings in Japanese-American men. Lab Invest 38:304–11

Ricardo Da Silva JM, Darmon N, Fernandez Y, Mitjavila S (1991) Oxygen free radical scavenger capacity in aqueous models of different procyanidins from grape seeds. J Agric Food Chem 39:1549–52

Rimm EB, Giovannucci E, Willet WC, et al. (1991a) Alcohol and mortality. Lancet 338:1073–74

Rimm EB, Giovannucci EL, Willet WC, et al. (1991b) Prospective study of alcohol consumption and risk of coronary disease in men. Lancet 338:464–68

Rissanen V (1974) Coronary and aortic atherosclerosis in chronic alcoholics. Z Rechtsmed 75:183–89

Rose G (1991) Ancel keys lecture. Circulation 84:1405–9

Rosenberg L, Slone D, Shapiro S, et al. (1981) Alcoholic beverages and myocardial infarction in young women. Am J Public Health 71:82–85

Ross RK, Mack TM, Paganini-Hill A, et al. (1981) Menopausal estrogen therapy and protection from death from ischaemic heart disease. Lancet 1:858–61

Rubin R (1989) Ethanol interferes with collagen-induced platelet activation by inhibition of arachidonic acid mobilization. Arch Biochem Biophys 270:99

Rudel LL, Leathers CW, Bond MG, Bullock BC (1981) Dietary ethanol-induced modifications in hyperlipoproteinemia and atherosclerosis in non human primates (Macaca nemestrina). Arteriosclerosis 1:144–55

Ruebner BH, Mikai H, Abbey H (1961) The low incidence of myocardial infarction in hepatic cirrhosis. Lancet 1:1435–36

Sackett L, Gibson RW, Bross IDJ, Pickren JW (1968) Relation between aortic atherosclerosis and the use of cigarettes and alcohol. an autopsy study. N Engl J Med 279:1413–20

Seigneur M, Bonnet J, Dorian B et al. (1990) Effect of the consumption of alcohol, white wine and red wine on platelet function and serum lipids. J Applied Cardiol 5:215–22

Shaper AG, Wannamethee G, Walter M (1988) Alcohol and mortality in British men: explaining the U-shaped curve. Lancet 2:1267–73

Sharp D (1993) Coronary disease: when wine is red. Lancet 341:27–28

Siskovick RK, Weiss NS, Fox N (1986) Moderate alcohol consumption and primary cardiac arrest. Am J Epidemiol 123:499–503

Smith GD, Shipley M (1991) Alcohol consumption and risk of coronary heart disease. Lancet 303:521

St Leger AS, Cochrane AL, Moore F (1979) Factors associated with cardiac mortality in developed countries with particular reference to the consumption of wine. Lancet 1:1017–20

Stampfer MJ, Colditz GC, Willett WC, et al. (1988) A prospective study of moderate alcohol consumption and the risk of coronary disease and stroke in women. N Engl J Med 319:267–73

Stampfer MJ, Sacks FM, Salvini S, et al. (1991) A prospective study of cholesterol, apolipoproteins, and risk of myocardial infarction. N Engl J Med 325:373–81

Stason WB, Neff RK, Miettinen OS, Jick H (1976) Alcohol consumption and non-fatal myocardial infarction. Am J Epidemiol 104:603–8

Steering Committee of the Physician's Health Study Research Group (1989) Final report on the aspirin component of the ongoing Physicians' Health Study. N Engl J Med 321:129–35

Suh I, Shaten BJ, Cutler JA, et al. (1992) Alcohol use and mortality from coronary heart disease: the role of high density lipoprotein cholesterol. Ann Intern Med 116:881–87

Suhonen O, Aromas A, Reunanen A, Knekt P (1987) Alcohol consumption and sudden coronary death in middle-aged Finnish men. Acta Med Scand 221:335–41

Tanaka H, Ueda Y, Hayashi M et al. (1982) Risk factors for cerebral hemorrhage and cerebral infarction in a Japanese rural community. Stroke 13:62–73

Thaulow E, Erikssen J, Sandvik L, et al. (1991) Blood platelet count and function are related to total and cardiovascular death in apparently healthy men. Circulation 84:613–17

Valimaki M, Taskinen MR, Ylikahri R, et al. (1988) Comparison of the effect of two different doses of alcohol on serum lipoproteins, HDL-subfractions and apolipoproteins A-I and A-II: a controlled study. Eur J Clin Invest 18:472:80

Veenstra J (1990c) Alcohol and fibrinolysis. Fibrinolysis 4(suppl 2):64–68

Veenstra J (1991) Moderate alcohol use and coronary heart disease: a U-shaped curve? In Simopoulos AP (ed), Impacts on nutrition and health. World Rev Nutr Diet, Karger, Basel, 65:38–71

Veenstra J (1992) Effects of alcohol on the cardiovascular system. Alcohol and Cardiovascular Disease, Pudoc, Wageningen, pp 87–113

Veenstra J, Kluft C, van de Pol H, Schaafsma G (1992) Acute effects of moderate alcohol consumption on fibrinolytic factors in healthy middle-aged men. Fibrinolysis, in press

Veenstra J, Ockhuizen Th, van de Pol H, et al. (1990a) Effects of a moderate dose of alcohol on blood lipids and lipoproteins postprandially and in the fasting state. Alcohol Alcohol 25:371–77

Veenstra J, van de Pol H, Schaafsma G (1990b) Moderate alcohol consumption and platelet aggregation in healthy middle-aged men. Alcohol: an International Biomedical Journal 7:547–49

Viel B, Donoso S, Salcedo D, et al. (1966) Alcoholism and socioeconomic status, hepatic damage and arteriosclerosis. Arch Intern Med 117:84–91

Wilhelmsen L, Wedel H, Tibblin G (1973) Multivariate analysis of risk factors for coronary heart disease. Circulation 48:950–58

Yano K, Rhoads GG, Kagan A (1977) Coffee, alcohol and risk of coronary heart disease among Japanese men living in Hawaii. N Engl J Med 297:405–9

Zucker MB, Peterson J (1968) Inhibition of adenosine diphosphate-induced secondary aggregation and other platelet functions by acetyl-salicylic acid ingestion. Proc Soc Exp Biol Med 127:547–51

5

Alcoholic Beverages and Cancers of the Digestive Tract and Larynx

R. Doll
Radcliffe Infirmary, Great Britain

D. Forman
Radcliffe Infirmary, Great Britain

C. La Vecchia
Institut Universitaire de Médicine Sociale et Preventive,
Lausanne, Switzerland, and Istituto di Ricerche
Farmacologiche "Mario Negri," Italy

R. Woutersen
TNO Toxicology and Nutrition Institute, The Netherlands

Abstract

Ethanol is not a carcinogen by standard laboratory tests. Animal experiments suggest, however, that, given by mouth, it may act as a cocarcinogen in the production of cancers in the oesophagus and possibly also in the nonglandular (fore)stomach, but not in the glandular stomach or pancreas. The evidence relating to the production of colorectal cancer is conflicting, and no conclusion can be drawn from it.

Epidemiological evidence shows that the consumption of alcoholic beverages increases the risk of developing cancers of the mouth (other than the salivary glands), pharynx (other than the nasopharynx), and larynx; that the risks are principally due to the presence of ethanol and increase with the amount consumed; that the risks are increased by increased smoking, each agent approximately multiplying the effect of the other; and that, in the absence of smoking, the risks in developed countries are small unless consumption is exceptionally heavy. The risks may be diminished by a diet rich in fruit and green vegetables, but the evidence is inconclusive. Whether the cocarcinogenic effects of different alcoholic beverages depend solely on the presence of ethanol and are unaffected by its concentration or by the presence of congeners is uncertain.

The epidemiological evidence also suggests that there may be some direct relationship between the consumption of alcohol and colorectal cancer. The apparent relationship is quantitatively moderate, and even with heavy consumption a doubling of the normal risk can be excluded. No apparent difference exists between the susceptibility of men and women or of the two sites (colon and rectum), or between the effect of different types of alcoholic beverage. The nature of the observed relationship remains in doubt. The relationship may be causal; it may be due to confounding between the consumption of alcoholic beverages and some other dietary factor that increases the risk of the disease, and it may be due, at least in part, to the selective publication of positive results.

The balance of the evidence suggests that alcoholic beverages do not cause cancers of the stomach or pancreas, but it does not rule out the possibility altogether. Alcohol may contribute specifically to the production of cancer of the gastric cardia and, indirectly through the production of chronic (calcifying) pancreatitis, to cancer of the pancreas; but the evidence is insufficient for any conclusion to be reached.

Introduction

A relationship between the heavy consumption of alcoholic beverages and the development of carcinoma of the oesophagus was recognized clinically before the First World War (Lamy 1910), but it was only with the publication of national occupational mortality statistics for England and Wales in the mid-1920s that evidence was obtained of a similar relationship with the development of cancers of the upper respiratory and digestive tracts as a group (Young and Russell 1926). No worthwhile evidence that these relationships were causal was obtained, however, until after the Second World War, when epidemiological techniques for investigating the aetiology of noninfectious diseases were developed. The evidence that has subsequently accrued relating to these and other cancers of the digestive tract has enabled some definitive conclusions to be reached about the role of alcoholic beverages in their production, but several important aspects of the observed relationships remain to be resolved. These are set out separately after the sections on animal experiments and after the four epidemiological sections dealing with (1) cancers of the mouth, pharynx, oesophagus, and larynx; (2) cancer of the stomach; (3) cancer of the pancreas; and (4) cancers of the large bowel.

For the purposes of this report, a carcinogen is defined as an agent that has initiating capacity and can induce tumours that seldom or never occur spontaneously; an agent that enhances the carcinogenic process without having initiating capacity is described as a cocarcinogen.

Evidence From Animal Experiments

Ethanol or alcoholic beverages have been tested for their carcinogenic potential in only a few adequately performed long-term studies with mice or rats. Most of the studies that have been described in the literature cannot be used for evaluation of the carcinogenicity of alcohol due to severe limitations in experimental design (International Agency for Research on Cancer 1988). In one adequate study, a group of 108 male and 42 female CF1 mice was given 43% ethanol in water for up to 1020 days (Horie et al. 1965). Another group of mice was given 14% ethanol, similarly, for up to 735 days, and a further group of 100 male mice was given 19.5% as the drinking fluid for a maximum of 664 days. No differences in the incidence of tumours was found.

Based on these rather limited data, it may be concluded that there is no experimental evidence that alcohol is a carcinogen. However, over the last 25 years several studies have been published reporting a cocarcinogenic or promoting effect of ethanol when administered to animals in combination with well-known chemical carcinogens. The present review concentrates on the effects of alcohol on digestive tract carcinogenesis in experimental animals.

Modifying Effects of Ethanol on the Activity of Known Carcinogens

Oesophagus and Stomach

When polycyclic hydrocarbons such as benzo(a)pyrene or dimethylbenzanthracene were applied locally to the oesophagus of mice, their carcinogenic potential was significantly enhanced when ethanol was used as a solvent (Horie et al. 1965). In this experiment, ethanol most likely has acted as a tumour promoter by its irritating effects on the tissue.

Mufti et al. (1989) demonstrated that ethanol, when administered to rats in an isocaloric diet after initiation by intraperitoneal injection with the oesophageal specific carcinogen N-nitrosomethylbenzylamine (NMBZA), increased the incidence of oesophageal tumours. When ethanol was administered before and during initiation with NMBZA, the incidence of oesophageal nodules and tumours was decreased in comparison with control. These results indicate that the occurrence of oesophageal tumours is inhibited by simultaneous ethanol administration but enhanced when ethanol is administered after initiation, most probably by allowing extensive dysplastic proliferation of the carcinogen-induced lesions.

Griciuté et al. (1982, 1984) exposed C57B mice by gastric intubation to N-nitrosodiethylamine (NDEA) or N-nitrosodi-n-propylamine (NDPA), either in tap water or in 40% aqueous ethanol, twice a week for 50 weeks. A statistically significant increase in incidence of squamous cell carcinomas of the oesophagus/forestomach was observed in the group given the carcinogens in ethanol in comparison with the group given the nitrosamines in tap water.

Gibel (1967) exposed Sprague-Dawley rats by intragastric intubation to NDEA or N,N'-dinitrosopiperazine (DNPIP) in tap water or 30% (v/v) ethanol. He found that the combination of NDEA plus ethanol increased the incidence of papillomas and carcinomas of the oesophagus/forestomach, whereas DNPIP plus ethanol caused an increase in numbers of oesophageal/forestomach papillomas but not of carcinomas in comparison with DNPIP alone.

Konishi et al. (1986) did not find a significant effect of ethanol on the incidence of oesophageal carcinomas induced by N-nitrosopiperidine (NPIP) in rats. In this study NPIP was given via the diet, and ethanol via a tube inserted into the pharynx, either followed or not by 10% ethanol in drinking water for 12 weeks.

Castonguay et al. (1984) did not find an effect of a liquid diet containing 6.6% (w/v) ethanol on the incidence of oesophageal tumours induced by subcutaneous injection of N'-nitrosonornicotine (NNN).

Takahashi et al. (1986) exposed rats via the drinking water to N-methyl-N'-nitro-N-nitrosoguanidine (MNNG) for 8 weeks followed by either tap water or 10% ethanol in water as drinking fluid. After 40 weeks, the incidence of adenocarcinomas in the glandular stomach of animals of the 10% ethanol group was similar to that in the controls.

Pancreas

The results of a long-term study with azaserine-treated rats (model for acinar adenocarcinomas of exocrine pancreas) demonstrated that ethanol caused an increase in multiplicity but not in incidence of malignant pancreatic tumours, pointing to an enhancing effect on the development of acinar adenocarcinomas in carcinoma-bearing animals (Woutersen et al. 1989).

In N-nitrosobis(2-oxopropyl)amine (BOP)-treated hamsters (model for ductular adenocarcinomas in exocrine pancreas), ethanol did not modulate pancreatic carcinogenesis (Woutersen et al. 1986b, 1989). These findings are in agreement with those of Pour et al. (1983), who found that ethanol given to outbred Syrian golden hamsters in drinking water at a 5% (w/v) concentration for life, beginning either before or after a single dose of BOP, had no effect on tumour induction. This observation was in contrast with the results of a previous study of this group (Tweedie et al. 1981) in which a higher concentration of ethanol (25% w/v) inhibited the development of BOP-induced pancreatic lesions. The observation of Pour et al. (1983), that hamsters treated with BOP and maintained on ethanol for life exhibited a few atypical acinar cell foci, might point to the pancreatic acinar cell as the main target cell for ethanol and not the centro-acinar or ductular cell. The results in the chronic studies performed by Woutersen et al. (1989) support this hypothesis, since ethanol influenced pancreatic carcinogenesis in azaserine-treated rats but not in BOP-treated hamsters.

The pancreatic tumours induced in the hamster pancreas by BOP are morphologically closely similar to the pancreatic cancers occurring in humans, and the absence of an enhancing effect of ethanol on pancreatic carcinogenesis in hamsters may be more relevant to the human situation than the enhancing effects found in the rat studies.

Long-term ethanol ingestion in rats (14–53 weeks) produced changes in acinar, centroacinar, and ductular cells. Microscopical changes comprised degeneration and atrophic changes of acinar cells, fibrosis, and intraductal protein precipitates (Sarles et al. 1971). The pseudoductular cysts are lined by cuboidal epithelium of ductal type, which may represent dedifferentiation of acinar structures or hyperplasia of centroacinar cells accompanied by atrophy of surrounding acini. A similar phenomenon has been observed in BOP-treated hamsters (Pour 1984, 1988, Meijers et al. 1989, Levitt et al. 1977, Takahashi et al. 1980, Flaks et al. 1980, 1981).

Colon and Rectum

Hamilton et al. (1987, 1988) studied the effects of chronic dietary ethanol consumption (Lieber–DeCarli-type liquid diet containing 33% of calories as ethanol) during the initiation phase in an azoxymethane (AOM)-treated rat model. They found a significantly lower incidence of tumours of the left colon when the liquid-ethanol diet was given prior to and during administration of carcinogen, whereas administration of the liquid-ethanol diet after injection of the carcinogen had no effect on the incidence of tumours of the colon. These findings suggest that inhibition of tumorigenesis may result from suppression of metabolic activation of AOM and the consequent reduced formation of DNA damage during the initiation phase of the model.

Seitz et al. (1984) studied the effect of chronic ethanol administration on 1,2-dimethylhydrazine (DMH; subcutaneously injected)-induced rectal carcinogenesis in male Sprague-Dawley rats fed a nutritionally adequate liquid diet containing 36% of total calories as ethanol or isocaloric carbohydrates. Chronic ethanol ingestion appeared to increase the total number of rectal tumours significantly (17 vs. 6; $p < 0.02$), whereas no cocarcinogenic effect of ethanol was observed in other parts of the intestine. Alcohol did not influence the size or type of the tumours.

Howarth and Pihl (1985) injected male inbred D/A rats subcutaneously with DMH and maintained the animals on tap water, commercially available beer, or 4.8% ethanol (v/v) in water as the drinking fluid. They found no significant difference in the incidence of intestinal cancer between the groups given ethanol or beer and the group given tap water. Nelson and Samelson (1985), who conducted a similar experiment with Sprague-Dawley rats exposed to DMH and maintained on either 5% ethanol (v/v) or tap water as the drinking fluid, also found no effect of ethanol on the development of colonic tumours.

Conclusion

It is generally accepted that alcohol per se is not a carcinogen. However, the available data on the effects of ethanol on digestive tract cancer induced in experimental animals by well-known chemical carcinogens suggest that chronic oral ethanol ingestion may have a cocarcinogenic effect on the oesophagus and possibly also the non-glandular (fore)stomach, but not on the glandular stomach or the pancreas. There has been very little work on the influence of ethanol on experimentally induced colorectal cancer, and the few results available have been conflicting; it is not possible to draw from them any conclusions about a possible cocarcinogenic effect of ethanol on the colon/rectum.

While a number of studies indicate that ethanol increases the incidence of some specific chemically-induced digestive tract tumours, other studies do not. One possible reason for these contradictory results may be that ethanol may have differing effects at various stages of the carcinogenic process. In fact, the controversial results obtained with various studies investigating the modifying effects of ethanol on the activity of known carcinogens can be explained by differences between the studies in their experimental design, such as the method (in drinking water, as liquid diet, intragastrically; prior to, with, or after carcinogen application), amount, concentration, and duration of ethanol administration as well as type, dose, duration, and method of carcinogen application.

The experimental work has so far failed to elucidate the underlying mechanism whereby excessive consumption of alcoholic beverages, which are complex solutions containing many compounds in addition to alcohol, may act as a cocarcinogen under certain conditions.

Epidemiological Evidence

Epidemiological evidence of the role of alcoholic beverages in the production of cancers of the digestive tract and larynx has been obtained from a few ecological studies, many cohort studies, and a very large number of case-control studies.

The best evidence has been obtained from cohort studies in which incidence or mortality rates for specific types of cancer have been observed in men and women who have previously been classified according to the amount of alcohol they habitually drink.[1] Even these studies, however, provide only imprecise evidence of the quantitative relationship between the amount consumed and the risk of cancer, partly because of the unreliability of the histories given by heavy drinkers and possibly also by light drinkers in communities where the consumption of alcohol is discouraged, as both groups may underestimate their consumption; and partly because of the rarity of the cancers most closely related to alcohol consumption in nondrinkers, who commonly tend also to be nonsmokers. The latter has meant that very large numbers of people have had to be recruited to the studies if adequate numbers of cases (or deaths) were to be observed.

Many aspects of the relationship between the consumption of alcohol and the risk of developing cancer have, therefore, had to be examined in case-control studies in which histories of alcohol consumption are obtained from cancer patients after the cancer has developed or, in some cases, from their relatives after the patients have died. This introduces a further element of uncertainty into the quantitative estimates of risk, as histories may not be given with equal reliability by the cancer patients and their controls (regardless of whether the controls are patients with other diseases or healthy members of the general population), and allowance has to be made for the possibility that "recall bias" may have influenced the results.

No useful quantitative evidence can be obtained from the few ecological studies: that is, from correlations between the incidence of or mortality from specific cancers in different populations and the average amounts of alcohol estimated to be consumed per person in these populations. Such studies have, however, occasionally suggested hypotheses for investigation by other methods (as was the case with the correlation observed between cancer of the rectum and the consumption of beer [Enstrom 1977]) and the results obtained from them contribute to the totality of the evidence that justifies the conclusion that an association observed in case-control and cohort studies implies cause and effect.

Cancers of the Mouth, Pharynx, Oesophagus, and Larynx

A massive amount of epidemiological evidence has been obtained to show (1) that in tobacco smokers, the consumption of alcoholic beverages increases the risk of cancers of the mouth, pharynx, oesopha-

---

[1]Throughout this section of the report, "drink" refers specifically to the consumption of alcohol, and alcohol implies alcohol beverages. When reference to the chemical C_2H_5OH is intended, it will be called "ethanol."

gus, and larynx (other than cancers of the salivary glands and naso-pharynx); (2) that the risk increases approximately in proportion to the amount drunk; (3) that, in each case, alcoholic beverages act syn-ergistically with smoking, each agent approximately multiplying the effects of the other; and (4) that the main component of alcoholic bev-erages that determines the risk of cancer is ethanol. Cancers of the salivary glands and nasopharynx are excluded from these statements, even though they have sometimes constituted a small proportion of the cancers of the mouth and pharynx in some series, because enough is known about their aetiology to be sure that other factors are more important and because no direct evidence has been obtained to indi-cate that they are related to the consumption of alcohol.

The evidence on which these statements are based has been ob-tained mainly from Europe and North America, where these diseases are rare in nonsmokers and nondrinkers; but very similar findings have also been recorded in South America (Franco et al. 1989, De Stefani et al. 1990b) and Asia (Sankaranarayanan et al. 1990, 1991, Choi and Kahyo 1991a,b). In some parts of Africa and Asia other fac-tors cause some of these diseases to be exceptionally common, and the role of alcohol and tobacco may be quite small. There is, however, no reason to suppose that alcoholic beverages do not have a similar qualitative effect in all societies.

Most of the many studies that have led to these conclusions have been summarized by the International Agency for Research on Can-cer (1988), in one of the Agency's series of monographs on the evalu-ation of carcinogenic risks to humans, and are not listed here. Studies reported subsequently have led to similar conclusions (Adami et al. 1992, Barra et al. 1990, Blot et al. 1988, Boffeta and Garfinkel 1990, Brown et al. 1988, Choi and Kahyo 1991a,b, De Stefani et al. 1990b, Falk et al. 1990, Franco et al. 1989, Kabat and Wynder 1989, La Vec-chia and Negri 1989, McLaughlin et al. 1988, Merletti et al. 1990, Sank-aranarayanan et al. 1990, 1991, Talamini et al. 1990, Tuyns et al. 1988, Zatonski et al. 1991, Zheng et al. 1990), and none has contradicted them. The results described below provide examples of the type of evidence obtained.

Dose-Response Relationship

An indication of the dose-response relationship for two types of upper digestive tract cancer, free from recall bias, is provided by the results of the American Cancer Society's cohort study of 1 million men and women over 30 years of age (Boffeta and Garfinkel 1990). Results relating to alcohol have been published so far for only 12 years

Table 1
Relative risk of developing oral[a]
or oesophageal cancer by drinking habit
(after Boffeta and Garfinkel 1990)

Drinks per day	Type of cancer	
	oral	oesophageal
0	1.0 (55)[b]	1.0 (59)
≤ 1	0.7 (16)	1.3 (29)
2–3	1.4 (25)	2.2 (37)
4–5	3.1 (18)	4.8 (25)
6+	6.2 (26)	5.8 (22)

[a]Including cancer of the salivary glands.
[b]Numbers of deaths in parentheses.

of observations on 276,802 men aged 40–59 years who had given detailed drinking histories. Mortality data have been given separately for oral cancer and for oesophageal cancer, standardized for age, smoking, and education. These are shown in Table 1. For both types of cancer, the mortality increases regularly (with one exception in the case of oral cancer) from that in nonsmokers through three categories of occasional or light drinkers to "heavy drinkers" (in the American sense) in whom the mortality is increased about sixfold.

Synergism With Smoking

In the above example, the effect of smoking was effectively eliminated by standardization. To see the way the two factors interact large numbers are needed, and these have been obtained only in case-control studies. Typical results were obtained by Rothman and Keller (1972) in a study of 598 men with squamous carcinomas of the mouth and pharynx, matched one-for-one with men of the same ages in the same hospital. The results given in Table 2 suggest that each factor contributes about equally, having perhaps a greater relative effect when the other is present than when it is absent.

For oesophageal cancer in Normandy, where much larger quantities of alcohol are consumed, the relative risk for heavy drinkers and heavy smokers rises to a much higher level, as is shown in Table 3.

Observations on laryngeal cancer are confused by the fact that, despite the small size of the larynx as defined for anatomical and clinical purposes, its different parts react differently to different aetiological factors. Aetiologically it is best divided into the glottis and subglottis, which lie wholly within the respiratory system, and the

Table 2
**Relative risk of oral or pharyngeal cancer
by level of smoking and drinking
(after Rothman and Keller 1972)**

Drinking: ml alcohol/day[a]	Smoking: cigarette equivalents/day			
	0	< 20	20–39	≥ 40
0	1.0	1.5	1.4	2.4
< 12	1.4	1.7	3.2	3.3
12–44	1.6	4.4	4.5	8.2
≥ 45	2.3	4.1	9.6	15.5

[a]The authors' "ounces per day" have been converted to ml
for comparison with other tables.

Table 3
**Relative risk of oesophageal cancer by level
of smoking and drinking (after Tuyns et al. 1977)**

Drinking: g alcohol/day	Smoking: tobacco in g/day		
	0–	10–	≥ 30
0–40	1.0	3.9	7.8
41–80	7.3	8.6	33.6
81–120	11.7	13.1	87.0
≥ 121	49.7	78.7	149.1

supraglottis and epilarynx, which border on the hypopharynx. Two
large case-control studies in France (Brugère et al. 1986) and in France,
Italy, Spain, and Switzerland (Tuyns et al. 1988) have obtained similar
results. These are summarized in Table 4. They show that cancers in
all parts of the larynx and the hypopharynx are closely related to the
amount smoked, but that the glottis is sharply distinguished from the
epilarynx in its relationship with alcohol, the latter being closely related to alcohol consumption, like the hypopharynx, while the former
is related to alcohol only when the consumption is what would be
regarded as exceptionally heavy in many other countries (that is, 100
g or more per day). The results for the supraglottic area differed, however, being more like those for the epilarynx in one series and more
like those for the glottis in the other. This is not easily explained by
the use of different definitions in the two series. The very different
relative risks for heavy consumption can be explained, however, as

Table 4

Relative risk of cancers of larynx and hypopharynx by level of drinking, divided by site within the larynx: standardized for smoking

Series	Drinking: g alcohol/day	Relative risk for cancer of:			
		Glottis	Supraglottis	Epilarynx	Hypopharynx
1	0–39	1.0	1.0	1.0	1.0
	40–99	0.8	2.6	1.9	3.3
	100–159	1.5	11.0	18.7	28.6
	≥ 160	6.1	42.1	101.4	143.1
	(no. of cancer patients)	(240)	(224)	(217)	(366)
2	0–20	1.0	1.0	1.0	1.0
	21–40	0.8	0.9	0.9	1.6
	41–80	1.1	1.1	1.5	3.2
	81–120	1.7	1.7	5.1	5.6
	≥ 121	3.4	2.0	10.6	12.5
	(no. of cancer patients)	(270)	(426)	(118)	(281)

1 Brugère et al. (1986)—alcohol measured as average daily current consumption.
2 Tuyns et al. (1988)—alcohol measured as average daily consumption in adult life.

Brugère et al. (1986) compared levels of current consumption, while Tuyns et al. (1988) compared average levels over all adult life.

Effect in the Absence of Smoking

In Europe and North America, all cancers of the upper respiratory and digestive tracts are rare in the absence of smoking, and only very few studies have included enough cases to provide any useful information about the effect of alcohol by itself. Groups of nonsmokers who are defined as not being current smokers (Elwood et al. 1984) or even as not having smoked for the past 20 years (Wynder et al. 1957a) are inadequate in view of the strong effect of tobacco, which is liable to persist for many years after smoking has been stopped.

The few data available for oropharyngeal, oesophageal, and laryngopharyngeal cancer are summarized in Tables 5A, 5B, and 5C. Little or no increase in risk with amount consumed is seen for oropharyngeal cancer in three out of five sets of data or in the one set for cancer of the endolarynx (glottis), but the increases seen for oesophageal cancer are substantial. The differences are difficult to explain by bias or confounding, but they can be explained by paucity of numbers and, if one drink is taken to equal approximately 10 g alcohol, by differ-

Table 5A
Relative risk of oropharyngeal cancer in nonsmokers by amount drunk

Alcohol drinks/week	Men		Women		
	Blot et al. 1988	Talamini et al. 1990[a]	Blot et al. 1988	Talamini et al. 1990[a]	Merletti et al. 1989[b]
<1	1.0 (12)[c]		1.0 (36)		
1–4	1.3 (12)	1.0 (1)	0.7 (11)	1.0 (10)	1.0 (6)
5–14	1.6 (15)		1.3 (7)		
15–29	1.4 (4)	1.2 (5)	0.0 (0)	1.6 (11)	1.1 (5)
≥ 30	5.8 (6)				0.8 (2)

[a]Data for nondrinkers and drinkers of less than 14 drinks/week grouped, and drinkers of 14–55 and 56 or more per week grouped. Authors gave relative risks for men and women combined (less than 14 per week 1.0, 14–55 per week 1.5, 56 or more per week 2.2) and calculated χ^2 for trend = 4.08 ($p = 0.04$) on four levels (0, less than 14, 14–55, and 56 or more).
[b]Oral cancer only. Authors gave 0–20, 21–40, and more than 40 g/day.
[c]Numbers of cases in parentheses.

Table 5B
Relative risk of oesophageal cancer in nonsmokers by amount drunk

Alcohol g/day[a]	Men		Women	
	Tuyns 1983a	La Vecchia and Negri 1989[a]	Tuyns 1983a	La Vecchia and Negri 1989[a]
0–40	1.0 (7)[b]	1.0 (5)	1.0 (25)	1.0 (22)
41–81	3.8 (15)	1.1 (3)	5.6 (8)	
81–120	10.2 (9)		11.0 (3)	4.3 (5)
≥ 121	101.0 (8)	3.3 (3)	———	

[a]Under 4, 4–8, and more than 8 drinks/day as reported by La Vecchia and Negri 1989. Relative risks calculated directly from published data. Authors gave relative risks for men and women combined adjusted for age and sex of 1.0 (less than 4 drinks per day, 2.1 for 4–8 per day, and 3.6 for more than 8 per day. χ^2 for trend .09).
[b]Numbers of cases in parentheses.

ences in the amount consumed. Acceptance of a causal relationship does not necessarily imply that ethanol is a complete carcinogen, however. There is no reason to suppose that tobacco smoke is the only carcinogenic agent to which the human upper respiratory and digestive tracts are exposed (indeed there is clear evidence that in parts of Asia and Africa it is not the only agent), and ethanol may be facilitating the effect of some other unrecognized carcinogenic agents in nonsmokers, just as it commonly facilitates the effect of tobacco smoke.

Table 5C
Relative risk of laryngopharyngeal cancer in male nonsmokers by amount drunk (after Tuyns et al. 1988)

Alcohol g/day	Epilarynx and hypopharynx	Endolarynx
0–39	1.0 (1)[a]	1.0 (7)
40–79	} 6.7 (8)	1.5 (3)
≥ 80		1.7 (6)

[a]Number of cases in parentheses.

Differential Effects of Different Alcoholic Beverages

Many attempts have been made to separate the effects of different types of alcoholic drink. Some authors have concluded that no separation is possible (e.g., Williams and Horm 1977, Breslow and Day 1980, Burch et al. 1981, Kabat and Wynder 1989, Merletti et al. 1990). Others have recorded greater risks with spirits, regardless of type, than with wine or beer (Wynder et al. 1956, 1957a, Wynder and Bross 1961, Hirayama 1979, Pottern et al. 1981). In Normandy, Tuyns et al. (1979) recorded a greater risk with apple-based drinks (digestives and cider) than with wine, beer, or aperitifs. In Italy, however, Barra et al. (1990) found greater risks of oropharyngeal and oesophageal cancer in wine drinkers than in wine drinkers who also drank spirits or beer after adjustment for amount consumed. It is doubtful, however, whether histories of the amount consumed can be equally accurate (or inaccurate) when described in tots of spirits, glasses of wine, and bottles of beer, and Barra et al. (1990) pointed out that the most frequently consumed beverage in each area tends to be the one with the highest estimated relative risk. It may be that "strong" drinks are more deleterious, gram for gram of alcohol, than other alcoholic beverages, but the evidence is weak and inconclusive.

That ethanol itself, independent of any congeners present in different alcoholic beverages, may act to increase the risk of cancer in mucosal tissues with which it comes into contact is also provided by the observation that the risk of oropharyngeal cancer is increased in both men and women who regularly use mouthwashes with a high content of ethanol (Winn et al. 1991).

Nutrition

The evidence that nutrition affects the incidence of a wide variety of cancers, if not of all, is mounting steadily. There is now reason to believe that the risks from exposure to many carcinogenic agents can be reduced by the regular consumption of fruit and green vegetables. Early evidence suggested that this might be particularly true for cancers of the hypopharynx, which have been associated with the Plummer-Vinson syndrome (Wynder et al. 1957b), and a deficiency of such foods seems to be a major cause of the exceptionally high risk of oesophageal cancer in parts of Asia (Day 1975). Heavy drinking is commonly associated with poor nutrition and poor nutrition may be held to increase the risk (particularly of pharyngeal and oesophageal cancers) in heavy drinkers. Direct evidence of the role of nutritional deficiency in increasing the risk of alcohol-associated cancers has been obtained for cancers of the mouth and pharynx by Winn et al. (1984), McLaughlin et al. (1988), La Vecchia et al. (1991), and Franco et al. (1989); for cancers of the larynx by Zatonski et al. (1991); and for cancers of the oesophagus by Ziegler et al. (1981), Tuyns (1983b), Decarli et al. (1987), Tuyns et al. (1987), and Brown et al. (1988).

Conclusion

There is consensus that the consumption of alcoholic beverages increases the risk of developing cancers of the mouth (other than the salivary glands), pharynx (other than the nasopharynx), oesophagus, and larynx; that the risks are principally due to the presence of ethanol and increase with the amount consumed; that the risks are increased by increased smoking, each agent approximately multiplying the effects of the other; and that, in the absence of smoking, the risks in developed countries are all small unless consumption is exceptionally heavy. There is also evidence that the risks are diminished by a diet rich in fruit and green vegetables.

Whether the cocarcinogenic effects of different alcoholic beverages depend solely on the presence of ethanol and are unaffected either by the concentration of ethanol or the presence of congeners is uncertain.

Cancer of the Stomach

As early as 1833 it was recognized that excessive alcohol consumption can cause an acute inflammation of the stomach lining (gastritis), and it is now believed that repeated insults of excess alcohol (in alcoholics, for example) leads to a persistent inflammatory response (chronic gastritis) (Taylor 1987). Because chronic gastritis is thought to predispose to later cancerous changes in the stomach (Correa 1988), it has been suggested that alcohol consumption might increase the risk of stomach cancer. Apart from the association with gastritis, alcohol might also affect stomach cancer risk by altering gastric juice physiology (e.g., by changing acidity), or by occasional contamination with cancer-causing substances (e.g., N-nitroso compounds in certain beers and whiskies) (Ministry of Agriculture, Fisheries, and Food 1987).

Stomach cancer is invariably more common in men than in women, by a factor of around two, and this has been attributed to comparable differences in alcohol consumption (Flamant et al. 1964). There has, however, been a dramatic worldwide decline in the incidence of stomach cancer (Muñoz 1988), a finding in contrast to the general increases in alcohol consumption and alcohol-related diseases such as cirrhosis of the liver. The male excess is much the same in different countries regardless of the level of consumption, and the attribution of the male excess to alcohol cannot be sustained.

Cohort Studies

The relationship between alcohol intake and cancer at a variety of sites has been assessed in several cohort studies, the results of which have been summarized in Table 6. In most studies, detailed information on type of beverage, amount consumed, and smoking habits was not available. Most of the cohort studies were of the retrospective (historical) type, comparing cancer incidence in groups with high alcohol intake with that of the general population.

In 11 studies, stomach cancer rates in groups with an established high intake of alcohol were compared with appropriate rates from the general population. Seven were groups of clinically diagnosed alcoholics (Adami et al. 1992, Adelstein and White 1976, Hakulinen et al. 1974, Monson and Lyon 1975, Robinette et al. 1979, Schmidt and Popham 1981, Sundby 1967), three were groups of brewery workers (Carstensen et al. 1990, Dean et al. 1979, Jensen 1980), and one a group of waiters (Andersen et al. 1989). The results are summarized in Table 6. Not one of these studies showed an increase in the stomach cancer rate that was statistically significant, and the small study of waiters showed a significant decrease. Combining the findings of all the studies, 325 cases of stomach cancer were observed, while 352 were expected from the comparison populations; that is, there was less stomach cancer than expected, overall, though not statistically significantly less.

There have also been seven published cohort studies in which alcohol consumption was recorded, by interview or questionnaire, in cross-sections of various populations (Gordon and Kannel 1984, Hirayama 1989, 1992, Kato et al. 1992, Klatsky et al. 1981, Kneller et al. 1991, Kono et al. 1987, Stemmermann et al. 1990). The subsequent rate of stomach cancer in alcohol consumers was then compared with

Table 6
Cohort studies of alcohol consumption in relation to cancers of the stomach, colon, rectum, and pancreas

Study, country	Stomach cancer	Colon cancer	Rectal cancer	Pancreas cancer	Comments
	Relative risk (no. of cancer cases or deaths)				
Studies of alcoholics					
Sundby 1967, Norway	1.3 (45)	1.0 (9)	1.9 (12)	0.9 (5)	1722 males compared with local rates
Hakulinen et al. 1974	0.8 (6)	1.8 (3)	—	1.8 (4)	16,000+ males compared with national incidence rates
and Hakulinen et al. 1974, Finland	—	1.0 (82)	—	—	205,000 males compared with national incidence rates
Monson and Lyon 1975, United States	1.0 (15)	0.6 (7)	0.7 (4)	0.6 (3)	1139 males, 143 females compared with national mortality rates
Adelstein and White 1976, United Kingdom	0.8 (8)	1.3 (9)	0.9 (4)	1.5 (7)	1595 males, 475 females compared with national mortality rates.
Robinette et al. 1979, United States	1.0 (9)	0.8 (7)	3.3 (6)	0.9 (4)	4401 males compared with national mortality rates
Schmidt and Popham 1981, Canada	1.0 (19)	1.0 (19)	1.0 (10)	1.2 (11)	9889 males (mean intake 200g/day) compared with local mortality rates

Table 6. *Continued*

Study, country		Stomach cancer	Colon cancer	Rectal cancer	Pancreas cancer	Comments
		Relative risk (no. of cancer cases or deaths)				
Studies of Alcoholics *continued*						
Adami et al. 1992, Sweden	M	0.9 (23)	1.2 (26)	0.8 (12)	1.4 (19)	8340 males, 1013 females compared with local incidence rates
	F	0.7 (1)	1.7 (4)	0.8 (1)	2.6 (3)	
Studies of brewery workers						
Dean et al. 1979, Ireland		0.8 (40)	1.3 (32)	1.6[a] (32)	1.2 (17)	3600 males (mean intake 58g/day) compared with local mortality rates
Jensen 1980, Denmark		0.9 (92)	1.1 (87)	1.0 (85)	1.1 (44)	14,313 males (allowance 78g/day) compared with national incidence rates
Carstensen et al. 1990, Sweden		1.1 (53)	1.2 (48)	1.7[a] (49)	1.7[a] (38)	6230 males (allowance 1 litre/day) compared with national incidence rates
Study of waiters						
Andersen et al. 1989, Norway		0.6[a] (14)	1.1 (24)	2.0 (28)	1.0 (11)	2413 males compared with national incidence rates
Follow-up studies of populations with known consumption						
Gordon and Kannel 1984, United States		sig[a] (18)	NS (36)	—	—	2106 males, 2641 females, RR not estimated, mortality study

Study					Comments
Kono et al. 1986, 1987, Japan (physicians)	1.2 (116)	combined with rectum	1.4 (39)	1.5 (14)	5130 males, RR for ≥ 2 drinks/day vs. nondrinkers mortality
Blackwelder et al. 1980, Stemmermann et al. 1990, Hawaii (Japanese)	1.2 (174)	1.4[a] (211)	1.9[a] (101)	N/A (13)	8006 males, RR for 40+ oz/month vs. nondrinkers incidence
Hirayama 1989, 1992, Japan	0.9 (5247)	1.7[a] (574)	1.4 (N/A)	1.0 (N/A)	122,261 males, 142,857 females, RR for daily vs. nondrinkers mortality, sig. for sigmoid colon only
Kneller et al. 1991, United States (mainly of European origin)	1.1 (75)	—	—	—	17,818 males, RR for 14+ drinks/month vs. nondrinkers mortality
Kato et al. 1992, Japan	2.8[a] (57)	—	—	—	9753 subjects, RR for ≥ 50g/day vs. nondrinkers mortality; trend not significant
Wu et al. 1987, United States	—	1.3 (76)	1.6 (51)	—	11,888 subjects, RR for > 30ml/day vs. nondrinkers, incidence
Klatsky et al. 1981, 1988, Hiatt et al. 1988, United States	NS (13)	1.6 (203)	2.5 (66)	0.9 (48)	100,000+ subjects, RR for daily vs. nondrinkers incidence; significant trend for rectum
Heuch et al. 1983, Norway	—	—	—	10.8[a] (18)	4995 males, RR for "frequent" vs. nondrinkers incidence; significant trend

[a]Statistically significant ($p < 0.05$).

that in nonconsumers. The results of these are also summarized in Table 6. Two studies (Gordon and Kannel 1984, Kato et al. 1992) reported a statistically significant excess with high alcohol consumption, of which one was based on a total of only 18 deaths from stomach cancer (Gordon and Kannel 1984). In contrast, the largest study, in Japan, was based on 5247 male deaths from stomach cancer and showed that the relative risk in daily alcohol drinkers was 0.92 compared with nondrinkers (Hirayama 1989, 1992).

Case-Control Studies

There have been at least 37 published case-control studies in which the relationship between alcohol consumption and stomach cancer has been reported. Of these, seven showed a significantly positive relationship (Agudo et al. 1992, Correa et al. 1985, De Stefani et al. 1990a, Hoey et al. 1981, Hu et al. 1988, Lee et al. 1990, Wu-Williams et al. 1990), while 30 did not (Acheson and Doll 1964, Armijo et al. 1981, Bjelke 1974, Boeing et al. 1991, Buiatti et al. 1989, 1990, Palli et al. 1992, Burr and Holliday 1989, Demirir et al. 1990, Ferraroni et al. 1989, Graham et al. 1967, 1972, Haenszel et al. 1972, 1976, Higginson 1966, Hoshiyama and Sasaba 1992, Jedrychowski et al. 1986, Kato et al. 1990, Kono et al. 1988, Modan et al. 1974, Risch et al. 1985, Stocks 1957, Tajima and Tominaga 1985, Tominaga et al. 1991, Trichopoulos et al. 1985, Tuyns et al. 1992, Unakami et al. 1989, Williams and Horm 1977, Wynder et al. 1963, You et al. 1988, Yu and Hseih 1991).

Among the negative studies, there were some that showed an effect in a particular subgroup. Thus, positive effects were reported for sake drinkers in a study of Japanese in Hawaii (Haenszel et al. 1972), beer drinkers in Germany (Boeing et al. 1991), and vodka drinkers (but only before breakfast) in Poland (Jedrychowski et al. 1986). None of these three studies showed a positive effect for overall alcohol consumption.

The seven positive studies were from a variety of countries: China (Hu et al. 1988), France (Hoey et al. 1981), Spain (Agudo et al. 1992), Taiwan (Lee et al. 1990), Uruguay (De Stefani et al. 1990a), and the United States (Correa et al. 1985, Wu-Williams et al. 1990). The relative risk for alcohol consumers compared with nonconsumers was reported in four studies (Agudo et al. 1992, Correa et al. 1985, Lee et al. 1990, Wu-Williams et al. 1990) and varied between 1.5 and 1.7. The results were all of borderline statistical significance. Five studies (Agudo et al. 1992, Correa et al. 1985, De Stefani et al. 1990a, Lee et al. 1990, Wu-Williams et al. 1990) reported on the trend in relative risk with increasing consumption of alcohol, which was statistically significant in all except one (Agudo et al. 1992), although in one U.S. study the significance was restricted to blacks and not to whites (Correa et al. 1985).

Two of the seven positive studies were made difficult to interpret by the grouping together of nonconsumers and "low" consumers of alcohol as a single baseline group. In one study (Hu et al. 1988) the "low" consumers consisted of individuals who drank up to the equivalent of 4000 g of ethanol per annum (equivalent to approximately one drink per day), while in the other study (Hoey et al. 1981) this cutoff point was 568 g/week (equivalent to seven litres of wine per week).

The type of alcohol consumed and relationship to risk was reported in four of the seven positive studies. In these studies, wine had the strongest effect in two studies (Agudo et al. 1992, De Stefani et al. 1990a), spirits in one (Correa et al. 1985), and beer in the fourth (Wu-Williams et al. 1990).

Two studies (Agudo et al. 1992, De Stefani et al. 1990a) had positive results for males but not for females.

Most of the positive results have been adjusted for tobacco smoking, but the extent to which other potential confounding factors (notably related to diet and socioeconomic status) were controlled for was variable. Many such confounding factors are related to both alcohol consumption and gastric cancer risk and could therefore have given rise to false-positive findings.

Cancer of the Gastric Cardia

The cardia region of the stomach is the uppermost area where the stomach adjoins the oesophagus. There has recently been interest in cancer at this site because, unlike the other more distal regions of the stomach, cardia cancer rates have been increasing. It has been suggested that this cancer resembles a specific type of cancer (adenocarcinoma) of the lower oesophagus and may share common risk factors, notably tobacco and alcohol exposure. Three of the case-control studies have analyzed alcohol consumption in relation to cardia cancer. One U.S. study (Wu-Williams et al. 1990) found an extremely strong effect of alcohol in the cardia, whereas the Italian (Palli et al. 1992) and Japanese (Unakami et al. 1989) studies found no effect in comparison with cancer elsewhere in the stomach. The U.S. study also found an increased effect of alcohol in the upper part of the noncardia stomach (the corpus) compared with the lower part (the antrum). A further study from Uruguay (De Stefani et al. 1990a), in which cardia and corpus cases were combined, found that the alcohol association with these was no stronger than that in the antrum. Finally, a

Canadian study (Gray et al. 1992), which did not have a control group, found no difference between alcohol use in patients with cardia cancer and those with cancer in other parts of the stomach, while both groups consumed less than oesophageal cancer patients.

Conclusion

The current evidence pertaining to the relationship between alcohol consumption and stomach cancer consists of 18 cohort and 37 case-control studies. The existing balance of the evidence indicates that alcohol consumption is unlikely to be involved in the aetiology of the disease. The absence of recall bias means that particular emphasis should be placed on the cohort studies, only two of which were positive. In addition, less than a quarter of the case-control studies reported positive findings and, in the majority of these, the size of the effect was relatively small and of borderline statistical significance.

Our conclusion is slightly less cautious than that reached by the International Agency for Research on Cancer (1988) that "there is little in the aggregate data to suggest a causal role for drinking of alcoholic beverages in stomach cancer." There is likely to be general consensus in favour of the IARC conclusion, but a minority of investigators might dissent from the present conclusion and suggest that alcohol could have an aetiological role in stomach cancer, albeit minor and unproven.

As yet there is insufficient evidence to draw conclusions about subsidiary hypotheses, such as whether alcohol consumption is a risk factor for cancer of the gastric cardia.

Cancer of the Pancreas

Pancreas cancer is reported to occur more frequently in men than in women, in blacks than in whites, and in urban rather than in rural populations. At present, epidemiological and toxicological studies have not consistently identified any specific factor responsible for the development of pancreatic cancer except cigarette smoking (Levison 1979, Morgan and Wormsley 1977, Wynder 1975). Consequently, it is believed that combinations of dietary and life-style factors such as fat, protein, and alcohol, which are thought to promote the effects of environmental carcinogens, may play a role in the pathogenesis of this highly fatal form of cancer. Alcohol as a possible cause of pancreas cancer was proposed for the first time by Dörken (1964) and has been extensively studied since then. The present review summarises the epidemiological data available to date about the role of alcohol in the development of pancreas cancer.

Cohort Studies

Heuch et al. (1983) reported a significant dose-response effect of alcohol (based on the frequency of consumption of beer and spirits) in a cohort of 16,713 Norwegians, which persisted after controlling for smoking of cigarettes in 18 cases with pancreas cancer. Based on these findings, the authors concluded that there exists a strong causal relationship between alcohol consumption and pancreatic cancer. However, the apparent high nonparticipation rate of heavy drinkers during the formative phase of the cohort, and the conflicting evidence derived from histologically confirmed and nonconfirmed pancreatic cancer cases (among the latter, the association with alcohol intake appears to be negative), makes a causal interpretation of the findings difficult (International Agency for Research on Cancer 1988). One of three studies of brewery workers (Carstensen et al. 1990) showed a significant 70% excess of pancreatic cancers, but none of the other cohort studies reviewed reported a significant association between consumption of alcoholic beverages and pancreatic cancer risk (Sundby 1967, Hakulinen et al. 1974, Monson and Lyon 1975, Adelstein and White 1976, Dean et al. 1979, Jensen 1979, 1980, Robinette et al. 1979, Hirayama 1992, Kono et al. 1983, 1986, Blackwelder et al. 1980, Schmidt and Popham 1981, Hiatt et al. 1988, Adami et al. 1992, Andersen et al. 1989).

Case-Control Studies

At least 23 case-control studies have been reported up to now in which patients with pancreas cancer or their relatives ("proxy respondents") were queried as to their life-style, and their responses were compared with those of people without the disease. The number of cases in the various studies ranged from 18 to 901. Controls were usually hospital-based. Occasionally population-based or community-based controls were used. Patients were usually classified into several categories according to alcohol intake, but the definition of these categories was not always explicitly stated. A significant positive association of alcohol consumption and pancreatic cancer was observed in five studies. Burch and Ansari (1968) reported that 54 (65%) of 83 patients with pancreatic cancer diagnosed in the New Orleans Veterans Hospital between 1960 and 1966 had an average daily consumption of 57–85 g of alcohol. Cuzick and Babiker (1989) reported evidence of a positive trend in risk of pancreatic cancer and total alcohol consumption. They found a threefold risk of pancreatic cancer among heavy beer drinkers and demonstrated a dose-response relationship. Moreover, they found that the effect of alcohol appeared to be largely confined to smokers. No significant trend with amount of alcohol was observed in nonsmokers. Furthermore, Durbec et al. (1983) found a positive association between total alcohol intake (especially in the case of wine with a high alcohol content) and pancreatic cancer risk (relative risk for drinkers versus nondrinkers was 2.4). The risk was reduced after controlling for fat and carbohydrate intake; there was no increased risk with regular drinking of aperitifs or spirits. Raymond et al. (1987) reported a significantly increased pancreatic cancer risk among beer drinkers. After pooling the data from the population-based case-control study performed by Raymond et al. (1987) and two negative hospital-based case-control studies conducted in Paris (Clavel et al. 1989) and Greater Milan (Ferraroni et al. 1989), no association with alcohol consumption was found (Bouchardy et al. 1990). Recently, Olsen et al. (1989) conducted a case-control study in the Minneapolis-St. Paul area and observed that heavy alcohol consumption (4 or more drinks per day), adjusted for several potential confounding variables, was positively associated with pancreatic cancer. All exposure data of this study, however, were obtained from proxy respondents, which may lead to misclassification of risk factors, as has recently been pointed out by Lyon et al. (1992).

Other investigators did not observe a consistent significant association between alcohol intake and cancer of the pancreas (Bueno de Mesquita et al. 1992, Clavel et al. 1989, Bouchardy et al. 1990, Wynder et al. 1973, 1983, Williams and Horm 1977, MacMahon et al. 1981, Manousos et al. 1981, Haines et al. 1982, Kodama and Mori 1983a,b, Gold et al. 1985a, Falk et al. 1988, Farrow and Davis 1990, Jain et al. 1991). Some investigators reported an inverse association between alcohol intake and the relative risk for pancreas cancer (Baghurst et al. 1991, Ghadirian et al. 1991, Gold et al. 1985b, Mack et al. 1986, Norell et al. 1986, Falk et al. 1988, Hiatt et al. 1988). The earliest report of an inverse relationship between pancreatic cancer and wine was that of Gold et al. (1985b). In a population-based case-control study in Los Angeles, Mack et al. (1986) found a nonsignificant inverse association between cancer of the pancreas and alcohol intake from any source; the inverse relationship was more pronounced for table wine consumption. Norell et al. (1986) performed a population-based case-control study in Sweden and found an inverse association with relative risks for frequent versus infrequent alcohol use of 0.5 (hospital controls) and 0.7 (population controls). Falk et al. (1988) found decreased risks for all types of alcoholic beverages among women and among the highest male consumers of beer. The pooled analysis of three case-control studies (Bouchardy et al. 1990) did not reveal a relationship with wine, although the data from the Paris study (Clavel et al. 1989) exhibited a significant inverse dose-response effect. No biologically plausible explanation for a protective effect of alcohol is apparent.

The Role of (Calcifying) Pancreatitis

It is generally accepted that chronic alcohol abuse, whether or not in combination with a high fat diet, is the most common cause of chronic (calcifying) pancreatitis (Ishii et al. 1973, Johnson and Zintel 1979, Sarles and Tiscornia 1974, Sarles et al. 1980, Singh 1986, Ammann et al. 1988, Singh and Simsek 1990).

Several mechanisms have been proposed for the pathogenesis of alcoholic pancreatitis. There is mounting evidence from studies on both experimental animals and humans that alcohol has a direct effect on the pancreatic cells. Light and electron microscopy of pancreatic tissue from alcoholic patients with chronic pancreatitis revealed dedifferentiation of acinar cells to tubular complexes (Singh 1986). In addition to the loss of acinar cells, there is loss of ductal cells.

The association between chronic pancreatitis and pancreatic cancer has been described by Mikal and Campbell (1950) in autopsies and by Paulino-Netto et al. (1960) and Becker (1978) in surgical patients. The data are inadequate to draw conclusions, however, especially since pancreatitis may be the consequence, but not the cause, of pancreatic cancer. Although chronic pancreatitis microscopically surrounding pancreatic carcinoma is common, cancer developing in chronic pancreatitis has rarely been shown. Recently, Haas et al. (1990) presented four male patients with pancreatic cancer who had had previous surgery for complications of chronic pancreatitis. Chronic pancreatitis, including calcifications, had been caused by alcohol in three cases.

Conclusion

Cohort studies of people with high alcohol intake provide no significant evidence for an association between alcohol consumption and the risk of pancreatic cancer. Population-based cohort studies as well as case-control studies provide inconsistent results. The amount of alcohol intake observed in the various studies does not account for the inconsistency. The average alcohol intake in the studies that reported a positive association was lower than in studies where no association between alcohol consumption and pancreatic cancer risk was reported.

It is generally accepted, however, that chronic alcohol abuse is associated with chronic (calcifying) pancreatitis. Recurrent tissue damage and repair is an important phenomenon in this disease. There is, moreover, substantial evidence that cancer may be associated with chronically injured tissue (Feron and Woutersen 1989). Colon cancer is frequently seen in patients with chronic colitis (Laroye 1974), skin cancer may occur in burn scars (Berenblum 1944), and many lung tumours grow in areas of scarring (Bennett et al. 1969). A large body of animal data also suggests that chronic tissue injury induced by chemical or physical agents could be a major factor in tumour development in connective tissue and epithelial tissues (Grasso 1987). For example, malignant tumours induced in the nasal epithelium by irritating substances such as acetaldehyde and formaldehyde have been found to arise only from epithelium that is severely damaged (Woutersen et al. 1986a, Kerns et al. 1983).

Taking into account all the epidemiological data now available it can be concluded that it is unlikely that a causal relationship between consumption of alcohol and the risk of pancreas cancer exists. An indirect association via the induction of chronic (calcifying) pancreatitis, however, cannot be completely excluded.

Cancer of the Large Bowel

A relationship between alcohol consumption and colorectal cancer was originally suggested, in the 1970s, by correlational studies in populations. At least five studies showed positive correlations between measures of alcohol disappearance or consumption and colorectal cancer incidence or mortality rates, both between populations (McMichael et al. 1979) and within them (Breslow and Enstrom 1974, Enstrom 1977, Kono and Ikeda 1979, Decarli and La Vecchia 1986). Such correlational studies, however, are of value only in formulating hypotheses worth further consideration in analytical studies.

Cohort Studies

At least 15 cohort studies gave some data on colorectal and large bowel cancer (International Agency for Research on Cancer 1988), the results of which have been summarized in Table 6. Of these, however, seven included fewer than 50 cases of (or deaths from) colorectal cancer combined and are not very informative. The main findings from the other eight cohort studies are described below (Hakulinen et al. 1974, Dean et al. 1979, Jensen 1979, Pollack et al. 1984, Stemmermann et al. 1990, Wu et al. 1987, Klatsky et al. 1988, Hirayama 1989, Carstensen et al. 1990).

The geographic area, the identification of the study cohorts, the main type of alcoholic beverage, and the pattern of drinking (i.e., regular versus binge) varied from study to study. It is thus remarkable that all the relative risk (RR) estimates for colon cancer varied within the relatively narrow range of 1.0 to 1.7, with most between 1.1 and 1.3. This overall consistency of results is only in apparent contrast with several heterogeneities observed within studies: for instance, in the large Japanese cohort (Hirayama 1989), the RR for daily alcohol drinking was 5.4 for sigmoid colon without any significant association for proximal colon or rectum. These apparent discrepancies are not surprising, however, since several combinations of alcoholic beverages and cancer subsites were examined.

For rectal cancer, the RRs for alcohol consumption in eight cohort studies (Hakulinen et al. 1974, Dean et al. 1979, Jensen 1979, Pollack et al. 1984, Stemmermann et al. 1990, Wu et al. 1987, Klatsky et al. 1988, Carstensen et al. 1990) ranged from 1.0 to 2.5, and in most studies were between 1.0 and 1.7. Beer drinking was a specific concern for rectal cancer because of the findings in some correlation studies, and three cohorts of brewery workers are, therefore, of particular interest: they gave RRs of 1.0, 1.6 (significant), and 1.7 (significant).

Thus, the overall evidence from these eight cohort studies providing data on alcohol and colorectal cancer risk excludes an excess risk among alcohol drinkers of a factor 2 or more. Inclusion of seven smaller studies (International Agency for Research on Cancer 1988, Adami et al. 1992) did not modify this conclusion: a total of 133 cases were observed in seven studies versus 115 expected, giving a summary RR of 1.2. The total evidence, therefore, indicates a weak positive association. The information from cohort studies is not easy to interpret, however, since several studies were based on highly selected populations, and most of them permitted only limited (or no) allowance for major covariates. In this respect, data from case-control studies may be more informative.

Case-Control Studies

At least 18 case-control studies (Wynder and Shigematsu 1967, Williams and Horm, 1977, Tuyns et al. 1982, Manousos et al. 1983, Miller et al. 1983, Potter and McMichael 1986, Kabat et al. 1986, Kune et al. 1987, Tuyns 1988, Freudenheim et al. 1990, Longnecker 1990, Slattery et al. 1990, Kato et al. 1990, Hu et al. 1991, Choi and Kahyo 1991a, Riboli et al. 1991, Barra et al. 1992, Peters et al. 1992) based on 100 or more cases of colorectal cancer provided information on the potential relationship of alcohol drinking and large bowel cancer. Eight were hospital-based studies, and 10 used community or neighbourhood controls. The number of cases ranged from 100 to over 1400.

Eight studies were from North America, five from Europe, two from Australia, and one each from Japan, China, and Korea.

Among these, four studies were totally negative and showed no evidence of association between cancer at any of the large bowel sub-sites or sex strata with alcohol or any type of alcoholic beverage (Wynder and Shigematsu 1967, Tuyns et al. 1982, Manousos et al. 1983, Slattery et al. 1990). Three others showed overall statistically significant direct associations. Of two from North America, one showed an association for beer (Kabat et al. 1986) with rectal cancer (RR = 2.7 for the highest consumption level), and one (Freudenheim et al. 1990) showed an association for total alcohol consumption again only for rectal cancer, but with RR estimates below 2 in both sexes. A third study from China showed significant trends in risk both for colon and rectum cancer (Hu et al. 1991), but numbers of regular alcohol drinkers were small, leaving open the possibility of some selection mechanisms. The remaining 11 studies showed no consistent and significant overall association, but the RRs were elevated in some specific strata. Also, these apparent associations were of moderate strength, the RRs being generally below 2 for the highest levels of alcoholic beverage intake.

In most case-control studies, and in particular in the most recent ones, the results were adjusted for major covariates, specifically for indicators of socioeconomic status and, in several, for intake of selected foods or nutrients as well. Even after these adjustments, however, the inherent problem remains that diet in alcohol drinkers is probably different in several aspects (including higher fat and total calorie consumption) from that of nondrinkers (La Vecchia et al. 1992). Persisting confounding is therefore possible and may partly or largely explain a pattern of risk characterized by several moderate and inconsistent associations.

Beer drinking, particularly in relation to rectal cancer, was a specific issue in several studies. While some North American investigations (Kabat et al. 1986, Freudenheim et al. 1990, Longnecker 1990) and one Australian investigation (Kune et al. 1987) found elevated risks, these were not confirmed by studies from Europe, including one from Belgium (Tuyns 1988), where beer is the main alcoholic beverage. It may be, therefore, that different correlates of beer drinking in different populations may account for some of the elevated risks, rather than there being a carcinogenic effect of beer itself on the rectal epithelium.

Conclusion

The majority of cohort and case-control studies suggest a positive relationship between alcohol consumption and colorectal cancer. A formal meta-analysis of published data (Longnecker et al. 1990) led to an estimate of overall relative risk of 1.1 (95%, CI 1.05–1.14) for total alcohol drinking, which was consistent for males and females and for colon and rectum. The relationship is quantitatively moderate, and there is consensus that a twofold risk for both colon and rectum cancer can be excluded, even with high levels of alcohol consumption. There is also consensus that there is no appreciable and consistent difference in risk between the sexes, cancer sites (colon and rectum), and type of alcoholic beverage. Apparent discrepancies in the results of the various studies can be easily accounted for by random variation.

Despite the large amount of epidemiological research, including the provision of data for several thousand cases, no consensus has emerged on the interpretation of the observations. The issue remains open and continues to attract research interest: almost half of all case-control studies of the subject were published during the last 3 years alone.

It is possible that alcohol causes some small risk of colorectal cancer. While some obvious biases and sources of confounding can be excluded, it is conceivable that some differences in diet between drinkers and nondrinkers may account for the observed association. Moreover, a moderate association may be produced, at least in part, by the selective publication of positive results. Thus, the epidemiological evidence regarding a causal role for alcoholic beverage consumption in the production of colorectal cancer remains inconclusive.

Recommendation for Research

The principal uncertainty in the relationship between alcoholic beverages and cancers of the digestive tract and larynx is whether the observed weak association between their consumption and the development of cancers of the large bowel is causal or a secondary effect of the type of diet commonly associated with the consumption of relatively large amounts of alcohol. It is recommended that research aimed at discovering whether the association can be explained by confounding with dietary habits should be encouraged.

References

Acheson ED, Doll R (1964) Dietary factors in carcinoma of the stomach: study of 100 cases and 200 controls. Gut 5:126–31

Adami HO, McLaughlin JK, Hsing AW, et al. (1992) Alcoholism and cancer risk: a population-based cohort study. Cancer Causes Control 3:419–25

Adelstein A, White G (1976) Alcoholism and mortality. Popul Trends 6:7–13

Agudo A, Gonzalez CA, Marcos G, et al. (1992) Consumption of alcohol, coffee, and tobacco, and gastric cancer in Spain. Cancer Causes Control 3:137–43

Ammann RW, Muench R, Otto R, et al. (1988) Evolution and regression of pancreatic calcification in chronic pancreatitis. A prospective long-term study of 107 patients. Gastroenterology 95:1018–28

Andersen AA, Bjelke E, Langmark F (1989) Cancer in waiters. Br J Cancer 60:112–15

Armijo R, Orellana M, Medina E, et al. (1981) Epidemiology of gastric cancer in Chile I: case-control study. Int J Epidemiol 10:53–56

Baghurst PA, McMichael AJ, Slavotinek AH, et al. (1991) A case-control study of diet and cancer of the pancreas. Am J Epidemiol 134:167–79

Barra S, Franceschi S, Negri E, et al. (1990) Type of alcoholic beverage and cancer of the oral cavity, pharynx and oesophagus in an Italian area with high wine consumption. Int J Cancer 46:1017–20

Barra S, Negri E, Franceschi S, et al. (1992) Alcohol and colorectal cancer: a case-control study from northern Italy. Cancer Causes Control 3:153–59

Becker V (1978) Cancer of the pancreas and chronic pancreatitis, a possible relationship. Acta Hepatogastroenterol 25:257–59

Bennett DE, Sasser WF, Ferguson TB (1969) Adenocarcinoma of the lung in men. Cancer 23:431–39

Berenblum I (1944) Irritation and carcinogenesis. Arch Pathol 38:233–44

Bjelke E (1974) Epidemiological studies of cancer of the stomach, colon, and rectum; with special emphasis on the role of diet. Scand J Gastroenterol 9:1–235

Blackwelder WC, Yano K, Rhoads GG, et al. (1980) Alcohol and mortality: the Honolulu Heart Study. Am J Cancer 68:164–69

Blot WH, McLaughlin JK, Winn DM, et al. (1988) Smoking and drinking in relation to oral and pharyngeal cancer. Cancer Res 48:3282–87

Boeing H, Frentzel-Beyme R, Berger M, et al. (1991) Case-control study on stomach cancer in Germany. Int J Cancer 47:858–64

Boffeta P, Garfinkel L (1990) Alcohol drinking and mortality among men enrolled in an American Cancer Society prospective study. Epidemiology 1:342–48

Bouchardy C, Clavel F, La Vecchia C, et al. (1990) Alcohol, beer and cancer of the pancreas. Int J Cancer 45:842–46

Breslow NE, Day N (1980) Statistical methods in cancer research, vol. 1. The analysis of case-control studies. IARC Sci Publ 32, pp 227–33.

Breslow NE, Enstrom JE (1974) Geographical correlations between cancer mortality rates and alcohol-tobacco consumption in the United States. J Natl Cancer Inst 53:631–39

Brown LM, Blot WJ, Schuman SH, et al. (1988) Environmental factors and high risk of esophageal cancer among men in coastal South Carolina. J Natl Cancer Inst 90:1620–25

Brugère J, Guenel P, Leclerc A, Rodriguez J (1986) Differential effects of tobacco and alcohol in cancer of the larynx, pharynx, and mouth. Cancer 57:391–95

Bueno de Mesquita HB, Maisonneuve P, Moerman CJ, et al. (1992) Lifetime consumption of alcoholic beverages, tea and coffee and exocrine carcinoma of the pancreas: a population-based case-control study in The Netherlands. Int J Cancer 50:514–22

Buiatti E, Palli D, Decarli A, et al. (1989) A case-control study of gastric cancer and diet in Italy. Int J Cancer 44:611–16

Buiatti E, Palli D, Decarli A, et al. (1990) A case-control study of gastric cancer and diet in Italy: II. Association with nutrients. Int J Cancer 45:896–901

Burch GE, Ansari A (1968) Chronic alcoholism and carcinoma of the pancreas: a correlative hypothesis. Arch Intern Med 122:273–75

Burch JD, Howe GR, Miller AB, Semenciw R (1981) Tobacco, alcohol, asbestos, and nickel in the etiology of cancer of the larynx: a case-control study. J Natl Cancer Inst 67:1219–24

Burr ML, Holliday RM (1989) Fruit and stomach cancer. J Hum Nutr Diet 2:273–77

Carstensen JM, Bygren LO, Hatschek T (1990) Cancer incidence among Swedish brewery workers. Int J Cancer 45:393–96

Castonguay A, Rivenson A, Trushin N, et al. (1984) Effects of chronic ethanol consumption on the metabolism and carcinogenicity of N'-nitrosonornicotine in F344 rats. Cancer Res 44:2285–90

Choi SY, Kahyo H (1991a) Effect of cigarette smoking and alcohol consumption in the aetiology of cancers of the digestive tract. Int J Cancer 49:381–86

Choi SY, Kahyo H (1991b) Effect of cigarette smoking and alcohol consumption in the aetiology of cancer of the oral cavity, pharynx, and larynx. Int J Epidemiol 20:845–51

Clavel F, Benhamou E, Auquier A, et al. (1989) Coffee, alcohol, smoking and cancer of the pancreas: a case-control study. Int J Cancer 43:17–21

Correa P (1988) A human model of gastric carcinogenesis. Cancer Res 48:3554–60

Correa P, Fontham E, Pickle LW, et al. (1985) Dietary determinants of gastric cancer in south Louisiana inhabitants. J Natl Cancer Inst 75:645–54

Cuzick J, Babiker AG (1989) Pancreatic cancer, alcohol, diabetes mellitus and gall-bladder disease. Int J Cancer 43:415–21

Day NE (1975) Some aspects of the epidemiology of esophageal cancer. Cancer Res 35:3304–07

Dean G, MacLennan R, McLoughlin H, Shelley E (1979) Causes of death of blue-collar workers at a Dublin brewery. Br J Cancer 40:581–89

Decarli A, La Vecchia C (1986) Environmental factors and cancer mortality in Italy: correlational exercise. Oncology 43:116–26

Decarli A, Liati P, Negri E, et al. (1987) Vitamin A and other dietary factors in the etiology of esophageal cancer. Nutr Cancer 10:39–47

Demirer T, Icli F, Üzunalimoglu O, Kucuk O (1990) Diet and stomach cancer incidence: a case-control study in Turkey. Cancer 65:2344–48

De Stefani E, Correa P, Fierro L, et al. (1990a) Alcohol drinking and tobacco smoking in gastric cancer: A case-control study. Rev Epidemiol Sante Publique 38:297–307

De Stefani E, Muñoz N, Esteve J, et al. (1990b) Male drinking, alcohol, tobacco, diet, and esophageal cancer in Uruguay. Cancer Res 50:426–31

Dörken H (1964) Einige Daten bei 280 Patienten mit Pancreaskrebs. Gastroenterologia 102:47–77

Durbec JP, Chevillotte G, Bidart JM, et al. (1983) Diet, alcohol, tobacco, and risk of cancer of the pancreas: a case-control study. Br J Cancer 47:463–70

Elwood JM, Pearson JCG, Skippen DH, Jackson SM (1984) Alcohol, smoking, social and occupational factors in the aetiology of cancer of the oral cavity, pharynx, and larynx. Int J Cancer 34:603–12

Enstrom JE (1977) Colorectal cancer and beer drinking. Br J Cancer 35:674–83

Falk RT, Pickle LW, Brown LM, et al. (1990) Effect of smoking and alcohol consumption on laryngeal cancer risk in coastal Texas. Cancer Res 49:4024–29

Falk RT, Williams PL, Fontham ET, et al. (1988) Life-style risk factors for pancreatic cancer in Louisiana: a case-control study. Am J Epidemiol 128:324–36

Farrow DC, Davis S (1990) Risk of pancreatic cancer in relation to medical history and the use of tobacco, alcohol and coffee. Int J Cancer 45:816–20

Feron VJ, Woutersen RA (1989) Role of tissue damage in nasal carcinogenesis. Feron VJ, Bosland MC (eds), In Nasal carcinogenesis in rodents: relevance to human health risk. Proceedings of the TNO-CIVO/NYU Nose Symposium, Veldhoven, Netherlands, 24–28 October 1988. Pudoc, Wageningen, pp 76–84

Ferraroni M, Negri E, La Vecchia C, et al. (1989) Socioeconomic indicators, tobacco and alcohol in the aetiology of digestive tract neoplasms. Int J Epidemiol 18:556–62

Flaks BJ, Moore MA, Flaks A (1980) Ultrastructural analysis of pancreatic carcinogenesis. I. Morphological characterization of N-nitroso-bis(2-hydroxopropyl)amine-induced neoplasms in Syrian hamster. Carcinogenesis 1:423–38

Flaks BJ, Moore MA, Flaks A (1981) Ultrastructural analysis of pancreatic carcinogenesis. IV. Pseudoductular transformation of acini in the hamster pancreas during N-nitroso-bis(2-hydroxopropyl)amine carcinogenesis. Carcinogenesis 2:1241–53

Flamant R, Lasserre O, Lazar P, et al. (1964) Differences in sex ratio according with use of tobacco and alcohol. Review of 65,000 cases. J Natl Cancer Inst 32:1309–16

Franco EL, Kowalski LP, Oliveira BV, et al. (1989) Risk factors for oral cancer in Brazil: a case-control study. Int J Cancer 43:992–1000

Freudenheim JL, Graham S, Marshall JR, et al. (1990) Lifetime alcohol intake and risk of rectal cancer in Western New York. Nutr Cancer 13:101–9

Ghadirian P, Simard A, Baillargeon J (1991) Tobacco, alcohol, and coffee and cancer of the pancreas. Cancer 67:2664–70

Gibel W (1967) Experimental studies on syncarcinogenesis in oesophageal carcinoma (Ger.). Arch Geschwulstforsch 30:181–89

Gold EB, Gordis L, Diener MD, et al. (1985a) Diet and other risk factors for cancer of the pancreas. Cancer 44:460–67

Gold EB, Gordis L, Diener MD, et al. (1985b) Diet and other risk factors for cancer of the pancreas: a case-control study. Cancer 55:460–67

Gordon T, Kannel WB (1984) Drinking and mortality: the Framingham study. Am J Epidemiol 120:97–107

Graham S, Lilienfeld AM, Tidings JE (1967) Dietary and purgation factors in the epidemiology of gastric cancer. Cancer 20:2224–34

Graham S, Schotz W, Martino P (1972) Alimentary factors in the epidemiology of gastric cancer. Cancer 30:927–38

Grasso P (1987) Persistent organ damage and cancer production in rats and mice. Arch Toxicol 11:75–83

Gray JR, Coldman AJ, MacDonald WC (1992) Cigarette and alcohol use in patients with adenocarcinoma of the gastric cardia or lower esophagus. Cancer 69:2227–31

Griciuté L, Castegnaro M, Béréziat J-C (1982) Influence of ethyl alcohol on the carcinogenic activity of N-Nitrosodi-n-propylamine. In Bartsch H, Castegnaro M, O'Neill IK, Okada M (eds), N-nitroso compounds: occurrence and biological effects. IARC Sci Publ 41, pp 643–48

Griciuté L, Castegnaro M, Béréziat J-C (1984) Influence of ethyl alcohol on carcinogenesis induced with N-Nitrosodiethylamine. In Börzsönyi M,

Day NE, Lapis K, Yamasaki H (eds), Models, mechanisms and aetiology of tumour promotion. IARC Sci Publ 56, pp 413–17

Haas O, Guillard G, Rat P, et al. (1990) Pancreatic carcinoma developing in chronic pancreatitis: a report of four cases. Hepatogastroenterology 37:350–51

Haenszel W, Kurihara M, Locke FB, et al. (1976) Stomach cancer in Japan. J Natl Cancer Inst 56:265–78

Haenszel W, Kurihara M, Segi M, Lee RKC (1972) Stomach cancer among Japanese in Hawaii. J Natl Cancer Inst 49:969–88

Haines AP, Moss AR, Whittemore A, Quivey J (1982) A case-control study of pancreatic carcinoma. J Cancer Res Clin Oncol 103:93–97

Hakulinen T, Lehtimäki L, Lehtonen M, Teppo L (1974) Cancer morbidity among two male cohorts with increased alcohol consumption in Finland. J Natl Cancer Inst 52:1711–14

Hamilton SR, Sohn OS, Fiala ES (1987) Effects of timing and quantity of chronic dietary ethanol consumption on azoxymethane-induced colonic carcinogenesis and azoxymethane metabolism in Fischer 344 rats. Cancer Res 47:4305–11

Hamilton SR, Sohn OS, Fiala ES (1988) Inhibition by dietary ethanol of experimental colonic carcinogenesis induced by high-dose azoxymethane in F344 rats. Cancer Res 48:3313–18

Heuch I, Kvale G, Jacobsen BK, Bjelke E (1983) Use of alcohol, tobacco and coffee, and risk of pancreatic cancer. Br J Cancer 48:637–43

Hiatt RA, Klatsky AL, Armstrong MA (1988) Pancreatic cancer, blood glucose, and beverage consumption. Int J Cancer 41:794–97

Higginson J (1966) Etiological factors in gastrointestinal cancer in man. J Natl Cancer Inst 37:527–45

Hirayama T (1979) Diet and cancer. Nutr Cancer 1:67–81

Hirayama T (1981) A large-scale cohort study on the relationship between diet and selected cancers of digestive organs. In Bruce WR, Correa P, Lipkin M, et al. (eds), Gastrointestinal cancer: endogenous factors; Banbury Report 7. Cold Spring Harbor Laboratory, New York, pp 409–26

Hirayama T (1989) Association between alcohol consumption and cancer of the sigmoid colon: observations from a Japanese cohort study. Lancet 2:725–27

Hirayama T (1992) Life-style and cancer: from epidemiological evidence to public behaviour change to mortality reduction of target cancers. J Natl Cancer Inst 12:65–74

Hoey J, Montvernay C, Lambert R (1981) Wine and tobacco: risk factors for gastric cancer in France. Am J Epidemiol 113:668–74

Horie A, Kohchi S, Kuratsune M (1965) Carcinogenesis in the esophagus. II. Experimental production of esophageal cancer by administration of ethanolic solution of carcinogens. Gann 56:429–41

Hoshiyama Y, Sasaba T (1992) A case-control study of stomach cancer and its relation to diet, cigarettes, and alcohol consumption in Saitama Prefecture, Japan. Cancer Causes Control 3:441–48

Howarth AE, Pihl E (1985) High-fat diet promotes and causes distal shift of experimental rat colonic cancer—beer and alcohol do not. Nutr Cancer 6:229–35

Hu J, Liu Y, Yu Y, et al. (1991) Diet and cancer of the colon and rectum: a case-control study in China. Int J Epidemiol 20:362–67

Hu J, Zhang S, Jia E, et al. (1988) Diet and cancer of the stomach: a case-control study in China. Int J Cancer 41:331–35

International Agency for Research on Cancer (1988) Alcohol Drinking. IARC Monogr Eval Carcinog Risks Hum 44

Ishii K, Takeuchi T, Hirayama T (1973) Chronic calcifying pancreatitis and pancreatic carcinoma in Japan. Digestion 9:429–37

Jain M, Howe GR, St Louis P, Miller AB (1991) Coffee and alcohol as determinants of risk of pancreas cancer: a case-control study from Toronto. Int J Cancer 47:384–89

Jedrychowski W, Wahrendorf J, Popiela T, Rachtan J (1986) A case-control study of dietary factors and stomach cancer risks in Poland. Int J Cancer 37:837–42

Jensen OM (1979) Cancer morbidity and causes of death among Danish brewery workers. Int J Cancer 23:454–63

Jensen OM (1980) Cancer morbidity and causes of death among Danish brewery workers. International Agency for Research on Cancer, Lyon. From: IARC Monograph on the Evaluation of Carcinogenic Risks for Humans, Vol. 44. "Alcohol Drinking," IARC, Lyon, France, 1988, p. 216

Johnson JR, Zintel HA (1979) Pancreatic calcification and cancer of the pancreas. Surg Gyn Obst 117:585–88

Kabat GC, Howson CP, Wynder EL (1986) Beer consumption and rectal cancer. Int J Epidemiol 15:494–501

Kabat GC, Wynder EL (1989) Type of alcoholic beverage and oral cancer. Int J Cancer 43:190–94

Kato I, Tominaga S, Ito Y, et al. (1990) A comparative case-control analysis of stomach cancer and atrophic gastritis. Cancer Res 50:6559–64

Kato I, Tominaga S, Matsumoto K (1992) A prospective study of stomach cancer among a rural Japanese population: A 6-year survey. Jpn J Cancer Res 83:568–75

Kato I, Tominaga S, Matsuura A, et al. (1990) A comparative case-control study of colorectal cancer and adenoma. Jpn J Cancer Res 81:1101–08

Kerns WD, Pavkov KL, Donofrio DJ, et al. (1983) Carcinogenicity of formaldehyde in rats and mice after long-term inhalation exposure. Cancer Res 43:4382–92

Klatsky AL, Armstrong MA, Friedman GD, Hiatt RA (1988) The relations of alcoholic beverage use to colon and rectal cancer. Am J Epidemiol 128:1007–15

Klatsky AL, Friedman GD, Siegelaub AB (1981) Alcohol and mortality: a ten-year Kaiser-Permanente experience. Ann Intern Méd 95:139–45

Kneller RW, McLaughlin JK, Bjelke E, et al. (1991) A cohort study of stomach cancer in a high-risk American population. Cancer 68:672–78

Kodama T, Mori W (1983a) Morphological behaviour of carcinoma of the pancreas. I. Histological classification and electron microscopical observation. Acta Pathol Jpn 33:467–81

Kodama T, Mori W (1983b) Morphological lesions of the pancreatic ducts. Significance of pyloric gland metaplasia in carcinogenesis of exocrine and endocrine pancreas. Acta Pathol Jpn 33:645–60

Konishi N, Kitahori Y, Shimoyama T, et al. (1986) Effects of sodium chloride and alcohol on experimental esophageal carcinogenesis induced by n-nitrosopiperidine in rats. Jpn J Cancer Res (Gann) 77:446–51

Kono S, Ikeda M (1979) Correlation between cancer mortality and alcoholic beverage in Japan. Br J Cancer 40:449–55

Kono S, Ikeda M, Ogata M, et al. (1983) The relationship between alcohol and mortality among Japanese physicians. Int J Epidemiol 12:437–41

Kono S, Ikeda M, Tokudome S, Kuratsune M (1988) A case-control study of gastric cancer and diet in northern Kyushu, Japan. Jpn J Cancer Res 79:1067–74

Kono S, Ikeda M, Tokudome S, et al. (1986) Alcohol and mortality: a cohort study of male Japanese physicians. Int J Epidemiol 15:527–32

Kono S, Ikeda M, Tokudome S, Nishizumi M (1987) Cigarette smoking, alcohol and cancer mortality: a cohort study of male Japanese physicians. Jpn J Cancer Res 78:4656–58

Kune S, Kune GA, Watson LF (1987) Case-control study of alcoholic beverages as etiological factors: the Melbourne colorectal cancer study. Nutr Cancer 9:43–56

Lamy L (1910) Statistical clinical study of 134 cases of cancer of the oesophagus and cardia (Fr.). Arch Mal Appar Dig Mal Nutr 4:451–75

Laroye GJ (1974) How efficient is immunological surveillance against cancer and why does it fail? Lancet 1:1097–1100

La Vecchia C, Negri E (1989) The role of tobacco in oesophageal cancer in non-smokers and of tobacco in non-drinkers. Int J Cancer 43:784–85

La Vecchia C, Negri E, d'Avonzo B, et al. (1991) Dietary indicators of oral and pharyngeal cancer. Int J Epidemiol 20:39–44

La Vecchia C, Negri E, Franceschi S, et al. (1992) Differences in dietary intake with smoking, alcohol and education. Nutr Cancer 17:297–304

Lee HH, Wu HY, Chuang YC, et al. (1990) Epidemiologic characteristics and multiple risk factors of stomach cancer in Taiwan. Anticancer Res 10:875–82

Levison DA (1979) Carcinoma of the pancreas. J Pathol 129:203–23

Levitt MH, Harris CC, Squire R, et al. (1977) Experimental pancreatic carcinogenesis. I. Morphogenesis of pancreatic adenocarcinoma in the

Syrian golden hamster induced by N-nitroso-bis(2-hydroxypro-pyl)amine. Am J Pathol 88:5–28

Longnecker MP (1990) A case-control study of alcoholic beverage consumption in relation to risk of cancer of the right colon and rectum in men. Cancer Causes Control 1:5–14

Longnecker MP, Orza MJ, Adams ME, et al. (1990) A meta-analysis of alcoholic beverage consumption in relation to risk of colorectal cancer. Cancer Causes Control 1:59–68

Lyon JL, Egger MJ, Robison LM, et al. (1992) Misclassification of exposure in a case-control study: the effects of different types of exposure and different proxy respondents in a study of pancreatic cancer. Epidemiol 3:223–31

Mack TM, Yu MC, Hanisch R, Henderson BE (1986) Pancreas cancer and smoking, beverage consumption, and past medical history. J Natl Cancer Inst 76:49–60

MacMahon B, Yen S, Trichopoulos D, et al. (1981) Coffee and cancer of the pancreas. New Engl J Med 304:630–33

Manousos O, Day NE, Trichopoulos D, et al. (1983) Diet and colorectal cancer: a case-control study in Greece. Int J Cancer 32:1–5

Manousos O, Trichopoulos D, Koutseliinis A, et al. (1981) Epidemiologic characteristics and trace elements in pancreatic cancer in Greece. Cancer Det Prev 4:439–42

McLaughlin JK, Gridley G, Block G, et al. (1988) Dietary factors in oral and pharyngeal cancer. J Nat Cancer Inst 80:1237–43

McMichael AJ, Potter JD, Hetzel BS (1979) Time trends in colo-rectal cancer mortality in relation to food and alcohol consumption: United States, United Kingdom, Australia and New Zealand. Int J Epidemiol 8:295–303

Meijers M, Bruijntjes JP, Hendriksen EGJ, Woutersen RA (1989) Histogenesis of early preneoplastic lesions induced by N-nitrosobis(2-oxopropyl)amine in exocrine pancreas of hamsters. Int J Pancreatol 4:127–37

Merletti F, Boffeta P, Ciccone G, et al. (1989) Role of tobacco and alcoholic beverages in the etiology of cancer of the oral cavity/oropharynx in Torino, Italy. Cancer Res 49:4919–24

Mikal S, Campbell A (1950) Carcinoma of pancreas: diagnostic and operative criteria based on 100 consecutive autopsies. Surgery 28:961–69

Miller AB, Howe GR, Jain M, et al. (1983) Food items and food groups as risk factors in a case-control study of diet and colo-rectal cancer. Int J Cancer 32:155–61

Ministry of Agriculture, Fisheries and Food (1987) Nitrate, nitrite and N-nitroso compounds in food. Food surveillance paper 20, London, HMSO

Modan B, Lubin F, Barell B, et al. (1974) The role of starches in the etiology of gastric cancer. Cancer 34:2087–92

Monson RR, Lyon JL (1975) Proportional mortality among alcoholics. Cancer 36:1077–79

Morgan GGH, Wormsley KG (1977) Cancer of the pancreas. Gut 18:580–96

Mufti SI, Becker G, Sipes IG (1989) Effect of chronic dietary ethanol consumption on the initiation and promotion of chemically-induced esophageal carcinogenesis in experimental rats. Carcinogenesis 10:303–09

Muñoz N (1988) Descriptive epidemiology of gastric cancer. In Reed PI, Hill MJ (eds), Gastric Carcinogenesis. 51–69. Amsterdam, Excerpta Medica, pp 51–69

Nelson RL, Samelson SL (1985) Neither dietary ethanol nor beer augments experimental colon carcinogenesis in rats. Dis Colon Rectum 28:460–62

Norell SE, Ahlbom A, Erwald R, et al. (1986) Diet and pancreatic cancer: a case-control study. Am J Epidemiol 124:894–902

Olsen GW, Mandel JS, Gibson RW, et al. (1989) A case-control study of pancreatic cancer and cigarettes, alcohol, coffee and diet. Am J Public Health 79:1016–19

Palli D, Bianchi S, Decarli A, et al. (1992) A case-control study of cancers of the gastric cardia in Italy. Br J Cancer 65:263–66

Paulino-Netto A, Dreiling DA, Boronofsky ID (1960) The relationship between pancreatic calcification and cancer of the pancreas. Ann Surg 151:530–37

Peters RK, Pike MC, Garabrant D, Mack TM (1992) Diet and colon cancer in Los Angeles County, California. Cancer Causes Control 3:457–73

Pollack ES, Nomoura AMY, Lance K, et al. (1984) Prospective study of alcohol consumption and cancer. N Engl J Med 310:617–21

Potter JD, McMichael AJ (1986) Diet and cancer of the colon and rectum: a case-control study. J Natl Cancer Inst 76:557–69

Pottern LM, Morris LE, Blot WJ, et al. (1981) Esophageal cancer among black men in Washington DC: Alcohol, tobacco, and other risk factors. J Natl Cancer Inst 71:1085–87

Pour PM (1984) Histogenesis of exocrine pancreatic cancer in the hamster model. Environ Health Perspect 56:229–43

Pour PM (1988) Mechanism of pseudoductular (tubular) formation during pancreatic carcinogenesis in the hamster model. An electron-microscopic and immuno-histochemical study. Am J Pathol 130:335–44

Pour PM, Reber HA, Stepan K (1983) Modification of pancreatic carcinogenesis in the hamster model. XII. Dose-related effect of ethanol. J Natl Cancer Inst 71:1085–87

Raymond L, Infante F, Tuyns AJ, et al. (1987) Diet and pancreatic cancer (Fr.). Gastroenterol Clin Biol 11:488–92

Riboli E, Cornée J, Macquart-Moulin G, et al. (1991) Cancer and polyps of the colorectum and lifetime consumption of beer and other alcoholic beverages. Am J Epidemiol 133:157–66

Risch HA, Jain M, Choi NW, et al. (1985) Dietary factors and the incidence of cancer of the stomach. Am J Epidemiol 122:947–59

Robinette CD, Hrubec Z, Fraumeni Jr, JF (1979) Chronic alcoholism and subsequent mortality in World War II veterans. Am J Epidemiol 109:687–700

Rothman K, Keller R (1972) The effect of joint exposure of alcohol and tobacco on risk of cancer of the mouth and pharynx. J Chron Dis 25:711–16

Sankaranarayanan R, Duffy SW, Nair MK, et al. (1990) Tobacco and alcohol as risk factors in cancer of the larynx in Kerala, India. Int J Cancer 45:879–82

Sankaranarayanan R, Duffy SW, Padmakumary G, et al. (1991) Risk factors for cancer of the oesophagus in Kerala, India. Int J Cancer 49:485–89

Sarles H, Figarella C, Tiscornia O, et al. (1980) Chronic calcifying pancreatitis (CCP). Mechanism of formation of the lesions. New data and critical study. In Fitzgerald PJ, Morrison AB, (eds), The pancreas. Williams and Wilkins, Baltimore, pp 48–66

Sarles H, Lebreuil G, Tasso F, et al. (1971) A comparison of alcoholic pancreatitis in rat and man. Gut 12:377–88

Sarles H, Tiscornia O (1974) Ethanol and chronic calcifying pancreatitis. Med Clin North Am 58:1333–46

Schmidt W, Popham RE (1981) The role of drinking and smoking in mortality from cancer and other causes in male alcoholics. Cancer 47:1031–41

Seitz HK, Czygan P, Waldherr R, et al. (1984) Enhancement of 1,2-dimethylhydrazine-induced rectal carcinogenesis following chronic ethanol consumption in the rat. Gastroenterology 86:886–91

Singh M (1986) Ethanol and the pancreas. In Go VLW, et al.(eds), The exocrine pancreas: biology, pathobiology, and disease. Raven Press, New York, pp 423–37

Singh M, Simsek H (1990) Ethanol and the pancreas: current status. Gastroenterology 98:1051–62

Slattery ML, West DW, Robison LM, et al. (1990) Tobacco, alcohol, coffee, and caffeine as risk factors for colon cancer in a low-risk population. Epidemiology 1:141–45

Stemmermann GN, Nomura AMY, Chyou PH, Yoshizawa C (1990) Prospective study of alcohol intake and large bowel cancer. Dig Dis Sci 35:1414–20

Stocks P (1957) Cancer in North Wales and Liverpool regions. In Thirty-Fifth annual report: supplement to part II London, British Empire Cancer Campaign, pp 51–113

Sundby P (1967) Alcoholism and mortality. Universitetsforlaget, Oslo

Tajima K, Tominaga S (1985) Dietary habits and gastro-intestinal cancers:

a comparative case-control study of stomach and large intestinal cancers in Nagoya, Japan. Jpn J Cancer Res 76:705–16

Takahashi M, Arai H, Kokubo T, et al. (1980) An ultrastructural study of precancerous and cancerous lesions of the pancreas in Syrian golden hamsters induced by N-nitroso-bis(2-oxopropyl)amine. Gann 71:825–31

Takahashi M, Hasegawa R, Furukawa F, et al. (1986) Effects of ethanol, potassium metabisulfite, formaldehyde and hydrogen peroxide on gastric carcinogenesis in rats after initiation with n-methyl-N'-nitro-N-nitrosoguanidine. Jpn J Cancer Res (Gann) 77:118–24

Talamini R, Franceschi S, Barra S, La Vecchia C (1990) The role of alcohol in oral and pharyngeal cancer in non-smokers and non-drinkers. Int J Cancer 46:391–93

Taylor KB (1987) Gastritis. In Weatherall DG, Ledingham JGG, Worrall, DA (eds), Oxford Textbook of Medicine, 2nd ed 12. Oxford University Press, 77–12.86.

Tominaga K, Koyama Y, Sasagawa M, et al. (1991) A case-control study of stomach cancer and its genesis in relation to alcohol consumption, smoking, and familial cancer history. Jpn J Cancer Res 82:974–79

Trichopoulos D, Ouranos G, Day NE, et al. (1985) Diet and cancer of the stomach: a case-control study in Greece. Int J Cancer 36:291–97

Tuyns AJ (1983a) Oesophageal cancer in non-smoking drinkers and in non-drinking smokers. Int J Cancer 32:443–44

Tuyns AJ (1983b) Protective effects of citrus fruit on esophageal cancer. Nutr Cancer 5:195–200

Tuyns AJ (1988) Beer consumption and rectal cancer. Rev Epidemiol Sante Publique 36:144–45

Tuyns AJ, Estève J, Raymond L, et al. (1988) Cancer of the larynx/hypolarynx, tobacco and alcohol. IARC International case-control study in Turin and Varese (Italy), Zaragoza and Navarra (Spain), Geneva (Switzerland) and Calvados (France). Int J Cancer 41:483–91

Tuyns AJ, Kaaks R, Haelterman M, Riboli E (1992) Diet and gastric cancer. A case-control study in Belgium. Int J Cancer 51:1–6

Tuyns AJ, Pequignot G, Abbatucci JS (1979) Oesophageal cancer and alcohol consumption: importance of type of beverage. Int J Cancer 23:443–47

Tuyns AJ, Pequignot G, Gignoux M, Valla A (1982) Cancers of the digestive tract, alcohol and tobacco. Int J Cancer 30:9–11

Tuyns AJ, Pequignot G, Jensen OM (1977) Les cancers de l'oesophage en Ille-et-Villaine en fonction des niveaux de consommation d'alcool et de tabac, Des risques qui se multiplient. Bull Cancer 64:45–60

Tuyns AJ, Riboli E, Doornbus G, Pequinot G (1987) Diet and esophageal cancer in Calvados (France). Nutr Cancer 9:81–92

Tweedie JH, Reber H, Pour PM, Ponder DM (1981) Protective effect of ethanol on the development of pancreatic cancer. Surg Forum 32:222–24

Unakami M, Hara M, Fukuchi S, Akiyama H (1989) Cancer of the gastric cardia and the habit of smoking. Jpn Soc Pathol 39:420–24

Williams RR, Horm JW (1977) Association of cancer sites with tobacco and alcohol consumption and socioeconomic status of patients: interview study from the Third National Cancer Survey. J Natl Cancer Inst 58:525–47

Winn DM, Blot WJ, McLaughlin JK, et al. (1991) Mouthwash use and oral conditions in the risk of oral and pharyngeal cancer. Cancer Res 51:3041–47

Winn DM, Ziegler RG, Pickle LW, et al. (1984) Diet in the etiology of oral and pharyngeal cancer among women from the Southern United States. Cancer Res 44:1216–22

Woutersen RA, Appelman LM, Wilmer JWGM, et al. (1986a) Inhalation toxicity of acetaldehyde in rats. III. Carcinogenicity study. Toxicology 41:213–31

Woutersen RA, Garderen-Hoetmer A van, Bax J, et al. (1986b) Modulation of putative preneoplastic foci in exocrine pancreas of rats and hamsters. I. Interaction of dietary fat and ethanol. Carcinogenesis 7:1587–93

Woutersen RA, Garderen-Hoetmer A van, Bax J, Scherer E (1989) Modulation of dietary fat-promoted pancreatic carcinogenesis in rats and hamsters by chronic ethanol ingestion. Carcinogenesis 10:453–59

Wu AH, Paganini-Hill A, Ross RK, Henderson BE (1987) Alcohol, physical activity and other risk factors for colorectal cancer: a prospective study. Br J Cancer 55:687–94

Wu-Williams AH, Yu MC, Mack TM (1990) Life-style, workplace, and stomach cancer by subsite in young men of Los Angeles County. Cancer Res 50:2569–76

Wynder EL (1975) An epidemiologic evaluation of the causes of cancer of the pancreas. Cancer Res 35:2228–33

Wynder EL, Bross IJ (1961) A study of etiological factors in cancer of the esophagus. Cancer 14:389–413

Wynder EL, Bross IJ, Day E (1956) A study of environmental factors in cancer of the larynx. Cancer 9:86–110

Wynder EL, Bross IJ, Feldman RM (1957a) A study of etiological factors in cancer of the mouth. Cancer 10:1300–1323

Wynder EL, Hall NEL, Polansky M (1983) Epidemiology of coffee and pancreatic cancer. Cancer Res 43:3900–3906

Wynder EL, Hultberg S, Jacobsen E, Bross IJ (1957b) Environmental factors in cancer of upper alimentary tract: Swedish study with special reference to Plummer-Vinson (Paterson-Kelly) syndrome. Cancer 10:470–87

Wynder EL, Kmet J, Dungal N, Segi M (1963) Epidemiological investigation of gastric cancer. Cancer 15:1461–96

Wynder EL, Mabuchi K, Maruchi N, Fortner JG (1973) A case-control study of cancer of the pancreas. Cancer 31:641–48

Wynder EL, Shigematsu T (1967) Environmental factors of cancer of the colon and rectum. Cancer 20:1520–63

You WC, Blot WJ, Chang YS, et al. (1988) Diet and high risk of stomach cancer in Shandong, China. Cancer Res 48:3518–23

Young M, Russell WT (1926) An investigation into the statistics of cancer in different trades and professions. Medical Research Council, special report series, London, HMSO 99

Yu GP, Hsieh CC (1991) Risk factors for stomach cancer: population-based case-control study in Shanghai. Cancer Causes and Control 2:169–74

Zatonski W, Becher H, Lissowska J, Wahrendorf J (1991) Tobacco, alcohol, and diet in the etiology of laryngeal cancer: a population-based case-control study. Cancer Causes Control 2:3–10

Zheng T, Boyle P, Hu H, et al. (1990) Tobacco smoking, alcohol consumption and risk of oral cancer: a case-control study in Beijing, People's Republic of China. Cancer Causes Control 1:173–79

Ziegler RG, Morris LE, Blot WJ, et al. (1981) Esophageal cancer among black men in Washington DC. II. Role of nutrition. J Natl Cancer Inst 67:1199–06

6

Alcohol and Liver Diseases

J. Rodés
Hospital Clinico i Provincial,
University of Barcelona, Spain

M. Salaspuro
University of Helsinki, Finland

T.I.A. Sorensen
Copenhagen Health Services, Denmark

Abstract

It is well established that excess alcohol consumption in man is associated with increased risk of developing liver disease. However, the pathogenesis of alcoholic liver injury is not well understood. At present, many questions still remain unanswered. In this report, an analysis of the knowledge on the effects of excess alcohol ingestion on the liver is made. For this purpose a critical review of the mechanisms involved in alcoholic liver damage, the clinical manifestations and pathology of alcoholic liver disease, the epidemiology of chronic alcoholism and liver disease, and a list of the associations between liver disease and chronic consumption of alcohol is performed.

At present there is strong evidence for the relation of the pathogenesis of alcohol-related liver damage to the direct toxicity of ethanol, its metabolism and, metabolites, obtained from experiments done with animal models. However, it is important to take into account that in these models the calories as ethanol vary from 30–50% of total calories. Therefore, nutritional deficiencies as major pathogenetic factors cannot be excluded in the development of liver injury.

The liver plays a dominant role in the metabolism of ethanol, with its main pathway for oxidation being alcohol dehydrogenase activity (ADH). By the action of ADH, ethanol is transformed to acetaldehyde, which in turn is rapidly oxidized in the liver to acetate by the action of aldehyde dehydrogenase. Acetaldehyde is a very potent and reactive compound, and it has been suggested that it is one of the major factors in the pathogenesis of alcoholic liver disease.

Excessive alcohol ingestion produces the development of hepatic steatosis. A key mechanism in the genesis of fatty liver is due to the ethanol-induced change in the redox state of the liver. It has also been suggested that excessive alcohol intake may produce liver damage by other mechanisms such as promotion of lipid peroxidation and toxicity associated with an activation of the microsomal ethanol-oxidizing system. Although there is some evidence that both mechanisms may play a role in the development of alcoholic liver injury, further studies are required to reach definitive consensus. Finally, nutritional factors have also been implicated in association with excessive alcohol ingestion; however, the data obtained until now are not sufficient to establish a critical role for nutritional factors.

It is considered that chronic alcoholics may exhibit a wide spectrum of hepatic lesions, the most frequent being fatty liver, alcoholic hepatitis, and hepatic cirrhosis. The deposition of fat in the hepatocytes is very frequent (90% of the cases) among chronic alcoholics. The deposition of a single large lipid droplet in hepatocytes is the histological lesion defining alcoholic fatty liver. A microvesicular form may also be observed, although less frequently. Chronic alcoholics may also develop an increase of collagen content, particularly in the perivenular area (perivenular fibrosis), and the association with steatosis (steatofibrosis) is relatively frequent. Alcoholic hepatitis is the most characteristic hepatic lesion found in heavy drinkers. This lesion is characterized by hepatocellular necrosis associated with an inflammatory cell infiltrate constituted by neutrophils and in many cases with Mallory bodies. The clinical picture starts with fatigue, anorexia, nausea, and vomiting. A few days later, abdominal pain, jaundice, and fever appear. Tender hepatomegaly may be detected. Biochemical tests reveal a moderate increase in transaminases; gammaglutamyl transpeptidase is very high and may be associated with hyperbilirubinemia and high alkaline phosphatase. It has recently been reported that chronic alcoholism may produce chronic hepatitis; however, it is possible that this lesion among alcoholics may be due to viral infection (hepatitis C virus). The prevalence of hepatic cirrhosis in chronic alcoholics varies from study to study and is usually the micronodular type. The clinical manifestations are identical to those observed in hepatic cirrhosis of other etiologies. It is important to point out that abstinence will reverse, improve, or delay progression of alcohol liver disease, depending on the stage of the lesion indicating that, in fact, alcohol in these cases is responsible for liver damage.

It is considered that chronic alcoholism presently constitutes a significant public health problem. The incidence of alcoholic cirrhosis has recently been estimated at 190 per million person-years in Danish males and 85 in Danish females, with the age-specific incidence rates peaking at 50–60 years. Similar results have been found in the United Kingdom and the United States. The gender difference in incidence of alcoholic liver disease may be due to the greater frequency of heavy drinkers among males, but it has also been suggested that females are more sensitive to develop liver injury due to chronic alcohol ingestion. Further prospective control studies are required to obtain a full consensus. The average duration of excessive alcohol ingestion until diagnosis of alcoholic cirrhosis may be between 10 and 20 years. Among excessive drinkers, the rate of development of cirrhosis may be at about 2–3% per year, and, accordingly, the prevalence of cirrhosis is greater the longer the duration of excessive alcohol consumption.

A large number of aggregate population studies have assessed the changes over time within populations and the differences between populations in mortality from cirrhosis in relation to total per-capita consumption of alcohol. These studies have shown very high correlations between mortality from cirrhosis and consumption. However, despite the strikingly high correlation, the risk function for development of cirrhosis cannot be clearly derived from these relationships. Several retrospective case-control studies have been conducted showing that the probability of becoming a hospitalized cirrhotic patient increases exponentially with increased daily alcohol consumption ranging from 20–160 g. However, the interpretation of these studies in terms of risk function for development of cirrhosis is very difficult. On the other hand, other retrospective, cross-sectional studies have been performed in which the study population was defined as alcoholics. One of these studies defined a threshold for cumulated consumption, below which there seemed to be no risk of cirrhosis (the theoretical amount of 1 g of alcohol/day/kg body weight during 15 years). The interpretation of these results, in terms of the risk function for cirrhosis, is also very difficult.

Five prospective studies of general populations have assessed the relationship between daily consumption reported at the start of the study and subsequent cirrhosis mortality during long-term follow-up. It was found that the risk increased steadily by increasing daily consumption. In one study it was found that the development of cirrhosis after 10–15 years with a minimum consumption of 50 g/day was about 2% per year. This study also showed that individuals drinking intermittently had a lower risk of liver damage. The studies performed so far do not allow a consensus about a precise threshold of safe alcohol consumption below which there is no risk of development of cirrhosis. On the other hand, there may be a levelling off of the risk at about 2–3% per year by increasing consumption above approximately 70 g/day.

There is firm consensus about the association between chronic alcohol consumption and the development of fatty liver, perivenular fibrosis, acute alcoholic hepatitis, and hepatic cirrhosis. This consensus implies that the probability of developing these conditions is higher in individuals who, for a period of time, have had a daily excessive consumption of alcohol. This is based on vast clinical experience and numerous systematic studies. In addition, the frequency of death attributed to liver disease in the general population is correlated across time and place with measures of the total consumption of alcohol by these populations. Whereas the consensus about the qualitative association between excessive alcohol consumption and the development of the above-mentioned hepatic lesions is well established, there is much uncertainly about the dose-effect relationship.

The fact that only a minor proportion of individuals consuming excessive amounts of alcohol develop the most severe forms of liver damage, cirrhosis in particular, indicates that other causal factors are involved. Despite years of research, no consensus has been achieved on any one such factor. Current research focuses on genetic factors, viral infections, and specific nutritional disturbances.

Mechanism of Liver Disease Induced by Chronic Alcoholism: General Overview

In the late 1940s the pathogenesis of alcoholic liver injury was assumed to be associated almost exclusively with a secondary protein and choline deficiency (Best et al. 1949). Since then, strong evidence has accumulated for the relation of the pathogenesis of alcohol-related liver damage to the direct toxicity of ethanol, its metabolism, and its metabolites (Lieber 1988b, 1991b, Lieber and DeCarli 1991, Lieber and Salaspuro 1992, French 1989, Salaspuro 1989, 1991). However, many questions still remain unanswered. Why do only a proportion of heavy drinkers or alcoholics develop liver injury? What is the basic mechanism behind the "cell death" caused by alcohol? What is the most important toxic factor: ethanol, its metabolism, or its metabolites? Can we indeed entirely exclude nutritional deficiency in the pathogenesis of alcoholic liver injury? During the past few decades, the pathways and principles of ethanol oxidation in the liver and other tissues have been extensively characterized. Numerous reviews and books cover epidemiological (Grant et al. 1988, Hall 1985a, Lelbach 1976, Paton 1988, Schmidt 1977, Sörensen 1989), metabolic, etiopathological (Agarwal and Goedde 1989, Bird and Williams 1988, French 1989, Goedde and Agarwal 1989, Hall 1985a, Israel and Orrego 1981, Lieber 1977a,b, 1984, 1988a,b, 1991a,b,c, 1992, Lieber and Salaspuro 1992, Mezey 1989, 1991, Salaspuro 1989, 1991, Seitz and Kommerell 1985), as well as clinical aspects of alcoholic liver disease (Burnett and Sorrell 1981, Diehl 1989, Fisher and Rankin 1977, Hall 1985a, Morgan 1981, 1991, Saunders 1989, Wallgren and Barry 1970). On the basis of expanding information, many hypotheses regarding the pathogenesis of alcoholic liver injury have been presented, but so far none of these many theories has gained general acceptance or solid scientific basis.

Animal Models of Alcohol-Related Organ Damage

A lot of evidence supporting the direct hepatotoxicity of ethanol has been obtained from experiments done with animal models of alcohol-induced organ damage (Salaspuro and Lieber 1980, Israel et al. 1984, Lieber and DeCarli 1986, 1991). One of the major advances has been the introduction of a technique of feeding ethanol to rats as a part of nutritionally adequate totally liquid diet (Lieber et al. 1965). However, even with the "liquid diet model," the rat will not consume more than 36% of total calories as ethanol. Consequently, liver lesions more advanced than fatty liver cannot be produced by "Lieber-DeCarli diet" in rats.

More advanced alcoholic liver disease has been produced in baboons by applying a liquid-diet feeding technique to this animal (Lieber and DeCarli 1974). The alcohol intake of baboons can be increased to 50% of total calories. Furthermore, the primates are phylogenetically close to man, and their lifespan is long enough for the development of cirrhosis to occur. In this animal model, the biochemical and morphological alterations in the liver (even liver cirrhosis) are comparable to those seen in humans, despite the fact that a complete histological spectrum of alcoholic hepatitis as seen in man has not been produced in baboons (Popper and Lieber 1980). However, the opinions vary greatly with regard to the respective roles of alcohol and/or nutritional deficiencies as major pathogenetic factors behind the liver injury of this animal model. Nevertheless, the establishment of the animal models of alcoholic liver injury has had its greatest contribution in the improved understanding of the multifactorial biochemical alterations produced in the liver during chronic feeding of alcohol.

Role of the Liver in the Metabolism of Ethanol

The importance of the liver in the elimination of ethanol was established in several studies in the 1930s (Chapheau 1934, Fiessinger et al. 1936, Mirsky and Nelson 1939), and subsequently the incomplete hepatic oxidation of ethanol to acetate was also demonstrated (Lundsgaard 1938, Leloir and Munoz 1938). Though the liver plays a dominant role in the metabolism of ethanol, other tissues such as the kidney (Leloir and Munoz 1938), the stomach (Carter and Isselbacher 1971), the intestine (Lamboeuf et al. 1981), and bone marrow cells (Bond and Wickramasinghe 1983) have also been shown to oxidize ethanol to a small extent. More recently, diminished gastric alcohol dehydrogenase (ADH) activity in females has been related to higher susceptibility to ethanol (DiPadova et al. 1988), but the magnitude and importance of the gastric metabolism of ethanol is still largely unknown.

Pathways of Ethanol Oxidation

ADH-mediated oxidation of ethanol to acetaldehyde represents the main pathway for ethanol oxidation. During the last two decades, the multiple molecular forms and characteristics of ADH have been established (Agarwal and Goedde 1989, Yoshida et al. 1991). Various ADH forms appear in different frequencies in different racial populations, which explains, at least in part, individual variations in the rate of ethanol elimination (Martin et al. 1985, Bosron et al. 1988). These have been related to the production of acetaldehyde and to the extent of the first-pass elimination of ethanol (von Wartburg and Bühler 1984). A possible relationship between ADH genotype and the susceptibility to alcoholism or alcohol-related organ injury, however, remains to be established.

Pathways of Acetaldehyde Oxidation

Over 90% of the acetaldehyde formed from ethanol is rapidly oxidized in the liver to acetate by aldehyde dehydrogenase (ALDH). Two major ALDH-isoenzymes exist in humans (Goedde and Agarwal 1989). Interestingly, the mitochondrial isoenzyme (ALDHI) has been found to be missing in about 50% of the Oriental population (Goedde et al. 1979, Agarwal et al. 1981). This loss of enzyme activity is due to a change of one amino acid in the enzyme molecule (Hsu et al. 1985, Yoshida et al. 1991). The deficiency of ALDHI in Orientals results in marked elevations of blood acetaldehyde concentrations following alcohol ingestion (Mizoi et al. 1979). These individuals then develop facial flushing and tachycardia as a direct consequence of acetaldehyde-induced catecholamine release (Ijiri 1974, Inoue et al. 1980). Accordingly, homozygotic Japanese with the atypical ALDHI allele are at a much lower risk of developing the alcoholic liver diseases than those with homozygotic-Caucasian ALDHI (Shibuya and Yoshida 1988).

Microsomal Ethanol-Oxidizing System

The existence of a distinct and adaptive microsomal ethanol-oxidizing system (MEOS) is, after two decades of lively debate, generally accepted (Lieber and DeCarli 1968, 1970a, Lieber 1988b, Lieber and Salaspuro 1992). Chronic ethanol consumption results in the induction of a unique cytochrome P450 that has been designated to P450IIE1 (Ohnishi and Lieber 1977, Lieber et al. 1988, Nebert et al. 1987). In addition to its role in ethanol metabolism, MEOS may have significant consequences for the pathogenesis of liver injury, either directly (through the production of active and potentially toxic acetaldehyde) or indirectly (through the microsomal activation of other xenobiotics).

Alterations in Metabolism of Ethanol and Acetaldehyde During Chronic Alcohol Consumption

Most studies show that chronic alcohol consumption enhances ethanol clearance, except in the presence of significant liver damage or severe food restriction. The biochemical background for the enhanced clearance is still the subject of debate and has variably been attributed to increased ADH activity (Hawkins et al. 1966), to increased mitochondrial reoxidation of NADH (Videla and Israel 1970), to a hypermetabolic state in the liver (Israel et al. 1975), to increased MEOS (Lieber and DeCarli 1970a, Alderman et al. 1989), and to catalase (Handler et al. 1987, 1988a,b). The theory on the hypermetabolic state of the liver produced by chronic alcohol consumption has been assumed to produce alcoholic liver injury via hypoxia-induced liver damage in the centrilobular area, and treatment by propylthiouracil has been suggested (Orrego et al. 1987).

Acetaldehyde is both pharmacologically and chemically a very potent and reactive compound, and accordingly it has been suggested as one of the major initiating factors in the pathogenesis of alcoholic liver damage (Salaspuro and Lindros 1985, Lieber 1988a,b, 1991b, Lauterburg and Bilzer 1988). Enhanced hepatic oxidation of ethanol associated with chronic alcohol consumption may lead to both increased blood and tissue acetaldehyde concentrations (Lindros et al. 1980). This may be further potentiated by a reduction in the capacity of mitochondria to oxidize acetaldehyde, at least in rats (Hasumura et al. 1975). In addition, hepatic aldehyde dehydrogenase activity has been shown to be decreased in chronic alcoholics as compared to nonalcoholic controls (Nuutinen et al. 1983).

Pathogenesis of Alcoholic Liver Injury: Specific Associations

Animal Models of Alcohol-Related Organ Damage

As previously stated, one of the major advances in the research on the pathogenesis of alcoholic liver injury has been the introduction of a technique of feeding ethanol to rats as a part of a nutritionally adequate totally liquid diet (Lieber et al. 1965, 1967, Salaspuro and Lieber 1980, Israel et al. 1984, Lieber and DeCarli 1986, 1991). With the Lieber-DeCarli diet, which in addition to ethanol (36% of total calories) contains rather large amounts of fat (35–43%), it is possible to produce fatty liver in rats (Lieber et al. 1965). However, if the fat content of the ethanol-containing liquid diet is decreased from 32 to 25%, hepatic triglyceride accumulation significantly decreases (Lieber and DeCarli 1970b). Accordingly, other authors have questioned the direct hepatotoxicity of ethanol in this animal model and have attributed the pathologic liver changes to nutritional factors (such as dietary proportions of protein, fat, and carbohydrate or lipotropic deficiency) rather than to ethanol itself (Porta et al. 1965, 1967, Patek et al. 1976, Barak and Beckenhauer 1988, Derr et al. 1990).

Severe and progressive steatosis with focal necrosis has been produced in rats by continuous intragastric infusion of ethanol and nutritionally defined low-fat liquid diet (Tsukamoto et al. 1986, French et al. 1986). Furthermore, this damage is potentiated with the development of early hepatic fibrosis by increasing the fat content of the diet to 25% of calories (Tsukamoto et al. 1986). In this animal model, the severity of alcohol-induced liver injury appeared to be related to high blood alcohol levels. Feeding an ethanol-containing liquid diet together with a small dose of 4-methylpyrazole (ADH-inhibitor) to rats potentiates alcoholic liver injury in this animal model (Lindros et al. 1983). By following blood alcohol levels, this effect could be related to uninterrupted and prolonged presence of alcohol in the animal. Alcohol feeding to rats subjected to jejunoileal bypass leads to marked liver injury, which mimics that of alcohol-induced liver disease in man but without zonal distribution (Bode et al. 1987).

With regard to rats as an animal model of alcoholic liver injury, two major conclusions can be drawn: (1) the Lieber-DeCarli diet has been accepted as a standard in the studies on alcoholic fatty liver in rats, but the degree of hepatic fatty infiltration in this animal model may be modified by dietary factors such as the fat and lipotropic

content of the diet; and (2) continuous intragastric infusion of ethanol and nutritionally-defined low-fat liquid diet to rats is a promising new experimental model of alcoholic liver injury. After confirmation in other laboratories, the use of this animal model should be
encouraged.

By feeding a totally liquid diet containing 50% of calories as ethanol, Lieber and co-workers have been able to produce significant hepatic fibrosis or cirrhosis in about one-third of baboons (Lieber and
DeCarli 1974, 1991). In this animal model, hepatitis is unusual and is
not necessary for the development of fibrosis and cirrhosis (Popper
and Lieber 1980). However, some other groups have not been able to
produce significant hepatic fibrosis or cirrhosis in primates, given large
amounts of ethanol and adequate diet up to 5 years (Rogers et al.
1981, Mezey et al. 1980, 1983, Ainley et al. 1988). The discrepancies in
these results have been attributed to the higher nutrient value of the
diet in the latter studies (Ainley et al. 1988) or to the much smaller
number of animals used by others as compared to Lieber and co-
workers (Lieber and DeCarli 1991).

It can be concluded that a consensus does not exist with respect
to the major pathogenetic factor (direct effect of ethanol or nutritional deficiency) behind the fibrosis and cirrhosis produced in baboons by the Lieber-DeCarli diet. Further studies on the topic are
warranted.

Hepatotoxic Factors Associated With Ethanol and its Oxidation

Toxicity of Ethanol to Liver Membranes

Hepatocytes isolated from ethanol-fed animals exhibit pronounced morphological alterations of their plasma membranes on scanning electron microscopy (Yamada et al. 1985). Ethanol directly "flu-
idizes" membrane lipid bilayers, and it has been proposed that
during chronic alcohol consumption, cell surface membranes may re-
sist this effect of ethanol (i.e., "adapt") by changing their membrane
lipid composition. Chronic ethanol feeding, however, has been shown
to increase—even when ethanol is not present—the fluidity of liver
plasma membranes of rats (Yamada et al. 1985), mice (Zysset et al.
1985), and in cell cultures (Polokoff et al. 1985). The membrane alterations are associated with a decrease in membrane vitamin A and an
increase in the cholesterol ester content (Kim et al. 1988).

Changes in the enzyme activities of liver plasma membrane include a decrease in cytochrome a and b, succinic dehydrogenase, cy-

tochrome oxidase, as well as in the total respiratory capacity of the mitochondria (Taraschi and Rubin 1985). Furthermore, chronic alcohol consumption potentiates the release of alkaline phosphatase from the liver plasma membranes (Yamada et al. 1985) and produces changes in the oligosaccharide chains of plasma membrane glycoproteins (Metcalf et al. 1987).

It can be concluded that ethanol may have direct effects on liver plasma membranes. However, the exact biochemical mechanisms behind the phenomenon are unknown, and the possible associations with the pathogenesis of alcoholic liver injury are still hypothetical.

Alcoholic Fatty Liver

Interactions of ethanol with lipids are multiple and complex (Lieber and Savolainen 1984, Lieber and Pignon 1989). Fatty liver can be produced by either acute or chronic administration of alcohol both in laboratory animals and man and is potentiated by increased fat content of the diet (Lieber and DeCarli 1970b, French et al. 1986).

Lipids accumulating in the liver may originate from dietary lipids or adipose tissue. Alcohol may increase peripheral fat mobilization, enhance hepatic triglyceride synthesis, decrease lipid oxidation in the liver, and increase hepatic lipoprotein release (Lieber and Salaspuro 1992). In each case the prevailing major mechanism is dependent on the experimental conditions.

The ethanol-induced increase in the NADH/NAD ratio (redox state) is a sign of major change in hepatic metabolism during ethanol oxidation. Many of the acute changes in the intermediary metabolism of the liver can be explained by the action of ethanol on the hepatic redox state. These include the inhibition of tricarboxylic acid cycle (Forsander et al. 1985) and gluconeogenesis. The redox-related inhibition of fatty acid oxidation (Lieber and Schmid 1961, Lieber et al. 1967) and the enhancement of triglyceride synthesis (Nikkilä and Ojala 1963) are important mechanisms in the development of alcoholic fatty liver. A major site of inhibition by this mechanism is 2-oxoglutarate dehydrogenase (Ontko 1973). After chronic ethanol consumption, the acute inhibition of fatty-acid oxidation is attenuated (Salaspuro et al. 1981), resulting in a levelling off in the accumulation of hepatic fat.

It can be concluded that consensus exists with respect to most of the pathogenetic mechanisms leading to alcoholic fatty liver. However, some conflicting results still exist and are most probably due to different experimental conditions.

The Role of Gastric ADH in the Hepatotoxicity of Ethanol

ADH is present in the mucosa of the stomach, and it has been suggested to be responsible for the gastric oxidation of ethanol (Hempel and Pietruszko 1979, Hempel et al. 1984, Lambouef et al. 1981, 1983, Pestalozzi et al. 1983). However, the magnitude of gastrointestinal ethanol metabolism was long assumed to be small or almost negligible (Lin and Lester 1980, Wagner 1986). It has recently been suggested, however, that a significant fraction (up to 20%) of alcohol ingested by rats (in doses in keeping with usual "social drinking") does not enter the systemic circulation in the rat, and is oxidized mainly in the stomach (Julkunen et al. 1985a,b, Caballeria et al. 1987, 1989b). This process was also shown to occur in man (DiPadova et al. 1987, 1988) and has been suggested to determine, in part, the bioavailability of alcohol and thus modulate its potential hepatotoxicity.

This gastric barrier may be low in females (DiPadova et al. 1988, Frezza et al. 1990) and may thereby contribute to their increased susceptibility to ethanol. Commonly used H2-antagonists such as cimetidine decrease the activity of gastric ADH (Caballeria et al. 1989a, Hernandez-Munoz et al. 1990) and may thereby enhance peripheral blood levels of ethanol. The existence of first-pass gastric metabolism of ethanol in the rat, however, has again been recently questioned (Smith et al. 1992). Moreover, the studies in man should be repeated, since it has been demonstrated that *Helicobacter pylori* also contains significant amounts of alcohol dehydrogenase (Roine et al. 1992a,b), which may obviously interfere with the gastric metabolism of ethanol in individuals carrying the bacteria (Salmela et al. 1993). The finding of "gastric" first-pass metabolism of ethanol is most interesting, but conflicting results and some new findings warrant further studies on the topic.

Hepatotoxicity of Acetaldehyde

Acetaldehyde is both pharmacologically and chemically a very potent and reactive compound and has accordingly been suggested to be a major initiating factor in the pathogenesis of alcoholic liver damage (Salaspuro and Lindros 1985, Lieber 1988a, 1991a, Sorrell and Tuma 1985, Lauterberg and Bilzer 1988).

Covalent Binding of Acetaldehyde—Acetaldehyde Adducts

In vitro, acetaldehyde has been shown to form adducts with phospholipids (Kenney 1982). However, the most probable target macromolecules are proteins (Gaines et al. 1977), including liver proteins such as hepatic microsomal proteins (Nomura and Lieber 1981), other hepatic proteins (Medina et al. 1985), and liver tubulin (Jennett et al.

1989, Tuma et al. 1991). Evidence for the formation of acetaldehyde adducts with liver proteins, also in vivo, has been recently presented (Barry and McGivan 1985, Lin et al. 1988). The target molecule for acetaldehyde binding can, for instance, be the microsomal ethanol-inducible P-450IIE1 (Behrens et al. 1988).

Acetaldehyde adducts may serve as antigens and generate an immune response in the centrilobular region of the liver of individuals consuming excessive amounts of alcohol (Niemelä et al. 1990). In addition, acetaldehyde adducts may (1) inhibit hepatic protein secretion produced by both acute and chronic ethanol administration (Matsuda et al. 1979, 1985, Valentine et al. 1987), (2) displace pyridoxal phosphate from its binding sites on proteins (Lumeng 1978), (3) impair biological functions of proteins (Mauch et al. 1984), or (4) combine with tissue macromolecules and thereby cause severe tissue injury, as in the case of acetaminophen.

Acetaldehyde has been related to hepatotoxicity of ethanol in many ways. After the establishment of reliable analytical methods for the determination of blood and tissue levels of acetaldehyde, consensus exists in most of the biochemical changes and associations observed to date. However, the true pathogenetic role of acetaldehyde in the genesis of alcoholic liver injury still remains hypothetical.

Hepatotoxicity Associated With MEOS

Theoretically, MEOS may cause enhanced hepatotoxicity by several means. MEOS contributes to the production of the potentially hepatotoxic agent acetaldehyde. MEOS may enhance oxygen consumption and provide so-called "empty calories" (Lieber 1991b), which may at least in part potentiate hypoxia. Both of these factors may be more crucial in the centrilobular (perivenous) areas of the hepatic acinus, since the ethanol-inducible microsomal cytochrome P-450IIE1 is predominantly localized in the perivenous region of the liver (Tsutsumi et al. 1989). MEOS may activate hepatotoxic agents such as carbon tetrachloride (Hasumura et al. 1974) or acetaminophen (Teschke et al. 1979). In accordance with this hypothesis, the history of ethanol consumption in humans has been shown to increase the hepatotoxicity of acetaminophen (Seeff et al. 1986).

Both in experimental animals and in man, chronic alcohol consumption has been shown to be associated with vitamin A depletion (Sato and Lieber 1981, Leo et al. 1982). This is caused by the induction of a new pathway of microsomal retinol oxidation that is inducible by ethanol and that may degrade an amount of retinol comparable to the daily intake (Leo and Lieber 1985). Decreased hepatic vitamin A levels may lead to some functional and structural abnormalities in the liver (Leo et al. 1983, Ray et al. 1988). However, the possible therapeutic use of vitamin A in alcohol-related liver disease may be complicated by its own potential hepatotoxicity (Leo et al. 1982, 1983).

Though the existence of MEOS is generally accepted, its role in the pathogenesis of alcoholic liver injury is still open for further studies.

Promotion of Lipid Peroxidation

Enhanced lipid peroxidation as a mechanism of alcoholic liver injury was proposed in 1966 by Kalish and DiLuzio. Free radicals (superoxide and hydroxyl radicals) may damage a wide range of cellular components via lipid peroxidation, including proteins, nucleic acids, free amino acids, and lipoproteins (Cross et al. 1987, Cederbaum 1987).

In addition to the cytochrome P-450 pathway, microsomes may oxidize ethanol by a separate pathway involving formation of hydroxyl radicals (Cederbaum 1987). Reactive oxygen intermediates are also produced when acetaldehyde is oxidized to acetate via xanthine oxidase (Lewis and Paton 1982). Free radicals are scavenged by superoxide dismutase and glutathione peroxidase. On the other hand, binding of acetaldehyde with cysteine or glutathione (GSH) may contribute to the depression of liver GSH (Shaw et al. 1981, 1983). Chronic ethanol feeding increases GSH turnover and the cellular requirements for GSH (Morton and Mitchell 1985). Furthermore, there is an increased loss of GSH from cells (Callans et al. 1987), especially from mitochondria (Fernandez-Checa et al. 1987). Evidence of GSH depletion and lipid peroxidation has also been found in human liver biopsies (Shaw et al. 1983).

In naive rats large amounts of ethanol (5–6g/kg) are required to produce lipid peroxidation (Di Luzio and Hartman 1967). After chronic alcohol consumption, however, even smaller doses of ethanol administered acutely produce lipid peroxidation, which can be partly prevented by the GSH precursor methionine (Shaw et al. 1981). Ethanol-induced microsomal induction and iron mobilization have been suggested as potentiating factors in lipid peroxidation reactions in rats (Shaw et al. 1988).

In chronic alcoholics there is an increase in both serum and liver lipoperoxide levels (Suematsu et al. 1981). The content of hepatic-reduced GSH is decreased, especially in patients with histological liver necrosis (Videla et al. 1984). As an integral part of the enzyme GSH peroxidase, selenium has a central role in the protection against the tissue damage caused by lipid peroxides. In this respect the decrease of selenium (not only in blood but also in liver) in patients with alcoholic liver injury may also play a significant role (Välimäki et al. 1987). Low vitamin E intake may also potentiate hepatic lipid peroxidation (Kawase et al. 1989).

There is consensus that lipid peroxidation is associated with the experimental models of alcoholic liver injury. Furthermore, there is some evidence supporting the existence of this damaging mechanism in man.

Perivenular Hypoxic Injury

A characteristic feature of liver injury in the alcoholic is the predominance of steatosis and other lesions in the perivenular (also called centrilobular) zone—zone 3 of the hepatic acinus. It has been postulated that the increased consumption of oxygen increases the gradient of oxygen tensions along the sinusoids to the extent of producing anoxic injury of perivenular hepatocytes (Israel et al. 1975, French et al. 1984). These findings have led to the theory of alcohol-induced liver necrosis secondary to a "hypermetabolic" state of the liver and consequently to therapeutic trials with propylthiouracil (Orrego et al. 1987, Orrego and Carmichael 1989).

Slight decreases in hepatic venous oxygen saturation and PO_2 have been reported both in experimental animals and in human alcoholics (Kessler et al. 1954, Jauhonen et al. 1982, Sato et al. 1983). However, results in baboons suggest that increased hepatic oxygen consumption is offset by increased blood flow, resulting in unchanged hepatic venous oxygen tension (Jauhonen et al. 1982). In baboons, defective O_2 utilization rather than lack of O_2 blood supply characterizes liver injury produced by high concentrations of ethanol (Lieber et al. 1989).

An alternative hypothesis to explain the selective perivenular hepatotoxicity of ethanol postulates that the low oxygen tensions normally prevailing in perivenular zones could exaggerate the redox shift produced by ethanol (Jauhonen et al. 1982, 1985).

Perivenular fibrosis has been suggested to be an early warning sign and a predictor of the development of more advanced liver fibrosis and cirrhosis, both in baboons and in man (Van Waes and Lieber 1977, Nasralah et al. 1980, Worner and Lieber 1985). No consensus exists with regard to the mechanism and pathogenetic significance of decreased oxygen tension in the perivenular area of the hepatic acinus. Consequently, confirming clinical studies with propylthiouracil in the treatment of alcoholic liver injury are still needed before it can be recommended for general use. Further studies are also needed to establish the true clinical significance of perivenular fibrosis.

Nutritional Factors

Excess weight has been shown to be a risk factor or a predictive sign of histological liver damage in alcoholics (Iturriaga et al. 1988). In epidemiological studies of populations at the aggregate level, the amount of pork consumed appears to correlate with mortality from cirrhosis (Nanji and French 1985). Further evaluation has suggested that both saturated fat and cholesterol may protect against alcoholic cirrhosis, while polyunsaturated fat may promote it (Nanji et al. 1986b). In accordance with these findings, high fat diet has been shown to potentiate, and beef fat to prevent, ethanol-induced hepatic fibrosis and alcoholic liver diseases in the rat (French et al. 1986, Nanji et al. 1989, Takahashi et al. 1991).

Deficiencies in lipotropic factors (choline and methionine) may produce fatty liver and cirrhosis in growing rats (Daft et al. 1941, Best et al. 1949). In later studies, hepatic injury induced by choline deficiency was suggested to be primarily an experimental disease of rats with little if any relevance to alcoholic liver injury, particularly in humans (Lieber 1982). More recently, rats have been shown to be more resistant to choline deficiency than humans, since humans have a reduced ability to produce betaine (main donor of methyl groups) from choline (Barak et al. 1985). Furthermore, choline has been suggested to be an essential nutrient for humans when excess methionine and folate are not available in the diet (Zeisel et al. 1991). Therefore betaine—the first metabolite of choline—has been suggested for the treatment of alcoholic liver injury in man (Barak and Beckenhauer 1988).

With respect to the protection of alcoholic liver injury in subhuman primates by choline, the results are controversial as stated previously (Lieber and DeCarli 1974, 1991, Popper and Lieber 1980, Rogers et al. 1981, Mezey et al. 1983, Ainley et al. 1988). The discrepancy in the results has also been related to the differences in the choline content of the diets. Accordingly, it has been suggested that chronic alcohol feeding may exaggerate choline requirements of monkeys (Mezey et al. 1983, Ainley et al. 1988). However, additional choline failed to prevent the development of fibrosis in baboons (Lieber et al. 1985). On the other hand, S-adenosyl-L-methionine (Lieber et al. 1990) and polyunsaturated lecithin (Lieber et al. 1990) have recently been shown to attenuate alcohol-induced hepatic injury in baboons. Because of the high phosphatidylcholine content of polyunsaturated lecithin, the preparation contained additional choline of 400mg/l, which is about four times more than the original "Lieber-DeCarli" diet.

From these studies it can be concluded that there is no consensus with respect to the role of choline in the prevention of alcoholic liver injury, either in experimental animals or in man. Accordingly, further controlled studies both in baboons and perhaps also in man are needed in order to establish the possible therapeutic value of choline, S-adenosyl-L-metionine, betaine, and polyunsaturated lecithin in the prevention of alcoholic liver injury.

It has been claimed that alcoholic liver disease is frequently recognized among well-nourished alcoholic individuals manifesting no nutritional deficiency. On the other hand, cirrhotic alcoholics have been reported to have a significantly lower total food calorie intake, and a significantly lower daily protein intake, than noncirrhotic chronic alcoholics (Patek et al. 1975). Using established criteria to diagnose and classify protein-calorie malnutrition, all 248 patients with alcoholic liver disease were shown to have some evidence of malnutrition (Mendenhall et al. 1984, Mendenhall 1985). The prevalence of the malnutrition correlated closely with the severity of the liver disease, with a prevalence of 72% of both kwashiorkor and marasmus in severe disease. It should be noted, however, that in neither study was the cause-relationship between malnutrition and liver disease established; malnutrition, at least in part, might have been secondary to the liver injury and not its cause.

Data on the nutritional status of heavy drinkers is also controversial. Only subtle nutritional alterations have been documented in several studies (Neville et al. 1986, Hurt et al. 1981, Goldschmith et al. 1983, Rissanen et al. 1987). Nevertheless, these drinkers also frequently develop laboratory signs of alcoholic liver injury (Rissanen et al. 1987). In some other studies, significantly decreased protein, fat, and cholesterol intake has been documented in heavy drinkers (Jones et al. 1982, Hillers and Massey 1985), and there is some epidemiological evidence pointing to the possible protective effect of a high-protein diet on alcohol-induced cirrhosis (Raymond et al. 1985).

It can be concluded that no firm consensus exist with regard to the occurrence of protein-calorie malnutrition among chronic alcoholics. In order to resolve this question, properly controlled prospective studies using modern nutritional techniques are needed.

Clinical Manifestations and Pathology of Alcoholic Liver Disease

Chronic alcoholics may present a wide spectrum of hepatic lesions, the most frequent being fatty liver, alcoholic hepatitis, and hepatic cirrhosis (Baptista et al. 1981, Hall 1985b, McSween and Burt 1986, Ishak et al. 1991). Other lesions more recently described, such as chronic hepatitis and fibrosis (Van Waes and Lieber 1977, Nasralah et al. 1980), are less frequent. These hepatic lesions may be found isolated or in combination, and the clinical manifestations are very variable, ranging from asymptomatic forms to severe hepatic failure. Therefore, to establish the exact diagnosis of hepatic diseases induced by chronic alcohol consumption, liver biopsy is required (Bruguera et al. 1977a).

Alcoholic Fatty Liver

The deposition of fat in the cytoplasm of hepatocytes is very frequent among chronic alcoholics (Edmondson et al. 1967, Christoffersen et al. 1971). This lesion may be seen isolated or in combination with more severe hepatic lesions (alcoholic hepatitis) (Morgan et al. 1978), particularly in those patients with recent and high alcohol intake. The incidence of fatty liver in alcoholic patients is about 90% of the cases (Edmondson et al. 1967).

The deposition of a single large lipid droplet in hepatocytes is the histological lesion defining alcoholic fatty liver. This lipid droplet may occupy all the hepatic cytoplasm, and the nucleous is displaced (macrovesicular steatosis) (Christoffersen et al. 1971). Occasionally, as a consequence of cellular damage secondary to cell distension induced by intracellular lipid deposition or to cell membrane alteration, an inflammatory response may occur with the presence of lymphocytes and macrophages, producing the development of lipogranulomas (Christoffersen et al. 1971). The degree of hepatic steatosis varies from patient to patient. In the moderate forms it is frequently localized in the perivenular areas, while in the massive forms lipid deposition occupies the entire hepatic acinus.

A microvesicular form of fatty liver has been described (Uchida et al. 1983). This lesion is characterized by the presence of multiple small droplets of fat in the hepatocellular cytoplasm. In these cases the nuclei of hepatic cells are not displaced. Microvesicular steatosis is usually present in the perivenular areas. The frequency of this lesion is very low and may be associated with other alcoholic liver lesions, such as alcoholic hepatitis, cholestasis, or fibrosis (Montull et al. 1989).

Fatty liver is usually asymptomatic, and in most cases the only sign is the presence of smooth, regular, and minimally tender hepatomegaly (Leevy et al. 1968). The biochemical tests are usually normal, and an overt increase of gammaglutamyltranspeptidase (GGT), a slight increase of serum aspartate transaminase activity (ASAT), and serum alanine transaminase activity (ALAT) is observed (Morgan 1991). In those patients in whom steatosis is associated with other hepatic lesions, the symptomatology observed is due to these latter lesions and not to fatty liver.

Massive hepatic steatosis is less common, and clinical manifestations are more evident. The development of severe hepatic failure with encephalopathy and marked decrease of prothrombin time has been described (Morgan et al. 1978). In these patients the development of cholestasis may take place.

Microvesicular steatosis usually presents with fatigue, anorexia, nausea, vomiting, and occasionally abdominal pain. Hepatomegaly is very frequent. There is a marked increase of plasma cholesterol and triglycerides, and in about half of the patients a decrease of prothrombin time and conjugated hyperbilirubinemia is observed (Montull et al. 1989).

Hepatic Fibrosis

Chronic alcoholics may exhibit an increase of collagen content in the space of Disse around the hepatocytes (pericellular fibrosis), particularly in the perivenular area (perivenular fibrosis) (Edmondson et al. 1963, Nakano et al. 1982). This lesion may be observed as isolated or in combination with fatty liver (fibrosteatosis) and alcoholic hepatitis (Van Waes and Lieber 1977). However, it has been found that chronic alcoholics may develop hepatic fibrosis without other associated hepatic lesions. This finding is a consequence of an increase in hepatic fibrogenetic activity. The prevalence of hepatic fibrosis is not known and probably varies from country to country; in Japan it is the most frequent lesion induced by chronic alcohol consumption (Takada et al. 1982).

Most patients are asymptomatic. Some cases may present hepatomegaly, with moderate abdominal pain and jaundice. These patients usually show a slight increase of transaminases and GGT.

There is no consensus in considering alcoholic fibrosis as a new form of alcoholic liver disease independent of steatosis, alcoholic hepatitis, and cirrhosis. Furthermore, the prognostic value of the different forms of alcoholic fibrosis must be further clarified (Nasralah et al. 1980, Worner and Lieber 1985, Parés et al. 1987).

Alcoholic Hepatitis

Alcoholic hepatitis is the most characteristic hepatic lesion found in chronic alcoholism, particularly in heavy drinkers. It is estimated that the prevalence of alcoholic hepatitis is about 40% of chronic alcoholics, although this figure may also vary from country to country (Hislop et al. 1983).

Histologically, the lesion is characterized by the presence of areas of hepatocellular necrosis associated with an inflammatory cell infiltrate constituted by neutrophil polymorphs (Baptista et al. 1981, McSween and Burt 1986). The lesion is generally located in the perivenular areas. In the necrotic areas hepatocytes are large and ballooned with a clear cytoplasm. Within the hepatocytes homogenous eosinophilic, perinuclear inclusion bodies with irregular appearance may be seen. This lesion constitutes the Mallory bodies or alcoholic hyaline. Ultrastructurally, the Mallory bodies are made up of clusters of proteinic fibrils with a special chemotactism for neutrophils (French 1981). This explains why neutrophils usually surround the Mallory bodies. Alcoholic hepatitis is usually associated with fatty liver and portal and pericellular fibrosis. Other lesions observed are giant mitochondria, acidophil bodies, and perivenular fibrosis (Bruguera et al. 1977a). This latter lesion may produce portal hypertension without the presence of cirrhosis. Perivenular fibrosis may be an important precursor of development of cirrhosis, although more studies are needed (Worner and Lieber 1985).

The clinical picture of alcoholic hepatitis is variable (Parés et al. 1978, Maddrey 1988). Alcoholic hepatitis usually develops when chronic alcoholics increases their alcohol intake. The most common clinical picture of this lesion initiates with fatigue, anorexia, nausea, and vomiting. A few days later, abdominal pain localized in the upper right abdominal quadrant, jaundice, and fever appear. Tender hepatomegaly and other signs of alcoholic liver disease (spider nevi, cutaneous telangiectasia, palmar erythema, parotid enlargement, gynecomastia, testicular atrophy, peripheral neuropathy, Dupuytren's contracture) may be detected. Biochemical tests reveal a moderate increase in transaminases, usually less than 300 U/l. Among patients with alcoholic hepatitis ASAT is usually greater than ALAT, and the ASAT/ALAT ratio is higher than 2 (Nanji et al. 1989). GGT are very high and may be associated with conjugated hyperbilirubinemia and high alkaline phosphatase. Macrocytosis is frequent and is probably due to the toxic effect of alcohol on developing erythrocytes (Morgan et al. 1981). Thrombocytopenia, leukocytosis, and neutrophilia are also frequent. Fever and leukocytosis could be secondary to hepatic necrosis and inflammation or bacterial infections (Parés et al. 1978). In a few cases the hepatic surface may be irregular, and a murmur may be detected. This is a consequence of intrahepatic arteriovenous anastomosis and an increase in hepatic arterial flow. These cases should be differentiated from hepatocellular carcinoma. A few patients may develop acute hepatic failure (Parés et al. 1978). Other patients may present clinical features similar to hepatic cirrhosis (ascites, gastrointestinal bleeding). To establish differential diagnosis in these patients, liver biopsy is required. Alcoholic hepatitis may also be asymptomatic, being detected by routine examination in chronic alcoholics (Bruguera et al. 1977b). Very few patients may develop acute hepatic failure with deep jaundice, encephalopathy, very low prothrombin time, and progressive renal failure. The prognosis of these patients is very poor, and death occurs within a short period of time. Acute alcoholic hepatitis may be associated with massive fatty liver, hemolysis, and hyperlipidemia (hypertriglyceridemia).

Chronic Alcoholic Hepatitis

It has been suggested that alcohol may produce chronic hepatitis (Goldberg et al. 1977, Crapper et al. 1983, Adelasco et al. 1987, Laskus et al. 1990, Corrao et al. 1991b). This suggestion was raised by the fact that chronic hepatitis among alcoholics improves after the suppression of alcohol ingestion (Takase et al. 1991). Clinical manifestations in these patients are very slight, with a moderate increase in transaminase levels being observed. At present there is no clear evidence indicating that chronic hepatitis may be due to chronic alcoholism. It is possible that chronic hepatitis described in chronic alcoholic patients may be due to viral infection, particularly the hepatitis C virus (Brillanti et al. 1989, Parés et al. 1990).

There is no consensus about the role of alcohol as an etiological agent of chronic hepatitis. The normalization of transaminases and liver lesions after alcohol abstinence suggests that this role could be important in some cases of chronic hepatitis, while in other cases the hepatitis C virus could be predominant. This point should be clarified in the future.

Hepatic Cirrhosis

The prevalence of hepatic cirrhosis in the chronic alcoholic population varies from study to study. Histologically, there are no differences between this and other types of cirrhosis. Alcoholics usually exhibit a micronodular type (McSween and Burt 1986). Other alcoholic hepatic lesions, particularly fatty liver and alcoholic hepatitis, are frequently observed in alcoholic cirrhosis. Clinical manifestations of these patients are identical to those observed in other cirrhotic patients. Portal hypertension, ascites, gastrointestinal bleeding by esophageal varices, and encephalopathy appear at the end stage of the disease. Symptoms and signs directly related to chronic alcoholism are also frequently observed.

Hepatocellular Carcinoma

It has been suggested that chronic alcohol consumption may lead to development of primary hepatocellular carcinoma (International Agency for Research on Cancer 1988). It is also considered that the development of hepatocellular carcinoma in patients with alcoholic cirrhosis is about 15% (Ishak et al. 1991). The role played by alcohol consumption in development of liver cancer seems complex, in that hepatic cirrhosis is definitely associated with increased risk of liver cancer; but when cirrhosis has developed, the role of alcohol in carcinogenesis is unclear (Colombo et al. 1992). It is also unknown whether cirrhosis caused by excessive alcohol carries a greater risk of cancer development than cirrhosis caused by other factors (except for chronic hepatitis B infection, which results in a very high cancer risk). The high prevalence of antibodies against hepatitis C virus in alcoholic patients with liver cirrhosis and hepatocellular carcinoma (Bruix et al. 1989, Colombo et al. 1989, Chiaramonte et al. 1990, Kaklamani et al. 1991) suggests that this virus is responsible for the tumour. A large Italian case-control study showed no influence on development of hepatocellular carcinoma of alcohol abuse per se, either among cirrhotics or noncirrhotics (Pagliaro et al. 1983). Another prospective Italian study also did not support the hypothesis that the alcoholic etiology is of particular importance for the development of carcinoma

(Colombo et al. 1991). Some studies suggest that the macronodular cirrhosis that develops in abstaining alcoholics is particularly prone to carcinogenesis (Lee 1966). However, the role of alcohol, hepatitis virus, or their association in the development of hepatocellular carcinoma in alcoholics needs further investigation.

Abstinence in the Treatment of Alcoholic Liver Disease

The main treatment for alcoholic liver disease is abstinence from alcohol. Abstinence will reverse, improve, or delay the progression of alcoholic liver disease, depending on the stage of the lesion. Even when cirrhosis is established, prognosis is improved with alcohol abstinence (D'Amico et al. 1986, Saunders et al. 1981b, Morgan 1977, Ginés et al. 1987, Orrego et al. 1987, Tygstrup and Juhl 1971).

Epidemiological Aspects of Chronic Alcoholism and Liver Disease

There is no doubt that alcohol consumption in humans is associated with a risk of liver disease with the characteristic features of the diagnostic categories of "alcoholic liver disease" (International Group 1981), which constitutes a significant public health problem (Grant et al. 1988). The incidence of the end-stage of alcoholic cirrhosis has recently been estimated at 190 per million person-years in Danish males and 85 in Danish females, with the age-specific incidence peaking at 50–60 years in both genders (Almdal and Sorensen 1991, Prytz and Skinhoj 1980). Comparable results have previously been obtained in the United Kingdom, the United States, and Canada (Garagliano et al. 1979, Saunders et al. 1981b, Hunter et al. 1988). The overall 5-year survival following diagnosis of cirrhosis is 50–35% but depends heavily on the degree of decompensation and continued drinking (Borowsky et al. 1981, Bouchier et al. 1992, Christensen et al. 1986, Orholm et al. 1985, Saunders et al. 1981b, Tygstrup and Juhl 1971).

Even among the heaviest drinkers, however, some remain free of liver disease throughout their lifetime (Klatskin 1961, Lelbach 1975, 1976). This means that alcohol consumption is not a sufficient cause of alcoholic liver disease. Alcohol consumption is also not a necessary cause: the morphological features of "alcoholic liver disease" are found—although very rarely—without preceding excessive alcohol consumption.

The Risk Function

The epidemiological analysis of the relationship between alcohol consumption and liver disease has three requirements: (1) measurement of alcohol consumption, (2) diagnosis of liver disease, and (3) estimation of their association implying estimation of the risk of liver disease following alcohol consumption. Since the amount of alcohol consumed differs between individuals and within individuals over time, the measure of the association is the risk for different given amounts of alcohol consumed for different given periods of time. The risk of liver disease should be specified as the risk or probability of occurrence of the liver disease at issue per unit of time from a given point in time (Sorensen 1989). The combination of this measure of alcohol consumption with the risk estimate is the risk function.

There are two important reservations to be made when applying the concept of the risk function to the relationship between alcohol consumption and liver disease. First, no data are—and will probably never become—available that allow a direct estimation of the values of the risk function as defined here. Second, even though data allowing proxy estimates of the risk function may be available from observations of populations of individuals with different alcohol consumption, the question of whether a given individual, by deliberately changing alcohol consumption, changes the affiliated risk of liver disease concordantly will remains unanswered. The scientific evidence for this link would require unfeasible and unethical large-scale human experiments with increases and decreases of alcohol consumption and no changes in other conditions for prolonged periods of time. The closest approximation to such evidence would be the conduct of large-scale, population-based longitudinal studies with repeated assessment of alcohol intake and recording of alcoholic liver disease development. In this design, the actual changes that do occur in alcohol consumption may be related to the subsequent risk of liver disease.

The Time Relationship

Using various epidemiological methods, a number of studies have approached an indirect estimation of the risk function. These studies have revealed two sets of specific problems: (1) the time relationship between alcohol consumption and the development of liver disease, and (2) the effect of alcohol consumption at the various stages of development and manifestation of liver disease (Sorensen 1989). The questions about time relationship deal with the minimum period of time of alcohol consumption required for development of liver injury, the duration of its damaging effect, and the possible time lag and cumulative effect of consumed alcohol.

The shortest period of time of excessive alcohol consumption reported to have caused fatty liver is a few days (Rubin and Lieber 1968), and three months for development of alcoholic hepatitis and cirrhosis (Lischner et al. 1971). Cirrhosis has been seen developing during a 12-month period of abstinence following excessive alcohol consumption (Galambos 1987), and the tendency to progress despite abstinence seems to be particularly strong in women (Parés et al. 1986).

The duration of excessive alcohol consumption until diagnosis of alcoholic cirrhosis has an average between 10 and 20 years, and the prevalence of cirrhosis is greater the longer the duration of excessive alcohol consumption. This has been interpreted as a combination of a time lag and a cumulative effect. However, this interpretation is probably wrong (Sorensen 1989). First, the distribution among patients of the duration of excessive alcohol consumption before diagnosis of cirrhosis is flat rather than bell-shaped (Lischner et al. 1971), indicating that the average has no meaning in terms of a shared characteristic among the patients. Second, even if there were no cumulative effect at all, but only a constant, short-lasting effect, the prevalence of the irreversible cirrhosis steadily increases just by the passage of time. Third, a prospective study of alcoholics has shown that the future risk of development of cirrhosis is independent of the duration of excessive alcohol consumption before entrance to the study (Sorensen et al. 1984). Finally, it seems unlikely that consumed alcohol in some individuals has no short-term damaging effect, but only damaging effects that suddenly emerge many years later.

Stage of Alcoholic Liver Disease

At the time of first diagnosis, alcoholic liver disease manifests itself in a variety of morphological changes in the liver, ranging from slight steatosis through end-stage macronodular cirrhosis with liver cancer; and a broad spectrum of clinical manifestations, from asymptomatic conditions through severe liver failure and death (Alves et al. 1982, Bruguera et al. 1977b, Lelbach 1967, Lischner et al. 1971). It is assumed that the more severe stages of the disease are reached by progression through less-severe forms (Galambos 1987, Junge et al. 1988, Lieber 1975, 1983, Maier et al. 1979, Parés et al. 1986, Sorensen et al. 1984). Most studies addressing the risk function have evaluated the development of cirrhosis, not necessarily applying to cirrhosis as such or clinical manifestations of cirrhosis. However, it is possible that the risk function is different for different stages and that the risk function for clinical manifestations at given stages of liver damage, including death, may be different from the risk function for developing these stages (Sorensen 1989). This means that a risk function estimated for the current and preceding stages, for example, the risk function for death from cirrhosis is a mixture of the risk function for cirrhosis and for death given that cirrhosis necessarily applies to cirrhosis as such. These problems have obvious consequences for the recommendations about alcohol consumption, both at the public health level and in the clinical setting.

Studies of the Risk Function

The studies addressing the risk function may be subdivided into those conducted at population aggregates and those based on examination of individual subjects.

Aggregate Population Studies

A large number of studies have assessed the changes over time within populations and differences between populations in mortality or morbidity from cirrhosis, assessed by national statistics, in relation to total per-capita consumption of alcohol, usually determined from sales statistics or population surveys (Capocaccia and Farchi 1988, Colón 1981, Colón et al. 1982, Coppéré and Audigier 1986, Gallagher and Elwood 1980, Hunter et al. 1988, 1989, Israel et al. 1991, Joliffe and Jellinek 1941, Klatskin 1961, McGlashan 1980, Norstrom 1987, Parrish et al. 1991, Prytz and Anderson 1988, Qiao et al. 1988, Romelsjo and Agren 1985, Sales et al. 1989, Schmidt 1977, Smart 1988, Smart and Mann 1987, 1991, Skinhoj and Prytz 1981, Skog 1985, Smith and Burwell 1985, Svendsen and Mosbech 1977, La Vecchia et al. 1986, Williams et al. 1988, Wilson 1984). With few exceptions, these studies have shown very high correlations between mortality or morbidity from cirrhosis and alcohol consumption.

Departures from this close direct relationship may be due to changes or differences (1) in gender and age composition of the populations (gender and age standardization may not always eliminate the problem); (2) in the procedures for recording death from cirrhosis, including distinction between alcoholic and nonalcoholic cirrhosis; (3) in nonregistered alcohol consumption; (4) in the distribution of consumption among the members of the populations including treatment of alcoholism; (5) in exposure of the populations to co-factors for development of cirrhosis or progression of a fatal course; and (6) to a time lag from changes in consumption until changes in mortality (Duffy and Latcham 1986, Furst and Beckman 1981, Graudal et al. 1991, Haberman and Weinbaum 1990, Halliday et al. 1991, Hyman 1981, Kreitman and Duffy 1989, Lint 1981a,b, Mann et al. 1988, 1991, Maxwell 1985, Nanji and French 1985, 1986a, Natta et al. 1985, Norstrom 1987, Parrish et al. 1991, Prytz and Anderson 1988, Qiao et al. 1988, Romelsjo and Agren 1985, Skinhoj and Prytz 1981, Skog 1980, 1984, 1985, Smart and Mann 1987, 1991, Williams et al. 1988, Wilson 1984).

Despite the strikingly high correlations, it is of note that the risk function for death from cirrhosis cannot be derived from such relationships. Thus, the mere existence of a risk function implying that there is no reduction in risk by increasing consumption by the individual will, regardless of the shape of the risk function, produce this kind of statistics at the aggregate level (Sorensen 1989).

Subject Population Studies

Proper interpretation of these studies requires a distinction between prospective studies and retrospective studies and, among the latter group, distinction between cross-sectional and case-control studies. In prospective studies, the assessment of alcohol consumption is carried out before development of liver disease in a study population, which then is followed with regard to development of liver disease. In the retrospective studies, alcohol consumption is assessed at the same time the diagnosis of liver disease is made or later. The cross-sectional study assesses alcohol consumption in a study population that is selected regardless of the presence of liver disease and in which the assessment of presence of liver disease takes place at the same time. In the case-control study, patients with liver disease are identified and their preceding alcohol consumption is compared with selected controls, usually matched to the cases by other characteristics possibly influencing the alcohol consumption (e.g., gender and age).

Retrospective Case-Control Studies

A large number of case-control studies have been conducted (Batey et al. 1992, Bourliere et al. 1991, Coates et al. 1986, Corrao et al. 1991a,b, Durbec et al. 1979, Norton et al. 1987, Pagliaro et al. 1982, Pequignot 1961, 1978, Rotily et al. 1990, Tuyns and Pequignot 1984). The controls have been either other hospitalized patients or various kinds of samples from the general populations. The studies showed that the probability of becoming a hospitalized cirrhotic patient increased exponentially by increasing daily alcohol consumption throughout a range from about 20–160 g. Some studies showed that women developing cirrhosis have had a smaller daily consumption and/or a shorter duration of excessive drinking than men developing cirrhosis. Interpretation of these studies in terms of risk function for development of cirrhosis is hampered for several reasons (Sorensen 1989). First, the risk function involves the risk of becoming hospitalized for symptomatic and even complicated cirrhosis and having this disease diagnosed (Corrao et al. 1991a). Second, the recorded intake may be a poor reflection of the alcohol intake before cirrhosis developed (Corrao et al. 1991b). The daily intake may not be constant, and there may very well be a recall bias in the reporting of previous consumption. The potential bias is accentuated by the fact that the liver disease probably developed at some unknown time before diagnosis, or the relevant time period of consumption cannot be identified. Third, daily consumption usually increases by duration of excessive consumption, so that the greater probability of cirrhosis at high daily consumption is at least to some extent due to the trivial explanation that the subjects have been at risk for a longer time.

These difficulties may also blur the comparison of men and women (Batey et al. 1992, Bourliere et al. 1991, Norton et al. 1987, Pagliaro et al. 1982, Tuyns and Pequignot 1984). It should be noted that the frequently made comparison between male and female patients with alcoholic liver disease (Morgan and Sherlock 1977, Saunders et al. 1981a, 1984) without including relevant male and female controls is not informative with regard to differences in the risk function (expressing different susceptibility) because of the great difference in distribution of alcohol consumption among men and women in the general population. If we assume that the risk function is the same for men and women, this difference in distribution would result in smaller and shorter excessive drinking by women than by men developing cirrhosis.

Retrospective Cross-Sectional Studies

Four such studies have been conducted in which the study population was defined as alcoholic, either identified in special clinics for alcoholics or in general hospitals (Eghöje and Juhl 1973, Lelbach 1967, 1975, 1976, Saunders et al. 1984, Wilkinson et al. 1969). In these populations, there was increasing prevalence of cirrhosis the longer the duration of the preceding excessive consumption, the greater the daily consumption, and therefore the greater the cumulated consumption. One of the studies defined a threshold for cumulated consumption below which there seemed to be no risk of cirrhosis (the theoretical amount of 15 g alcohol/day per kg body weight during 1 year, or 1 g during 15 years, in a man of 70 kg).

The reservation that must be made before interpreting these results in terms of the risk function for cirrhosis is the same as those for the case-control study, except that the possible effect of alcohol on the manifestation of cirrhosis is less likely to confound the result (Sorensen 1989).

An important difference between the case-control studies and the cross-sectional studies conducted among alcoholics is that the former group can address the relationship between consumption and cirrhosis at lower daily consumption than seen among subjects identified as alcoholics.

Prospective Studies

Several studies of general populations or special subpopulations defined according to criteria not related to their alcohol consumption have assessed the relationship between daily consumption reported at the start of the study to subsequent cirrhosis mortality during long-term follow-up (Blackwelder et al. 1980, Farchi et al. 1992, Klatsky 1981, Kono et al. 1983, 1989). They found that the risk increased steadily by increasing daily consumption up to 30 and 60 g more alcohol, respectively. A recent study of 129,000 subjects followed for up to 10 years with regard to mortality from cirrhosis showed that, compared to nondaily drinking, those drinking 1–2 drinks/day, 3–5 drinks/day, and 6 or more drinks/day had relative risk ratios of 3.5, 6.1, and 23.6, with no consistent differences between men and women (Klatsky et al. 1992).

In none of the studies was the absence of liver diseases histologically verified at the start of the study, and the development of cirrhosis during follow-up was not recorded. The estimated risk function is thus a mixture of the risk function for development of cirrhosis and death from cirrhosis.

In one study (Sorensen et al. 1984), alcoholics reporting a minimum consumption of 50 g/day for at least 1 year had liver biopsy performed in addition to an inquiry about the duration and amount of their previous alcohol consumption at the start of the observation. Development of cirrhosis during the subsequent 10–13 years was observed and occurred at a rate of about 2% per year, regardless of the amount and duration of alcohol consumption before start of the study. This finding indicates that there are no long-term cumulative effects of previous alcohol consumption.

This study also showed that those who were drinking intermittently at start of the study later exhibited a lower risk of liver damage than those drinking continuously. This is in accordance with an interpretation implying that the risk of damage exists when drinking, vanishes while drinking is interrupted, and emerges again when drinking is resumed. The evidence is rather weak, however, because the intermittent drinkers and the continuous drinkers may not be comparable in terms of other aspects of their alcohol consumption.

Another study (Marbet et al. 1987) among hospitalized alcoholics, which was prospective with regard to recent development of cirrhosis among patients proven to be noncirrhotic at the start of the study but retrospective with regard to quantitative assessment of the alcohol consumption (at the follow-up), found no relationship between the amount of daily intake and the development of cirrhosis.

These two studies did not allow assessment of the relationship between alcohol consumption and risk of cirrhosis on a short-term basis or at daily consumption below 50 g/day. None of the prospective studies addresses the risk of other types of alcoholic liver disease or the possible difference between men and women in risk of liver disease at given consumption.

List of Specific Associations Between Liver Disease and Consumption of Alcohol

Progress in Achievement of Scientific Consensus

Existing Current Consensus

There is a firm consensus about the association between excessive alcohol consumption and the development of the following conditions: fatty liver, hepatic centrilobular fibrosis, alcoholic hepatitis, and hepatic cirrhosis.

Specific Content of the Consensus

Consensus about the qualitative association between excessive alcohol consumption and the development of fatty liver, hepatic centrilobular fibrosis, alcoholic hepatitis, and hepatic cirrhosis implies that the likelihood that these conditions develop is much higher in individuals who, for a period of time, have had a daily excessive consumption of alcohol as compared to individuals who have had little or no consumption, or excessive consumption only for a short period of time. It is also implied that, for a given consumption over a given period of time, the likelihood is greatest for development of fatty liver and decreased for the other above conditions. There is consensus about these associations being only one of likelihood, since some individuals may consume huge amounts of alcohol for decades without developing any of the conditions.

Research Allowing Consensus

The consensus about the qualitative association between excessive alcohol consumption and the development of fatty liver, hepatic centrilobular fibrosis, alcoholic hepatitis, and hepatic cirrhosis is based on vast clinical experience and numerous systematic studies showing either a higher frequency of these conditions among individuals who have consumed excessive amounts of alcohol than among other individuals, or a much higher frequency of excessive alcohol consumption among patients with these diseases than among individuals without the diseases.

In addition, the frequency of death attributed to liver disease in the general population is correlated over time and place with measurement of the total consumption of alcohol by these populations.

These four types of liver damage may have distinct causes other than alcohol consumption. However, they exhibit a variety of histopathological features, of which sets can be defined, that are very rarely seen in patients in whom there is no excessive alcohol consumption.

Although the studies may have methodological problems of various sorts in the selection of the study populations, in the diagnosis of the liver disease, and in the assessment of alcohol consumption, none of these problems provides grounds for raising doubt about the qualitative association between the diseases and alcohol consumption.

Most of these studies are retrospective in design, in that the diagnosis of liver disease at one point in time has been related to reports on alcohol consumption during preceding periods of time. Since development of the conditions precedes the diagnosis by some unknown time interval, this kind of evidence leaves open the question about the time sequence of excessive alcohol consumption and the development of the condition. The main argument supporting that the liver disease develops after excessive alcohol consumption is the observation that the specific histopathological changes, as mentioned, are very rarely seen without excessive alcohol consumption, and that symptoms and signs associated with the conditions appear some time after the patients have undertaken excessive alcohol consumption.

Accepting that excessive alcohol consumption is followed by increased risk of liver damage, the association may be either a direct cause-effect relationship or an indirect apparent relationship resulting from confounding by another factor causing the liver damage and occurring together with excessive alcohol consumption. Such a confounding effect, itself being of merely methodological and not genuine scientific interest, must be clearly distinguished from a possible mediation of the damaging effect of alcohol through some other consequences of the excessive consumption, or the possible requirement of other causal factors, acting together with alcohol in damaging the liver. Mediating or co-acting factors are of great scientific interest and could be, for example, specific nutritional disturbances.

No convincing confounding factors have yet been identified. As reflected in the synonym of alcoholic cirrhosis—nutritional cirrhosis—poor nutrition has been suspected of being involved. Severe malabsorption, probably mainly of protein, induced by intestinal bypass surgery for massive obesity may rarely result in liver damage of a similar type (Peters 1977). This is an extreme situation, and exposure to alcohol, perhaps by intestinal production, has not been definitely excluded. There is no evidence indicating that poor nutrition by itself without alcohol consumption is associated with development of the type of liver damage seen after excessive alcohol consumption. Moreover, the association of alcohol and liver damage has been observed in many different populations of different genetic background and life-style under such diverse conditions that it is extremely unlikely that confounding is responsible.

For fatty liver, the observational studies have been supplemented by a few controlled experimental studies in humans that confirm the direct causal relationship with alcohol consumption (Rubin and Lieber 1968).

Consensus on Dose-Effect Relationships

Whereas consensus about the qualitative association between excessive alcohol consumption and the development of fatty liver, hepatic centrilobular fibrosis, acute alcoholic hepatitis, and hepatic cirrhosis is quite well-established, there is much uncertainty about the more complex issue of a dose-effect relationship, including a possible threshold effect or safe limit (Anderson et al. 1984), and no clear operational conclusion can be drawn from the available evidence.

Missing Scientific Consensus and Need of Research

The lack of consensus on the quantitative association (i.e., the dose-effect relationships) between excessive alcohol consumption and the development of fatty liver, hepatic centrilobular fibrosis, alcoholic hepatitis, and hepatic cirrhosis is due to several substantial, both theoretical and practical, difficulties in the study of this matter.

To identify the problems, it is important to specify the question further in order to interpret the results of the available studies as answers to the question. Existence of a dose-effect relationship will imply that the current risk per unit of time of development of any of the conditions is dependent on the current or the preceding dose of alcohol consumed by the individual. Denoting this as the "risk function" we may proceed by asking about its position or shape in relation to particular measures of alcohol consumption.

Most studies have dealt with hepatic cirrhosis. The information on dose-effect relationship for the other three conditions is scarce. This is particularly regrettable in view of their role as possibly reversible precursor states of cirrhosis. A dose-effect relationship has been found in one study of fatty liver (Coates et al. 1986). Another case-control study of asymptomatic "chronic hepatitis" (Corrao et al. 1991b) showed a clear dose-effect relationship, the strength of which declined, however, by increasing duration of consumption and disappeared at durations exceeding 30 years, possibly suggesting a selection effect.

The measure of alcohol consumption involves the fundamental question about the possible effect on the current risk of liver damage of previous alcohol consumption. The studies relating reported previous alcohol consumption to the current diagnosis of liver damage indicate that the damage does not occur unless the individual has been consuming alcohol daily for at least a number of days, the minimum reported for fatty liver being 10 days, and for alcohol hepatitis and cirrhosis being about 3 months. This demonstrates that a "memory" spanning at least 3 months is implicit in the risk function, in that the risk may be related to the consumption up until 3 months back in time. In agreement with this interpretation, intermittent or binge drinking seems to be associated with a lower risk of liver damage than steady drinking (Brunt et al. 1974, Grant et al. 1988, Sorensen et al. 1984).

Whether the consumption before this minimum period of time also influences the current risk of liver damage is still disputed. It is a common finding in the retrospective studies that the longer the duration of excessive alcohol consumption, the greater is the proportion of individuals who suffer from liver damage. This has been taken as evidence of a cumulative effect of alcohol consumption. It does not necessarily imply, however, that current risk is greater in those who have consumed excess alcohol for a long time as compared to those who have consumed alcohol only during the minimum time required for the risk to be established (Sorensen 1989). The finding may be a simple consequence of studying individuals subject to a constant risk induced by the current or immediately preceding consumption for variable periods of time. Even if the risk is constant per unit of time, it is obvious that the longer the individuals are at this risk, the greater is the number that will suffer from liver damage. The resolution of the problem requires prospective studies, of which only one addressing this problem has so far been conducted (Sorensen et al. 1984). The results suggested that how long alcohol-abusing men had been drinking in the past had no influence on their future risk of developing alcoholic cirrhosis.

The next question is about the relationship between the shape of the risk function and the amount of alcohol consumed per day over the minimum period of time required for the risk to be manifest. Implicit in this question is the special question about whether a threshold of consumption exists below which there is no risk of liver damage.

Several studies based on retrospective assessment of alcohol consumption at the time of diagnosis of liver damage, particularly liver cirrhosis, have addressed this question. Most of them found that the risk of liver damage increased by amount of alcohol consumed throughout the range reported. The amount below which no cirrhosis was found varied considerably between the studies and ranged from 20–160 g.

There are, as previously mentioned, several difficulties in interpreting these studies as answers to the question about the risk function, and about the safe limits in particular. In principle, the prospective study design, including longitudinal monitoring, will escape the difficulties.

The fact that only a minor proportion of individuals consuming excessive amounts of alcohol do develop the most severe form of liver damage, cirrhosis in particular, indicates that differences exist in exposure to other causal factors, among which at least one must be time-dependent and thereby determine the occasion at which the damage begins. Despite years of research, no consensus has been achieved on any one such factor (Bird and Williams 1988, Brunt 1988, Galambos 1987, Grant et al. 1988, Johnson and Williams 1985, Lieber 1991, Saunders 1984). Current research focuses on genetic factors (Devor et al.

1988, Hrubec and Omenn 1981), viral infections (Fong et al. 1988, Pagliaro et al. 1982, Parés et al. 1990, Saunders et al. 1983), and specific nutritional disturbances (Ainley et al. 1988, Derr et al. 1990, Nanji and French 1985, 1986b, Qiao et al. 1988, Rao et al. 1986, 1989, Rotily et al. 1990).

Type of alcoholic beverage (beer, wine, spirits) consumed has in several studies been excluded as vehicle of such a co-factor (Tuyns and Pequignot 1984). One exception is that the proportion of females among cirrhotics is higher in beer-drinking countries than in spirit- and wine-drinking countries (Nanji and French 1984).

To achieve progress in most of the areas lacking scientific consensus, we need substantial investment in prospective studies with proper assessment of alcohol consumption and liver pathology and, where appropriate, subsequent experimental intervention studies (Grant et al. 1988).

References

Adelasco L, Monarca A, Dantes M, et al. (1987) Features of chronic hepatitis in alcoholics. A survey in Milan. Liver 7:283–89

Agarwal DP, Goedde HW (1989) Enzymology of alcohol degradation. In Goedde HW, Agarwal DP (eds), Alcoholism. Biomedical and genetic aspects. Pergamon Press, New York, 3–20

Agarwal DP, Harada S, Goedde HW (1981) Racial differences in biological sensitivity to ethanol: the role of alcoholdehydrogenase and aldehyde dehydrogenase isoenzymes. Alcohol Clin Exp Res 5:12–16

Ainley CC, Senapati A, Brown IMH, et al. (1988) Is alcohol hepatotoxic in the baboon? J Hepatol 7:85–92

Alderman J, Kato S, Lieber CS (1989) The microsomal ethanol oxidizing system mediates metabolic tolerance to ethanol in deermice lacking alcohol dehydrogenase. Arch Biochem Biophys 271:33–39

Almdal TP, Sorensen TIA (1991) Incidence of parenchymal liver disease in Denmark, 1981 to 1985: analysis of hospitalization registry data. Hepatology 13:650–55

Alves PS, Correia JP, Borda d'Agua C, et al. (1982) Alcoholic liver diseases in Portugal. Clinical and laboratory picture, mortality and survival. Alcohol Clin Exp Res 6:216–24

Anderson P, Cremona A, Wallace P (1984) What are safe levels of alcohol consumption? Bri Med J 289:1657–58

Baptista A, Bianchi L, De Groote J (1981) Alcoholic liver disease: Morphological manifestations. Review by an international group. Lancet 1:707–11

Barak AJ, Beckenhauer HC (1988) The influence of ethanol on hepatic transmethylation. Alcohol Alcohol 23:73–77

Barak AJ, Tuma DJ, Beckenhauer HC (1985) Ethanol, the choline requirement, methylation and liver injury. Life Sci 37:789–91

Barry RE, McGivan JD (1985) Acetaldehyde alone may initiate hepatocellular damage in acute alcoholic liver disease. Gut 26:1065–69

Batey RG, Burns T, Benson RJ, Byth K (1992) Alcohol consumption and the risk of cirrhosis. Med J Aust 153:413–16

Behrens UJ, Hoerner M, Lasker JM, Lieber CS (1988) Formation of acetaldehyde adducts with ethanol-inducible P450IIE1 in vivo. Biochem Biophys Res Commun 154:584–90

Best CH, Hartroft WS, Lucas SS, Ridout JH (1949) Liver damage produced by feeding alcohol or sugar and its prevention by choline. Br Med J 2:1001–6

Bird GLA, Williams R (1988) Factors determining cirrhosis in alcoholic liver disease. Mol Aspects Med 10:97–105

Blackwelder WC, Yano K, Rhoads GG, et al. (1980) Alcohol and mortality: the Honolulu Heart Study. Am J Med 68:164–69

Bode C, Gast J, Zelder O, et al. (1987) Alcohol-induced liver injury after jejunoileal bypass operation in rats. J Hepatol 5:75–84

Bond AN, Wickramasinghe SN (1983) Investigations into the production of acetate from ethanol by human blood and bone marrow cells in vitro. Acta Haematol 69:303–13

Borowsky SA, Strome S, Lott E (1981) Continued heavy drinking and survival in alcohol cirrhotics. Gastroenterology 80:1405–9

Bosron WF, Lumeng L, Li T-K (1988) Genetic polymorphism and susceptibility to alcoholic liver disease. Mol Aspects Med 10:147–58

Bouchier IAD, Hislop WS, Prescott RJ (1992) A prospective study of alcoholic liver disease and mortality. J Hepatol 16:290–97

Bourliere M, Barthet H, Berthenzene P, et al. (1991) Is tobacco a risk factor for chronic pancreatitis and alcoholic cirrhosis? Gut 32:1392–95

Brillanti S, Barbara L, Miglioli M, Bonino F (1989) Hepatitis C virus: a possible cause of chronic hepatitis in alcoholics. Lancet 2:1390–91

Bruguera M, Bertrán A, Bombí JA, Rodés J (1977a) Giant mitochondria in hepatocytes. A diagnostic hint for alcoholic liver diseases. Gastroenterology 73:1383–87

Bruguera M, Bordas JM, Rodés J (1977b) Asymptomatic liver disease in alcoholics. Arch Pathol Lab Med 101:644–47

Bruix J, Barrera JM, Calvet X, et al. (1989) Prevalence of antibodies to hepatitis C virus in Spanish patients with hepatocellular carcinoma and cirrhosis. Lancet 2:1004–6

Brunt P (1988) The liver and alcohol. J Hepatol 7:377–83

Brunt PW, Kew MC, Scheuer PJ, Sherlock S (1974) Studies in alcoholic liver disease in Britain. Gut 15:52–58

Burnett, DA, Sorrell, MF (1981) Alcoholic cirrhosis. Clin Gastroenterol 10:443–55

Caballeria J, Baraona E, Lieber CS (1987) The contribution of the stomach to ethanol oxidation in the rat. Life Sci 41:1021–27

Caballeria J, Baraona E, Rodmilans M, Lieber CS (1989a) Effects of cimetidine on gastric alcohol dehydrogenase activity and blood ethanol levels. Gastroenterology 96:388–92

Caballeria J, Frezza M, Hernandez-Munoz R, et al. (1989b) The gastric origin of the first pass metabolism of ethanol in man: effect of gastrectomy. Gastroenterology 97:1205–9

Callans DJ, Wacker LS, Mitchell MC (1987) Effects of ethanol feeding and withdrawal on plasma glutathione elimination in the rat. Hepatology 7:496–501

Capocaccia R, Farchi G (1988) Mortality from liver cirrhosis in Italy: proportion associated with consumption of alcohol. J Clin Epidemiol 41:347–57

Carter EA, Isselbacher KJ (1971) The metabolism of ethanol to carbon dioxide by stomach and small intestinal slices. Proc Soc Exp Biol Med 138:817–19

Cederbaum AI (1987) Microsomal generation of hydroxyl radicals: its role in microsomal ethanol oxidising system (MEOS) activity and requirement for iron. Ann N Y Acad Sci 492:35–49

Chapheau M (1934) Action de la phlorizine et de l'acide iodoacetique sur la combustion de l'alcool ethylique chez le lapin. C R Soc Biol 116:887–89

Chiaramonte M, Farinati F, Fagiouli S, et al. (1990) Antibody to hepatitis C virus in hepatocellular carcinoma. Lancet 1:301–2

Christensen E, Schlichting P, Andersen PK, et al. (1986) Updating prognosis and therapeutic effect evaluation in cirrhosis with Cox's multiple regression model for time-dependent variables. Scand J Gastroenterol 21:163–74

Christoffersen P, Braendstrup O, Juhl E (1971) Lipogranulomas in human liver biopsies with fatty liver. A morphological, biochemical and clinical investigation. Acta Pathol Microbiol Scand 79:150–58

Coates RA, Halliday ML, Rankin JG, et al. (1986) Risk of fatty infiltration or cirrhosis of the liver in relation to ethanol consumption: a case-control study. Clin Invest Med 9:26–32

Colombo M (1992) Hepatocellular carcinoma. J Hepatol 15:225–36

Colombo M, Franchis Rd, Ninno ED, et al. (1991) Hepatocellular carcinoma in Italian patients with cirrhosis. New Engl J Med 325:675–80

Colombo M, Kwo G, Choo QL, et al. (1989) High prevalence of antibody to hepatitis C virus in patients with hepatocellular carcinoma. Lancet 2:1006–8

Colón I (1981) Alcohol availability and cirrhosis mortality rates by gender and race. Am J Public Health 71:1325–28

Colón I, Citter HSG, Jones WC (1982) Prediction in alcoholism from available alcohol consumption and demographic data. J Stud Alcohol 43:1199–1213

Coppéré H, Audigier JC (1986) Evolution de la mortalité par cirrhose en France entre 1925 et 1982. Gastroenterol Clin Biol 10:468–74

Corrao G, Arico S, Carle F (1991a) A case-control study on alcohol consumption and the risk of chronic liver disease. Rev Epidemiol Sante Publique 39:333–43

Corrao G, Arico S, Russo R (1991b) Alcohol consumption and non-cirrhotic chronic hepatitis: a case-control study. Int J Epidemiol 20:1037–42

Crapper RM, Bhathaland PS, Mackay IR (1983) Chronic active hepatitis in alcoholic patients. Liver 3:327–37

Cross CE, Halliwell B, Borish ET, et al. (1987) Oxygen radicals and human disease. Ann Int Med 107:526–45

Daft FS, Sebrell WH, Lillie RD (1941) Production and apparent prevention of a dietary liver cirrhosis in rats. Proc Soc Exp Biol Med 48:228–29

D'Amico G, Morabito VS, Pagliaro L, Marubini E (1986) Survival and prognostic indicators in compensated and decompensated cirrhosis. Dig Dis Sci 5:468–75

Derr RF, Porta EA, Larkin CA, Rao GA (1990) Is ethanol per se hepatotoxic? J Hepatol 10:381–86

Devor EJ, Reich T, Cloninger CR (1988) Genetics of alcoholism and related end-organ damage. Semin Liv Dis 8:1–11

Diehl AM (1989) Alcoholic liver disease. Med Clin North Am 73:815–30

DiLuzio NR, Hartman AD (1967) Role of lipid peroxidation on the pathogenesis of the ethanol-induced fatty liver. Fed Proc 26:1436–42

DiPadova C, Frezza M, Lieber CS (1988) Gastric metabolism of ethanol; implications for its bioavailability in men and women. In Kuriyama K, Takada A, Ishii H (eds), Biomedical and social aspects of alcohol and alcoholism. Elsevier, Barking, pp 81–84

DiPadova C, Worner TM, Julkunen RJK, Lieber CS (1987) Effects of fasting and chronic alcohol consumption on the first-pass metabolism of ethanol. Gastroenterology 92:1169–73

Duffy JC, Latcham RW (1986) Liver cirrhosis mortality in England and Wales compared to Scotland: an age-period-cohort analysis 1941–81. J R Statis Soc A 149:45–49

Durbec JP, Bidart JM, Sarles H (1979) Etude des variations du risque de cirrhose du foie en function de la consommation d'alcool. Gastroenterol Clin Biol 3:725–34

Edmondson HA, Peters RL, Frankel HH (1967) The early stage of liver injury in the alcoholic. Medicine 46:119–20

Edmondson HA, Peters RL, Reynolds TB (1963) Sclerosing hyaline necrosis of the liver in the chronic alcoholic. Ann Intern Med 59:646–53

Eghöje KN, Juhl E (1973) Factors determining liver damage in chronic alcoholics. Scand J Gastroenterol 8:505–12

Farchi G, Fidanza F, Mariotti S, Menotti A (1992) Alcohol and mortality in the Italian rural cohorts of the Seven Countries Study. Int J Epidemiol 21:74–82

Fernandez-Checa JC, Ookhtens M, Kaplowitz N (1987) Effect of chronic ethanol feeding on rat hepatocyte glutathione. Compartmentation, afflux and response to incubation with ethanol. J Clin Invest 80:57–62

Fiessinger N, Bernard H, Courtial J, Dermer L (1936) Combustion de l'alcool ethylique au cours de la perfusion du foie. C R Soc Biol 122:1255–58

Fisher MM, Rankin JG, eds (1977) Alcohol and the Liver. Plenum Press, New York, vol 3

Fong TL, Govindarajan S, Valinluck B, Redeker AG (1988) Status of hepatitis B virus DNA in alcoholic liver disease: a study of a large urban population in the United States. Hepatology 8:1602–4

Forsander OA, Räihä N, Salaspuro M, Mäenpää P (1985) Influence of ethanol on the liver metabolism of fed and starved rats. Biochemical J 94:259–65

French SW (1981) The Mallory body: structure composition and pathogenesis. Hepatology 1:76–83

French SW (1989) Biochemical basis for alcohol-induced liver injury. Clin Biochem 22:41–49

French SW, Benson NC, Sun PS (1984) Centrilobular liver necrosis induced by hypoxia in chronic ethanol-fed rats. Hepatology 4:912–17

French SW, Miyamoto K, Tsukamoto H (1986) Ethanol-induced hepatic fibrosis in the rat: role of the amount of dietary fat. Alcohol Clin Exp Res 10:13S–19S

Frezza M, DiPadova C, Pozzata G, et al. (1990) High blood alcohol levels in women: role of decreased gastric alcohol dehydrogenase activity and first pass metabolism. New Engl J Med 322:95–99

Furst CJ, Beckman LJ (1981) Alcohol-related mortality and alcohol consumption statistics. Stability of estimates for small areas. J Stud Alcohol 42:57–63

Gaines KC, Sakhany JM, Tuma DJ, Sorrell MF (1977) Reaction of acetaldehyde with human erythrocyte membrane proteins. FEBS Lett 74:115–19

Galambos JT (1987) Natural history of cirrhosis due to alcohol. In Tygstrup N, Orlandi F (eds), eds. Cirrhosis of the liver: methods and fields of research. Elsevier, Amsterdam, pp 307–22

Gallagher RP, Elwood JM (1980) Increase in alcohol related mortality in Canada, 1965–77 (letter). Lancet 2:775–76

Garagliano CF, Lilienfeld AM, Mendeloff AI (1979) Incidence rates of liver cirrhosis and related diseases in Baltimore and selected areas of the United States. J Chron Dis 32:543–53

Ginés P, Quintero E, Arroyo V, et al. (1987) Compensated cirrhosis: natural history and prognostic factors. Hepatology 7:122–28

Goedde HW, Agarwal DP (1989) Acetaldehyde metabolism: genetic variation and physiological implications. In Goedde HW, Agarwal DP (eds), Alcoholism. Biomedical and genetic aspects. Pergamon Press, New York, pp 21–56

Goedde HW, Harada S, Agarwal DP (1979) Racial differences in alcohol sensitivity: a new hypothesis. Hum Genet 51:331–34

Goldberg SJ, Mendenhall CL, Connell AM, Chedid A (1977) "Non-alcoholic" chronic hepatitis in the alcoholic. Gastroenterology 72:598–604

Goldschmith RH, Iber FL, Miller BA (1983) Nutritional status of alcoholics of different socioeconomic class. J Am Coll Nutr 2:215–20

Grant BF, Dufour MC, Harford TC (1988) Epidemiology of alcoholic liver disease. Semin Liv Dis 1:12–25

Graudal N, Leth P, Marbjerg L, Galloe AM (1991) Characteristics of cirrhosis undiagnosed during life: a comparative analysis of 73 undiagnosed cases and 149 diagnosed cases of cirrhosis, detected in 4929 consecutive autopsies. J Int Med 230:165–71

Haberman PW, Weinbaum DF (1990) Liver cirrhosis with and without mention of alcohol as cause of death. Br J Addict 85:217–22

Hall P, ed (1985a) Alcoholic Liver Disease. Edward Arnold, London

Hall PM (1985b) Pathological spectrum of alcoholic liver disease. Pathology 17:209–18

Halliday ML, Coates RA, Rankin JG (1991) Changing trends of cirrhosis mortality in Ontario, Canada, 1911–1986. Int J Epidemiol 20:199–208

Handler JA, Bradford BU, Glassman EB, et al. (1987) Inhibition of catalase-dependent ethanol metabolism in alcohol dehydrogenase-deficient deermice by fructose. Biochem J 248:415–21

Handler JA, Forman DT, Glassman EB, et al. (1988a) Hepatic catalase-dependent ethanol oxidation. In Kuriyama K, Takada A, Ishii H (eds), Biomedical and social aspects of alcohol and alcoholism. Elsevier, Excerpta Medica, Amsterdam, New York, pp 71–75

Handler JA, Koop DR, Coon MJ, et al. (1988b) Identification of P-450ALC in microsomes from alcohol dehydrogenase-deficient deermice: contribution to ethanol elimination in vivo. Arch Biochem Biophys 264:114–24

Hasumura Y, Teschke R, Lieber CS (1974) Increased carbon tetrachloride hepatotoxicity, and its mechanism, after chronic ethanol consumption. Gastroenterology 66:415–22

Hasumura Y, Teschke R, Lieber CS (1975) Acetaldehyde oxidation by hepatic mitochondria. Decrease after chronic ethanol consumption. Science 189: 727–29

Hawkins RD, Kalant H, Khanna JM (1966) Effects of chronic intake of ethanol on rate of ethanol metabolism. Can J Physiol Pharmacol 44:241–57

Hempel J, Bühler R, Kaiser R, et al. (1984) Human liver alcohol dehydrogenase. 1. The primary structure of the B1B1 isoenzyme. Eur J Biochem 145:437–45

Hempel JD, Pietruszko R (1979) Human stomach alcohol dehydrogenase: isoenzyme composition and catalytic properties. Alcohol Clin Exp Res 3:95–98

Hernandez-Munoz R, Caballeria J, Baraona E, et al. (1990) Human gastric alcohol dehydrogenase: its inhibition by H2-receptor antagonists, and its effect on the bioavailability of ethanol. Alcohol Clin Exp Res 14:946–50

Hillers VN, Massey LK (1985) Interrelationships of moderate and high alcohol consumption with diet and health status. Am J Clin Nutr 41:356–62

Hislop WS, Bouchier IA, Allan JG, et al. (1983) Alcoholic liver disease in Scotland and Northeastern England: presenting features in 510 patients. Q J Med 206:232–43

Hodges JR, Millward GH, Wright R (1982) Chronic active hepatitis: the spectrum of disease. Lancet 1:550–55

Hrubec Z, Omenn GS (1981) Evidence of genetic predisposition to alcoholic cirrhosis and psychosis: twin concordances for alcoholism and its biological end points by zygosity among male veterans. Alcohol Clin Exp Res 5:207–15

Hsu LC, Tani K, Fujiyoshi T, et al. (1985) Cloning of cDNAs for human aldehyde dehydrogenases 1 and 2. Proc Natl Acad Sci U S A 82:3771–75

Hunter DJW, Halliday ML, Coates RA, Rankin JG (1988) Hospital morobidity from cirrhosis of the liver and per capita consumption of absolute alcohol in Ontario, 1978 to 1982: a descriptive analysis. Can J Public Health 79:243–48

Hunter DJW, Halliday ML, Coates RA, Rankin JG (1989) Mortality and hospital morbidity from cirrhosis of the liver in relation to per capita consumption of absolute alcohol, education and native status, Ontario; 1978 to 1982. Clin Invest Med 12:230–34

Hurt RD, Higgins JA, Nelson RA, et al. (1981) Nutritional status of a group of alcoholics before and after admission to an alcoholism treatment unit. Am J Clin Nutr 34:386–92

Hyman MM (1981) "Alcoholic", "unspecified" and "other specified" cirrhosis mortality: a study in validity. J Stud Alcohol 42:336–43

Ijiri I (1974) Studies on the relationship between the concentrations of blood acetaldehyde and urinary catecholamine and the symptoms after drinking alcohol. Jpn J Stud Alcohol 9:35–39

Inoue K, Fukunaga M, Yamasawa K (1980) Correlation between human erythrocyte aldehyde dehydrogenase activity and sensitivity to alcohol. Pharmacol Biochem Behav 13:295–97

International Agency for Research on Cancer (1988) Alcohol drinking. IARC Monogr Eval Carcinog Risks Hum vol 44

International Group (1981) Alcoholic liver disease: morphological manifestations. Lancet 2:707–11

Ishak KG, Zimmerman HJ, Ray MB (1991) Alcoholic liver disease: pathologic, pathogenetic and clinical aspects. Alcohol Clin Exp Res 15:45–66

Israel Y, Oporto B, Macdonald AD (1984) Simultaneous pair-feeding system for the administration of alcohol-containing liquid diets. Alcohol Clin Exp Res 8:505–8

Israel Y, Orrego H (1981) Hepatocyte demand and substrate supply as factors in the susceptibility to alcoholic liver injury. Clin Gastroenterol 10:355–73

Israel Y, Orrego H, Schmidt W, et al. (1991) Trauma in cirrhosis: an indicator of the pattern of alcohol abuse in different societies. Alcohol Clin Exp Res 15:3:433–37

Israel Y, Videla L, Bernstein J (1975) Liver hypermetabolic state after chronic ethanol consumption: hormonal interrelationships and pathogenic implications. Fed Proc 34:2052–59

Iturriaga H, Bunout D, Hirsch S, Ugarte G (1988) Overweight as a risk factor or a predictive sign of histologic liver damage in alcoholics. Am J Clin Nutr 47:235–38

Jauhonen P, Baraona E, Lieber CS, Hassinen IE (1985) Dependence of ethanol-induced redox shift on hepatic oxygen tensions prevailing in vivo. Alcohol 2:163–67

Jauhonen P, Baraona E, Miyakawa H, Lieber CS (1982) Mechanism of selective perivenular hepatotoxicity of ethanol. Alcohol Clin Exp Res 6:350–57

Jennett RB, Sorrell MF, Saffar-Fard A, et al. (1989) Preferential covalent binding of acetaldehyde to the alpha-chain of purified rat liver tubulin. Hepatology 1:57–62

Johnson RD, Williams R (1985) Genetic and environmental factors in the individual susceptibility to the development of alcoholic liver disease. Alcohol Alcohol 20:137–60

Joliffe N, Jellinek EM (1941) Vitamin deficiencies and liver cirrhosis in alcoholics. Part VII. Cirrhosis of the liver. J Stud Alcohol 2:544–83

Jones BR, Barrett-Connor E, Criqui MH, Holdbrook MJ, (1982) A community study of calorie and nutrient intake in drinkers and nondrinkers of alcohol. Am J Clin Nutr 35:135–39

Julkunen RJK, DiPadova C, Lieber CS (1985a) First pass metabolism of ethanol—a gastrointestinal barrier against the systemic toxicity of ethanol. Life Sci 37:567–73

Julkunen RJK, Tannenbaum L, Baraona E, Lieber CS (1985b) First pass metabolism of ethanol: an important determinant of blood levels after alcohol consumption. Alcohol 2:437–41

Junge J, Bentsen KD, Christoffersen P, et al. (1988) Fibronectin as predictor of development of cirrhosis in alcohol abusing men. Br Med J 296:1629–30

Kaklamani E, Thrichopoulus D, Tzonou A, et al. (1991) Hepatitis B and C viruses and their interaction in the origin of hepatocellular carcinoma. JAMA 256:1974–76

Kalish GH, Di Luzio NR (1966) Peroxidation of liver lipids in the pathogenesis of the ethanol-induced fatty liver. Science 152:1390–92

Kawase T, Kato S, Lieber CS (1989) Lipid peroxidation and antioxidant defence system in rat liver after chronic ethanol feeding. Hepatology 10:815–21

Kenney WC (1982) Acetaldehyde adducts of phospholipids. Alcohol 6:412–16

Kessler BJ, Liebler JB, Bronfin GJ, Sass M (1954) The hepatic blood flow and splanchnic oxygen consumption in alcoholic fatty liver. J Clin Invest 33:1338–45

Kim C-I, Leo MA, Lowe N, Lieber CS (1988) Effects of vitamin A and ethanol on liver plasma membrane fluidity. Hepatology 4:735–41

Klatskin G (1961) Alcohol and its relation to liver damage. Gastroenterology 41:443–51

Klatsky AL, Friedman GD, Siegelaub AB (1981) Alcohol and mortality. A ten-year Kaisser-Permanente experience. Ann Int Med 95:139–45

Klatsky AL, Friedman GD, Siegelaub AB (1992) Alcohol and mortality. Ann Int Med 117:646–54

Kono S, Ikeda M, Ogata M, et al. (1989) The relationship between alcohol and mortality among Japanese physicians. Int J Epidemiol 12:437–41

Kono S, Ikeda M, Tokudome S, et al. (1989) Alcohol and mortality: a cohort study of male Japanese physicians. Int J Epidemiol 15:527–32

Kreitman N, Duffy J (1989) Alcoholic and non-alcoholic liver disease in relation to alcohol consumption in Scotland, 1978–84. Part I: epidemiology of liver diseases. Br J Addict 84:607–18

Lamboeuf Y, de Saint Blanquat G, Derache R (1981) Mucosal alcohol dehydrogenase- and aldehyde dehydrogenase- mediated ethanol oxidation in the digestive tract of the rat. Biochem Pharmacol 30:542–45

Lambouef Y, la Droitte P, De Saint DP (1983) The gastrointestinal metabolism of ethanol in the rat. Effect of chronic alcoholic intoxication. Arch Int Pharmacodyn Ther 261:157–69

Laskus T, Slusarczyk J, Lupa E, Cianciara J (1990) Liver disease among Polish alcoholics. Contribution of chronic active hepatitis to liver pathology. Liver 10:221–28

Lauterburg BH, Bilzer M (1988) Mechanism of acetaldehyde hepatotoxicity. J Hepatol 7:384–90

La Vecchia CL, DeCarli A, Mezzanotte G, Cislaghi C (1986) Mortality from alcohol related disease in Italy. J Epidemiol Community Health 40:257–61

Lee FI (1966) Cirrhosis and hepatoma in alcoholics. Gut 7:77–85

Leevy CM (1968) Fatty liver: a study of 270 patients with biopsy proven fatty liver and a review of the literature. Medicine 41:1445–51

Lelbach WK (1967) Leberschäden bei chronischem Alkoholismus. Teil III: Bioptisch-Histologische Ergebnisse. Teil IV: Diskussion und Schlussfolgerungen. Acta Hepatosplenol 14:9–39

Lelbach WK (1975) Cirrhosis in the alcoholic and its relation to the volume of alcohol abuse. Ann N Y Acad Sci 252:85–105

Lelbach WK (1976) Epidemiology of alcoholic liver disease. In Popper H, Schaffner F (eds), Progress in Liver Diseases. Grune & Stratton, New York, pp 494–515

Leloir LF, Munoz JM (1938) Ethyl alcohol metabolism in animal tissues. Biochem J 31:299–307

Leo MA, Lieber CS (1982) Hepatic vitamin A depletion in alcoholic liver injury in men. N Engl J Med 37:597–601

Leo MA, Lieber CS (1985) New pathway for retinol metabolism in liver microsomes. J Biol Chem 260:5228–31

Leo MA, Sato M, Lieber CS (1983) Effect of hepatic vitamin A depletion on the liver in humans and rats. Gastroenterology 84:562–72

Lewis KO, Paton A (1982) Could superoxide cause cirrhosis? Lancet 2:188–89

Lieber CS (1975) Liver disease and alcohol: fatty liver, alcoholic hepatitis, cirrhosis, and their interrelationships. Ann N Y Acad Sci 252:63–84

Lieber CS (1977a) Metabolism of ethanol. In Lieber CS (ed), Metabolic aspects of alcoholism. University Park Press, Baltimore, pp 1–29

Lieber CS (1977b) Pathogenesis of alcoholic liver disease: an overview. In Fisger MM, Rankin JG (eds), Alcohol and the liver. Plenum Press, New York, pp 197–225

Lieber CS (1982) Medical disorders of alcoholism: Pathogenesis and treatment. W.B. Saunders Company, Philadelphia

Lieber CS (1983) Precursor lesions of cirrhosis. Alcohol Alcohol 18:5–20

Lieber CS (1984) Alcohol and the liver: 1984 update. Hepatology 6:1243–60

Lieber CS (1988a) Metabolic effects of ethanol and its interaction with other drugs, hepatotoxic agents, vitamins, and carcinogens: a 1988 update. Semin Liv Dis 8:47–68

Lieber CS (1988b) Biochemical and molecular basis of alcohol-induced injury to liver and other tissues. New Engl J Med 319:1639–50

Lieber CS (1991a) Perspectives: do alcohol calories count? Am J Clin Nutr 54:976–82

Lieber CS (1991b) Hepatic, metabolic and toxic effects of ethanol: 1991 update. Alcohol Clin Exp Res 15:573–92

Lieber CS (1991c) Alcohol, liver and nutrition. J Am Coll Nutr 10:602–32

Lieber CS (1992) Alcoholic liver injury. Curr Opin Gastroenterol 8:449–57

Lieber CS, Baraona E, Hernandez-Munoz R, et al. (1989) Impaired oxygen utilization: a new mechanism for the hepatotoxicity of ethanol in subhuman primates. J Clin Invest 83:1682–90

Lieber CS, Casini A, DeCarli LM, et al. (1990) S-adenosyl-L-methionine attenuates alcohol-induced liver injury in the baboon. Hepatology 11:165–72

Lieber CS, DeCarli LM (1968) Ethanol oxidation by hepatic microsomes: adaptive increase after ethanol feeding. Science 162:917–918

Lieber CS, DeCarli LM (1970a) Hepatic microsomal ethanol-oxidizing system: *in vitro* characteristics and adaptive properties *in vivo*. J Biol Chem 245:2505–12

Lieber CS, DeCarli LM (1970b) Quantitative relationship between amount of dietary fat and severity of alcoholic fatty liver. Am J Clin Nutr 23:474–78

Lieber CS, DeCarli LM (1974) An experimental model of alcohol feeding and liver injury in the baboon. J Med Primatol 3:153–63

Lieber CS, DeCarli LM (1986) The feeding of ethanol in liquid diets: 1986 update. Alcohol Clin Exp Res 10:550–53

Lieber CS, DeCarli LM (1991) Hepatotoxicity of ethanol. J Hepatol 12:394–401

Lieber CS, DeCarli LM, Mak KM, et al. (1990a) Attenuation of alcohol-induced hepatic fibrosis by polyunsaturated lecithin. Hepatology 12:1390–98

Lieber CS, Jones DP, DeCarli LM (1965) Effects of prolonged ethanol intake: production of fatty liver despite adequate diets. J Clin Invest 44:1009–21

Lieber CS, Lasker JM, DeCarli LM, et al. (1988) Role of acetone, dietary fat and total energy intake in the induction of the hepatic microsomal ethanol oxidizing system. J Pharm Exp Ther 247:792–95

Lieber CS, Lefevre A, Spritz N, et al. (1967) Difference in hepatic metabolism of long- and medium-chain fatty acids: the role of fatty acid chain length in the production of the alcoholic fatty liver. J Clin Invest 46:1451–60

Lieber CS, Leo MA, Mak K, et al. (1985) Choline fails to prevent liver fibrosis in alcohol-fed baboons but causes toxicity. Hepatology 5:561–72

Lieber CS, Pignon J-P (1989) Ethanol and lipids. In Fruchart JC, Shepherd J (eds), Human plasma lipoproteins: chemistry, physiology and pathology. Walter De Gruyter, New York, pp 245–80

Lieber CS, Salaspuro M (1992) Alcoholic liver disease. In Millward-Sadler GH, Wright R, Arthur MJP (eds), Wright's liver and biliary disease. Saunders, London, pp 900–64

Lieber CS, Savolainen M (1984) Ethanol and lipids. Alcohol Clin Exp Res 8:409–23

Lieber CS, Schmid R (1961) The effect of ethanol on fatty acid metabolism: stimulation of hepatic fatty acid synthesis *in vitro*. J Clin Invest 40:394–99

Lin GWJ, Lester D (1980) Significance of the gastrointestinal tract in the in vivo metabolism of ethanol in the rat. Adv Exp Med Biol 131:281–86

Lin RC, Smith RS, Lumeng L (1988) Detection of a protein-acetaldehyde adduct in the liver of rat fed alcohol chronically. J Clin Invest 81:615–19

Lindros KO, Stowell A, Pikkarainen P, Salaspuro M (1980) Elevated blood acetaldehyde in alcoholics with accelerated ethanol elimination. Pharmacol Biochem Behav 13 (suppl 1):119–24

Lindros KO, Stowell A, Väänänen H, et al. (1983) Uninterrupted prolonged ethanol oxidation as a main pathogenetic factor of alcoholic liver damage: evidence from a new liquid diet animal model. Liver 3:79–91

Lint JD (1981a) Alcohol consumption and liver cirrhosis mortality. The Netherlands, 1950–78. J Stud Alcohol 42:48–56

Lint JD (1981b) The influences of much increased alcohol consumption on mortality rates: The Netherlands between 1950 and 1975. Br J Addict 76:77–83

Lischner MW, Alexander JF, Galambos JT (1971) Natural history of alcoholic hepatitis. 1. The acute disease. Dig Dis Sci 16:481–94

Lumeng L (1978) The role of acetaldehyde in mediating the deleterious effect of ethanol on pyridoxal 5-phosphate metabolism. J Clin Invest 62:286–93

Lundsgaard E (1938) Alcohol oxidation as a function of the liver. Compt Rend des Trav Lab Carlsberg (Kobenhavn) 22:333–37

Maddrey WC (1988) Alcoholic hepatitis: clinicopathologic features and therapy. Semin Liv Dis 8:91–102

Maier KP, Seitzer D, Haag G, et al. (1979) Verlaufsformen alkoholischer Lebererkrankungen. Klin Wochenschr 57:311–17

Mann RE, Smart RG, Anglin L, Adlaf EM (1991) Reductions in cirrhosis deaths in the United States: associations with per capita consumption and AA membership. J Stud Alcohol 52:361–65

Mann RE, Smart RG, Anglin L, Rush BR (1988) Are decreases in liver cirrhosis rates a result of increased treatment for alcoholism? Br J Addict 83:683–88

Marbet UA, Bianchi L, Meury U, Stadler GA (1987) Long-term histological evaluation of the natural history and prognostic factors of alcoholic liver disease. J Hepatol 4:364–72

Martin NG, Perl J, Oakshott JG, et al. (1985) A twin study of ethanol metabolism. Behav Genet 15:93–109

Matsuda Y, Baraona E, Salaspuro M, Lieber CS (1979) Effects of ethanol on liver microtubules and Golgi apparatus. Possible role in altered hepatic secretion of plasma proteins. Lab Invest 41:455–63

Matsuda Y, Takada A, Sato H, et al. (1985) Comparison between ballooned hepatocytes occurring in human alcoholic and nonalcoholic liver diseases. Alcohol Clin Exp Res 9:366–70

Mauch TJ, Donuhue TM, Zetterman RK, et al. (1984) Covalent binding of acetaldehyde to purified enzymes. Fed Proc 43:960–64

Maxwell JD (1985) Effect of coroner's rules on death certification for alcoholic liver disease. Br Med J 291:708

McGlashan ND (1980) The social correlates of alcohol-related mortality in Tasmania, 1971–1978. Soc Sci Med 14D:191–203

McSween RNM, Burt AD (1986) Histological spectrum of alcoholic liver disease. Semin Liv Dis 6:221–32

Medina VA, Donohue Jr TM, Sorrell MF, Tuma DJ (1985) Covalent binding of acetaldehyde to hepatic proteins during ethanol oxidation. J Lab Clin Med 105:5–10

Mendenhall CL (1985) VA Cooperative Study Group on Alcoholic Hepatitis: Clinical and therapeutic aspects of alcoholic liver disease. In Seitz HK, Kommerell B (eds), Alcohol related diseases in gastroenterology. Springer-Verlag, Berlin, pp 304–23

Mendenhall CL, Anderson S, Weesner RE, et al. (1984) Protein-calorie malnutrition associated with alcoholic hepatitis. Veterans Administration Cooperative Study Group on Alcoholic Hepatitis. Am J Med 76:211–22

Metcalf JP, Casey CAS, Sorrell MF, Tuma DJ (1987) Chronic ethanol administration alters hepatic surface membranes as evidenced by decreased concavalin A binding. Proc Soc Exp Biol Med 185:1–5

Mezey E (1989) Animal models for alcoholic liver disease. Hepatology 9:904–5

Mezey E (1991) Interaction between alcohol and nutrition in the pathogenesis of alcoholic liver disease. Semin Liver Dis 11:340–48

Mezey E, Potter JJ, French SW, et al. (1983) Effect of chronic ethanol feeding on hepatic collagen in monkeys. Hepatology 3:41–44

Mezey E, Potter JJ, Slusser RJ, et al. (1980) Effect of ethanol feeding on hepatic lysosomes in the monkey. Lab Invest 43:88–93

Mirsky IA, Nelson N (1939) The role of the liver in ethyl alcohol oxidation. Am J Physiol 126:P587–P588

Mizoi Y, Ijiri I, Tatsuno Y, et al. (1979) Relationship between facial flushing and blood acetaldehyde levels after alcohol intake. Pharmacol Biochem Behav 10:303–11

Montull S, Parés A, Bruguera M, et al. (1989) Alcoholic foamy degeneration in Spain. Prevalence and clinico-pathological features. Liver 9:79–85

Morgan MY (1981) Alcoholic liver disease: its clinical diagnosis, evaluation and treatment. Br J Alc Alcoholism 16:62–76

Morgan MY (1991) Alcoholic liver disease: natural history, diagnosis, clinical features, evaluation, management, prognosis, and prevention. In McIntyre N, Benhamou J-P, Bircher J, et al. (eds), Oxford Textbook of Clinical Hepatology. Oxford University Press, Oxford, pp 815–55

Morgan M, Camilo ME, Luck W (1981) Macrocytosis in alcohol related liver disease. Its value for screening. Clin Lab Haemat 3:35–44

Morgan MY, Sherlock S (1977) Sex-related differences among 100 patients with alcoholic liver disease. Br Med J 1:939–41

Morgan MY, Sherlock S, Scheuer PJ (1978) Acute cholestasis, hepatic failure and fatty liver in the alcoholic. Scand J Gastroenterol 13:299–303

Morton S, Mitchell MC (1985) Effects of chronic ethanol feeding on glutathione turnover in the rat. Biochem Pharmacol 34:1559–63

Nakano M, Worner TM, Lieber CS (1982) Perivenular fibrosis in alcoholic liver injury: ultrastructure and histologic progression. Gastroenterology 83:777–85

Nanji AA, French SW (1984) Increased susceptibility of women to alcohol: is beer the reason? (letter). N Engl J Med 311:1075–80

Nanji AA, French SW (1985) Relationship between pork consumption and cirrhosis. Lancet 1:681–83

Nanji AA, French SW (1986a) Correlations between deviations from expected cirrhosis mortality and serum uric acid and dietary protein intake. J Stud Alcohol 47:253–55

Nanji AA, French SW (1986b) Dietary factors and alcoholic cirrhosis. Alcohol Clin Exp Res 10:271–73

Nanji AA, Mendenhall CL, French AW (1989) Beef fat prevents alcoholic liver disease in the rat. Alcohol Clin Exp Res 13:15–19

Nasralah SM, Nassar VH, Galambos JT (1980) Importance of terminal hepatic venule thickening. Arch Pathol Lab Med 104:84–86

Natta PV, Malin H, Bertolucci D, Kaelber C (1985) The influence of alcohol abuse as a hidden contributor to mortality. Alcohol 2:535–39

Nebert DW, Adesnik M, Coon MJ, et al. (1987) The P450 gene superfamily: recommended nomenclature. DNA 6:1–11

Neville JN, Eagles JA, Samson G, Olson RE (1986) Nutritional status of alcoholics. Am J Clin Nutr 21:1329–40

Niemelä O, Juvonen T, Parkkila S (1990) Immunohistochemical demonstration of acetaldehyde-modified epitopes in human liver after alcohol consumption. J Clin Invest 87:1367–74

Nikkilä EA, Ojala K (1963) Role of hepatic l-glycerophosphate and triglyceride synthesis in the production of fatty liver by ethanol. Proc Soc Exp Biol Med 113:814–17

Nomura F, Lieber CS (1981) Binding of acetaldehyde to rat liver microsomes: enhancement after chronic alcohol consumption. Biochem Biophys Res Commun 100:131–37

Norstrom T (1987) The impact of per capita consumption on Swedish cirrhosis mortality. Br J Addict 82:67–75

Norton R, Batey R, Dwyer T, McMahon S (1987) Alcohol consumption and the risk of alcohol related cirrhosis in women. Br Med J 295:80–82

Nuutinen H, Lindros KO, Salaspuro M (1983) Determinants of blood acetaldehyde level during ethanol oxidation in chronic alcoholics. Alcohol Clin Exp Res 7:163–68

Ohnishi K, Lieber CS (1977) Reconstitution of the microsomal ethanol oxidizing system: qualitative and quantitative changes of cytochrome P-450 after chronic ethanol consumption. J Biol Chem 252:7124–31

Ontko JA (1973) Effects of ethanol on the metabolism of free fatty acids in isolated liver cells. J Lipid Res 14:78–85

Orholm M, Sorensen TIA, Bentsen KD, et al. (1985) Mortality of alcohol abusing men prospectively assessed in relation to history of abuse and degree of liver injury. Liver 5:253–60

Orrego H, Blake JE, Blendis LM, et al. (1987) Long-term treatment of alcoholic liver disease with propylthiouracil. N Engl J Med 312:1921–27

Orrego H, Carmichael FJ (1989) Alcohol, liver hypoxia and treatment of alcoholic liver disease with propylthiouracil. Alcohologia 1:15–30

Pagliaro L, Saracci R, Bardelli D, Filippazzo MG (1982) Chronic liver disease, alcohol consumption and HBsAg antigen in Italy: a multiregional case-control study. Ital J Gastroenterol 14:90–95

Pagliaro L, Simonetti RG, Craxi A (1983) Alcohol and HBV infection as risk factors for hepatocellular carcinoma In Italy: a multicentric, controlled study. Hepatogastroenterol 30:48–50

Parés A, Barrera JM, Caballería J, et al. (1990) Hepatitis C virus antibodies in chronic alcoholic patients: association with severity of liver injury. Hepatology 12:1295–99

Parés A, Bosch J, Bruguera M, Rodés J (1978) Características clínicas y criterios pronósticos en la hepatitis alcohólica. Gastroenterol Hepatol 1:118–23

Parés A, Caballería J, Bruguera M, et al. (1986) Histological course of alcoholic hepatitis: influence of abstinence, sex and extent of hepatic damage. J Hepatol 2:33–42

Parés A, Prats E, Bruguera M, et al. (1987) Predictive value of histological features in the progression of alcoholic fatty liver. J Hepatol 5:S177

Parrish KM, Higuchi S, Muramatsu T, et al. (1991) A method for estimating alcohol-related liver cirrhosis mortality in Japan. Int J Epidemiol 20:921–26

Patek AJ, Bowry SC, Sabesin SM (1976) Minimal hepatic changes in rats fed alcohol and high casein diet. Arch Pathol Lab Med 100:19–24

Patek Jr AJ, Toth IG, Saunders MG, et al. (1975) Alcohol and dietary factors in cirrhosis. An epidemiological study of 304 alcoholic patients. Arch Intern Med 135:1053–57

Paton A (1988) Alcohol: lessons from epidemiology. Proc Nutr Soc 47:79–83

Pequignot G (1961) Die Tolle des Alkohols bei der Atiologie von Leberzirrhosen in Frankreich. Munch Med Wochenschr 31:1464–68

Pequignot G, Tuyns AJ, Berta JL (1978) Ascitic cirrhosis in relation to alcohol consumption. Int J Epidemiol 7:113–20

Pestalozzi DM, Bühler R, von Wartburg JP, Hess M (1983) Immunohistochemical localization of alcohol dehydrogenase in the human gastrointestinal tract. Gastroenterology 85:1011–16

Peters RL (1977) Patterns of hepatic morphology in jejunoileal bypass patients. Am J Clin Nutr 30:53–57

Polokoff MA, Simon TJ, Harris A, et al. (1985) Chronic ethanol increases liver plasma membrane fluidity. Biochem 24:3114–20

Popper H, Lieber CS (1980) Histogenesis of alcoholic fibrosis and cirrhosis in the baboon. Am J Pathol 98:695–716

Porta EA, Hartroft WS, Comez-Dunn CLA, Koch OR (1967) Dietary factors in the progression and regression of hepatic alterations associated with experimental chronic alcoholism. Fed Proc 26:1449–57

Porta EA, Hartroft WS, De la Iglesia FA (1965) Hepatic changes associated with chronic alcoholism in rats. Lab Invest 14:1437–55

Prytz H, Anderson H (1988) Underreporting of alcohol-related mortality from cirrhosis is declining in Sweden and Denmark. Scand J Gastroenterol 23:1035–43

Prytz H, Skinhoj P (1980) Morbidity, mortality and incidence of cirrhosis in Denmark, 1976–1978. Scand J Gastroenterol 16:839–44

Qiao ZK, Halliday ML, Coates RA, Rankin JG (1988) Relationship between liver cirrhosis death rate and nutritional factors in 38 countries. Int J Epidemiol 17:414–18

Rao GA, Larkin EC, Porta EA (1986) Two decades of chronic alcoholism research with the misconception that liver damage occurred despite adequate nutrition. Biochem Arch 2:223–27

Rao GA, Larkin EC, Porta EA (1989) Is alcohol itself hepatotoxic independent of nutritional factors in nonalcoholic humans? Biochem Arch 5:1–9

Ray MB, Mendenhall CL, French SW, Gartside PS (1988) Serum vitamin A deficiency and increased intrahepatic expression of cytokeratin antigen in alcoholic liver disease. Hepatology 8:1019–26

Raymond L, Infante F, Voirol M, et al. (1985) Interaction des facteurs alcool et nutrition dans l'étiologie de la cirrhose hépatique, chez les hommes. Schweiz Med Wochenschr 115:998–1000

Rissanen A, Sarlio-Lähteenkorva S, Alfthan G, et al. (1987) Employed problem drinkers: a nutritional risk group? Am J Clin Nutr 45:456–61

Rogers AE, Fox JG, Gottlieb LS (1981) Effect of ethanol and malnutrition on nonhuman primate liver. In Berk PD, Chalmers T Ch (eds), Frontiers in liver disease. Georg Thieme Verlag, New York, pp 167–75

Roine RP, Salmela KS, Höök-Nikanne J, et al. (1992a) Alcohol dehydrogenase mediated acetaldehyde production by Helicobacter pylori—a possible mechanism behind gastric injury. Life Sci 51:1333–37

Roine RP, Salmela KS, Höök-Nikanne J, et al. (1992b) Colloidal bismuth subcitrate and omeprazole inhibit alcohol dehydrogenase mediated acetaldehyde production by Helicobacter pylori. Life Sci 51:195–200

Romelsjo A, Agren G (1985) Has mortality related to alcohol decreased in Sweden? Br Med J 291:167–70

Rotily M, Durbec JP, Berthezene P, Sarles H (1990) Diet and alcohol in liver cirrhosis: a case-control study. Eur J Clin Nutr 44:595–603

Rubin E, Lieber CS (1968) Alcohol induced hepatic injury in non-alcoholic volunteers. N Engl J Med 278:869–76

Salaspuro M (1989) The organ pathogenesis of alcoholism: liver and gastrointestinal tract. In Goedde HW, Agarwal DP (eds), Alcoholism: biomedical and genetic aspects. Pergamon Press, New York, pp 133–66

Salaspuro M (1991) Epidemiological aspects of alcohol and alcoholic liver disease, ethanol metabolism, and pathogenesis of alcoholic liver injury. In McIntyre N, Benhamou J-P, Bircher J, et al. (eds), Oxford textbook of clinical hepatology. Oxford University Press, Oxford, pp 791–810

Salaspuro MP, Lieber CS (1980) Comparison of the detrimental effects of chronic alcohol intake in humans and animals. In Eriksson K, Sinclair JD, Kiianmaa K (eds), Animal models in alcohol research. Academic Press, London, New York, pp 359–76

Salaspuro M, Lindros K (1985) Metabolism and toxicity of acetaldehyde. In Seitz HK, Kommerell B (eds), Alcohol related diseases in gastroenterology. Springer-Verlag, Berlin, Heidelberg, New York, Tokyo, pp 106–23

Salaspuro MP, Shaw S, Jayatilleke E, et al. (1981) Attenuation of the ethanol induced hepatic redox change after chronic alcohol consumption in baboons: metabolic consequences *in vivo* and *in vitro*. Hepatology 1:33–38

Sales J, Duffy J, Peck D (1989) Alcohol consumption, cigarette sales and mortality in the United Kingdom: an analysis of the period 1970–1985. Drug Alcohol Depend 24:155–60

Salmela KS, Roine RP, Koivisto T, et al. (1993) Characteristics of helicobacter pylori alcohol dehydrogenase. Gastroenterology, in press

Sato N, Kamada T, Kawano S, et al. (1983) Effect of acute and chronic ethanol consumption on hepatic tissue oxygen tension in rats. Pharmacol Biochem Behav 18:443–47

Sato M, Lieber CS (1981) Hepatic vitamin A depletion after chronic ethanol consumption in baboons and rats. J Nutr 111:2015–23

Saunders JB (1989) Treatment of alcoholic liver disease. Baillieres Clin Gastroenterol 3:39–65

Saunders JB, Davis M, Williams R (1981a) Do women develop alcoholic liver disease more readily than men? Br Med J 282:1140–43

Saunders JB, Walters JRF, Davies P, Paton A (1981b) A 20 year prospective study of cirrhosis. Br Med J 282:263–66

Saunders JB, Wodak AD, Morgan-Capner P, et al. (1983) Importance of markers of hepatitis B virus in alcoholic liver disease. Br Med J 286:1851–54

Saunders JB, Wodak AD, Williams R (1984) What determines susceptibility to liver damage from alcohol? (discussion paper). J R Soc Med 77:204–16

Schmidt, W (1977) The epidemiology of cirrhosis of the liver: a statistical analysis of mortality data with special reference to Canada. In Fisher MM, Rankin JG (eds), Alcohol and the liver. Plenum Press, New York, pp 1–26

Seeff LB, Cuccherini BA, Zimmerman HJ, et al. (1986) Acetaminophen hepatotoxicity in alcoholics (clinical review). Ann Int Med 106:399–404

Seitz HK, Kommerell B, eds (1985) Alcohol related diseases in gastroenterology. Springer-Verlag, Berlin

Shaw S, Jayatilleke E, Lieber CS (1988) Lipid peroxidation as a mechanism of alcoholic liver injury: role of iron mobilization and microsomal induction. Alcohol 5:135–40

Shaw S, Jayatilleke E, Ross WA, et al. (1981) Ethanol induced lipid peroxidation: potentiation by long-term alcohol feeding and attenuation by methionine. J Lab Clin Med 98:417–24

Shaw S, Rubin K, Lieber CS (1983) Decreased hepatic glutathione and increased diene conjugates in alcoholic liver disease: evidence of lipid peroxidation. Dig Dis Sci 28:585–89

Shibuya A, Yoshida A (1988) Genotypes of alcohol-metabolizing enzymes in Japanese with alcohol liver diseases: a strong association of the usual Caucasian-type aldehyde dehydrogenase gene (ALDH) with the disease. Am J Hum Gen 43:744–48

Skinhoj P, Prytz H (1981) Changing mortality from cirrhosis in Denmark 1965–1978. Scand J Gastroenterol 16:833–37

Skog OJ (1980) Liver cirrhosis epidemiology: some methodological problems. Br J Addict 75:227–43

Skog OJ (1984) The risk function for liver cirrhosis from lifetime alcohol consumption. J Stud Alcohol 45:199–208

Skog OJ (1985) The wetness of drinking cultures: a key variable in epidemiology of alcoholic liver cirrhosis. Acta Med Scand 703(suppl):157–84

Smart RG (1988) Recent international reductions and increases in liver cirrhosis deaths. Alcohol Clin Exp Res 12:239–42

Smart RG, Mann RE (1987) Large decreases in alcohol-related problems following a slight reduction of alcohol consumption in Ontario 1975–83. Br J Addict 82:285–91

Smart RG, Mann RE (1991) Factors in recent reductions in liver cirrhosis deaths. J Stud Alcohol 52:232–40

Smith DI, Burwell PW (1985) Epidemiology of liver cirrhosis morbidity and mortality in Western Australia, 1971–82: some preliminary findings. Drug Alcohol Depend 15:35–45

Smith T, DeMaster EG, Furne JK, et al. (1992) First-pass gastric mucosal metabolism of ethanol is negligible in the rat. J Clin Invest 89:1801–06

Sorensen TIA (1989) Alcohol and liver injury: dose-related or permissive effect. Br J Addict 84:581–89

Sorensen TIA, Bentsen KD, Eghoje K, et al. (1984) Prospective evaluation of alcohol abuse and alcoholic liver injury in men as predictors of development of cirrhosis. Lancet 2:241–44

Sorrell MF, Tuma DJ (1985) Hypothesis: alcoholic liver injury and the covalent binding of acetaldehyde. Alcohol Clin Exp Res 9:306–09

Suematsu T, Matsumura T, Sato N, et al. (1981) Lipid peroxidation in alcoholic liver disease in humans. Alcohol Clin Exp Res 5:427–36

Svendsen HO, Mosbech J (1977) Alcoholic cirrhosis of the liver in the Scandinavian countries 1961–1974. Int J Epidemiol 6:345–47

Takada A, Nei J, Matsuda Y (1982) Clinicopathological study of alcoholic fibrosis. Am J Gastroenterol 77:660–66

Takahashi H, Wong K, Jui L, et al. (1991) Effect of dietary fat on Ito cell activation by chronic ethanol intake: a long-term serial morphometric study on alcohol-fed and control rats. Alcohol Clin Exp Res 15:1060–66

Takase S, Takada N, Enomoto N, et al. (1991) Different types of chronic hepatitis in alcoholic patients: Does chronic hepatitis induced by alcohol exist? Hepatology 13:876–81

Taraschi TF, Rubin E (1985) Biology of disease. Effects of ethanol on the chemical and structural properties of biologic membranes. Lab Invest 52:120–31

Teschke R, Stutz G, Strohmeyer G (1979) Increased paracetamol-induced hepatoxicity after chronic alcohol consumption. Biochem Biophys Res Commun 91:368–74

Tsukamoto H, Towner SJ, Ciofalo LM, French SW (1986) Ethanol-induced hepatic fibrosis in the rat: role of the amount of dietary fat. Hepatology 6:814–22

Tsutsumi M, Lasker JM, Shimizu M, et al. (1989) The intralobular distribution of ethanol-inducible P450IIE1 in rat and human liver. Hepatology 10:437–46

Tuma DJ, Smith SL, Sorrell MF (1991) Acetaldehyde and microtubules. Ann N Y Acad Sci 625:786–92

Tuyns AJ, Esteve J, Pequignot G (1984) Ethanol is cirrhogenic, whatever the beverage. Br J Addict 79:389–93

Tuyns AJ, Pequignot G (1984) Greater risk of ascitic cirrhosis in females in relation to alcohol consumption. Int J Epidemiol 13:53–57

Tygstrup N, Juhl E (1971) The treatment of alcoholic cirrhosis. The effect of continued drinking and prednisone on survival. In Gerok W, Sicknger K, Hennekeuser HH (eds), Alcohol and the liver. FK Schattauer Verlag, Stuttgart, New York, pp 519–36

Uchida T, Kao H, Quispe-Sjogren M (1983) Alcoholic foamy degeneration. A pattern of acute alcoholic injury of the liver. Gastroenterology 84:683–92

Valentine GD, Ogden KA, Kortje DK, et al. (1987) Role of acetaldehyde in the ethanol-induced impairment of hepatic glycoprotein secretion in the rat in vitro. Hepatology 7:490–95

Välimäki M, Alfthan G, Pikkarainen J, et al. (1987) Blood and liver selenium concentrations in patients with liver diseases. Clin Chim Acta 166:171–76

Van Waes LV, Lieber CS (1977) Early perivenular sclerosis in alcoholic fatty liver, an index of progressive liver injury. Gastroenterology 73:646–50

Videla L, Israel Y (1970) Factors that modify the metabolism of ethanol in rat liver and adaptive changes produced by its chronic administration. Biochem J 118:275–81

Videla LA, Iturriaga H, Pino ME, et al. (1984) Content of hepatic reduced glutathione in chronic alcoholic patients: influence of the length of abstinence and liver necrosis. Clin Sci 66:283–90

von Wartburg JP, Bühler R (1984) Biology of disease. Alcoholism and aldehydism: new biomedical concepts. Lab Invest 50:5–15

Wagner JG (1986) Lack of first-pass metabolism of ethanol at blood concentrations in the social drinking range. Life Sci 39:407–14

Wallgren H, Barry III H, (1970) Prolonged exposure to alcohol. In Wallgren H, Barry H (eds), Actions of alcohol. Elsevier Publishing, Amsterdam, London and New York, vol II, pp 480–583

Wilkinson P, Santamaria JN, Rankin JG (1969) Epidemiology of alcoholic cirrhosis. Australas Ann Med 18:222–26

Williams GD, Grant BF, Stinson FS, et al. (1988) Trends in alcohol-related morbidity and mortality. Public Health Rep 103:592–97

Wilson RA (1984) Changing validity of the cirrhosis mortality-alcoholic beverage sales construct: U.S. trends, 1970–1977. J Stud Alcohol 45:53–58

Worner TM, Lieber CS (1985) Perivenular fibrosis as precursor lesion of cirrhosis. JAMA 253:627–30

Yamada S, Mak KM, Lieber CS (1985) Chronic ethanol consumption alters rat liver plasma membranes and potentiates release of alkaline phosphatase. Gastroenterology 88:1799–1806

Yoshida A, Hsu LC, Yasunami M (1991) Genetics of human alcohol-metabolizing enzymes. Prog Nucleic Acid Res Mol Biol 40:255–87

Zeisel SH, Da Costa K-A, Franklin PD, et al. (1991) Choline, an essential nutrient for humans. FASEB J 5:2093–98

Zysset T, Polokof MA, Simon FR (1985) Effect of chronic ethanol administration on enzyme and lipid properties of liver plasma membranes in long and short sleep mice. Hepatology 5:531–37

7

Breast Cancer

K. McPherson
University of London, United Kingdom

E. Engelsman
Amsterdam, The Netherlands

D. Conning
The British Nutrition Foundation, United Kingdom

Abstract

Some biological theory concerning mechanisms of breast cancer initiation suggests the potential for an association between the consumption of alcohol and increased breast cancer risk. While no such unambiguous and compelling biological mechanism suggests itself, this hypothesis has been the subject of some 30 epidemiological studies. In this report we seek to present the consensus of this research by reviewing the epidemiological evidence for a causative association between alcohol consumption and the risk of breast cancer.

The accumulated evidence suggests that there is possibly a weak association between alcohol consumption and breast cancer. Some studies seem to show a relationship with increasing amounts of consumption, but this is not necessarily a linear one. The possibilities of this association, however, seem not to be a cause of concern among the public in Europe.

Since the evidence of association is all nonexperimental, and since breast cancer is known to have an aetiology that remains unexplained in large measure, the definitive interpretation of this evidence is problematic. This is because the opportunities for important unknown confounding are large. In particular, aspects of diet (mostly regarding dietary fat but also other dietary patterns) have been shown to be associated with breast cancer risk, and these are likely to be associated independently with alcohol consumption.

Determining relevant exposures to foods that may be implicated in the risk of breast cancer is difficult. It is often past exposures, possibly decades previously, that are important, and recall or memory of these past exposures may be unreliable and possibly biased. In such circumstances of poorly identified possible risk factors that could be expected to correlate with alcohol use, the patterns of epidemiological findings reviewed are entirely consistent with no causative effect but show varying amounts of residual, possibly unmeasured, confounding.

Since experimental studies in which such confounding could be minimised are unlikely, the resolution of this question must await the ability to better adjust for such dietary or other confounding by knowing more about their roles as primary risk factors for breast cancer. This will involve prospective studies in which the consequences of contemporary dietary patterns are observed in the future.

In the meantime, any recommendation that women should limit their alcohol consumption specifically in order to reduce their risk of breast cancer cannot be supported or justified by the existing epidemiological evidence.

Introduction

Alcohol or ethanol is unlikely to be carcinogenic to the breast per se, but may facilitate the process of carcinogenesis by a number of recognised mechanisms. The main metabolite of ethanol, acetaldehyde, is carcinogenic in animal studies and during prolonged exposure might exhibit that effect in man. This is likely to occur only with heavy and prolonged consumption. Although heavy drinkers do carry an increased burden of cancer in general, there is no evidence that this can be attributed to increased exposure to acetaldehyde.

If ethanol is accepted as having promotional or cocarcinogenic properties, it is conceivable that it would enhance a cancerous response to any direct-acting carcinogens also present in alcoholic beverages. These have been identified, but their occurrence is variable and always at low concentrations. On a geographical basis, certain beverages produced and consumed to excess in certain localities have been associated with increased incidence of cancer, mainly of the oesophagus, larynx, and pharynx. Usually, however, the increase is small except in subjects who also smoked cigarettes. The coincidence of these tumour sites with those observed experimentally with diethylnitrosamine and dimethylnitrosamine has suggested to some that these volatile nitrosamines might be the prime carcinogens in specific alcoholic beverages. The available evidence falls far short of proof (Tuyns et al. 1979), and the evidence on the association of alcohol and these other cancers is being reviewed elsewhere by the relevant panel. Any extrapolation of such a mechanism to the breast would therefore be conjectural.

Since breast cancer clearly has, in part, a hormonal aetiology (Key and Pike 1988), any effect that alcohol may have on a woman's endogenous hormonal milieu might therefore indirectly affect risk. Such a postulate must remain imprecise, however, since the exact role of endogenous hormones remains poorly understood. Thus, in principle, such a mechanism could reduce, increase, or have no aggregate effect on risk.

Interest in any possible association between alcohol use and breast cancer was aroused empirically in 1977 in a report by Williams and Horm. From the population-based Third National Cancer Survey, 7518 incident cases had been interviewed about their lifetime use of tobacco and alcohol, as well as their socioeconomic status (SES). Associations were found for breast cancer and alcohol use and for breast cancer and SES. Comparisons of breast cancer patients and patients with other cancers were made, acknowledging the reasonable suspicion that tobacco, alcohol, and SES are sufficiently correlated to be powerful confounding variables in the observed association. Breast cancer exhibited a weak association with alcohol consumption.

Since then, a large number of epidemiological studies have been published, many confirming this association, but a substantial number failing to find any association, significant or otherwise. We have reviewed 11 cohort studies and 36 case-control studies, of which 7 cohort studies and 27 case-control studies supplied sufficient data to look for a dose-response relationship (see Figure 1). Around 40 articles commenting on the association, and about 40 articles suggesting and discussing biological mechanisms to explain any possible causal association, have been reviewed.

Possible Specific Associations

From these studies a large number of detailed possible specific associations between the consumption of alcohol and breast cancer emerge. These consist of any plausible combination of the following factors:

(1) Nature of consumption:
    (a) type of alcohol (e.g., beer, spirits, or wine);
    (b) quantity of consumption per week or per day; and
    (c) age at consumption, possibly relative to diagnosis of breast cancer.
(2) Nature of breast cancer:
    (a) premenopausal or
    (b) postmenopausal.
(3) Nature of the association:
    (a) causative or
    (b) associative only.

The dominant associations suggested consist of quite general but weak hypotheses of the effect of increasing daily alcohol consumption with increasing breast cancer risk. Nothing in the literature predicts a strong association of alcohol consumption with breast cancer. Since the consumption of alcohol is common and the incidence of breast cancer is high, this does not imply that the public health consequences of even

Figure 1

Relative risk of breast cancer by daily alcohol consumption in epidemiological studies

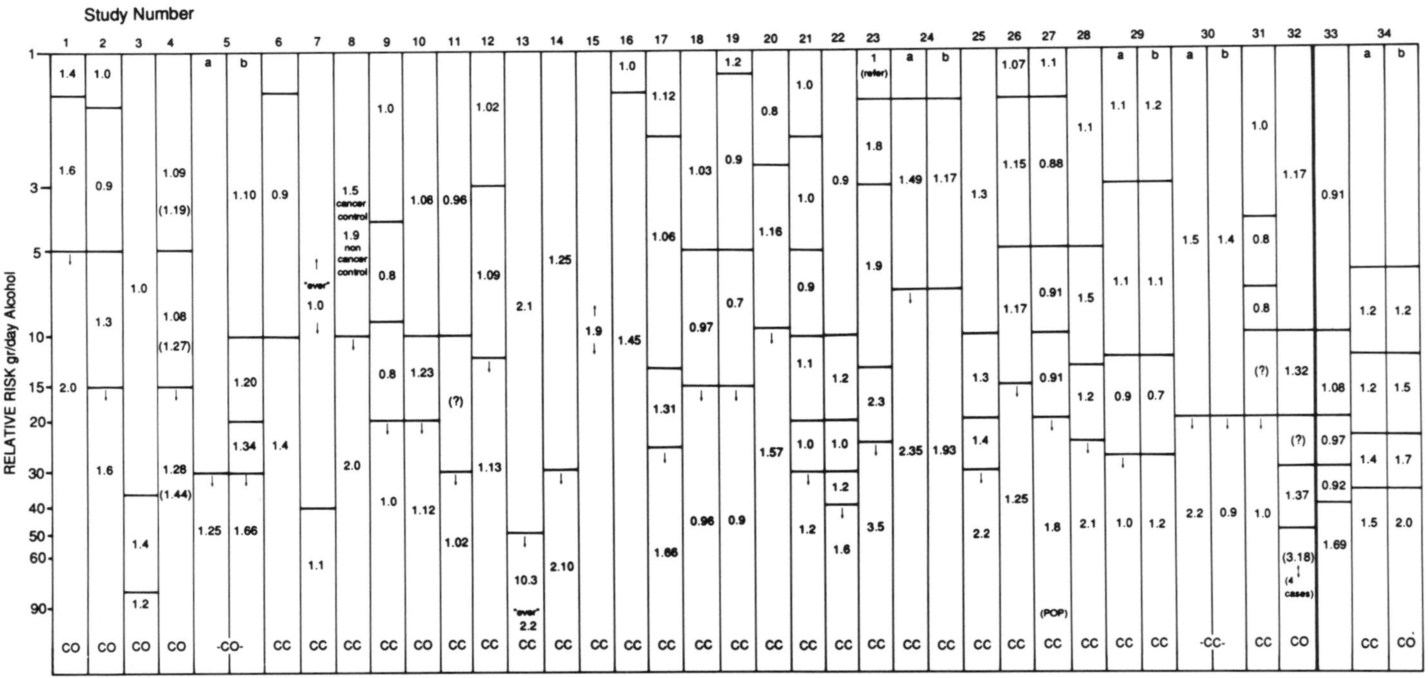

Studies listed: (1) Schatzin et al. 1989, (2) Willet et al. 1987a, (3) Hiatt and Bawol 1984, Hiatt et al. 1988a, (4) Gapstur et al. 1992, (5) Friedenreich et al. 1992 (a = overall, b = premenopausal breast cancer), (6) Begg et al. 1983, (7) Webster et al. 1983, (8) Rosenberg et al. 1982, (9) Rosenberg et al. 1990, (10) Simon et al. 1991, (11) Paganini-Hill and Ross 1983, (12) Byers and Funch 1982, (13) Talamini et al. 1984, (14) La Vecchia et al. 1985, (15) Lê et al. 1986, (16) O'Connel et al. 1987, (17) Harvey et al. 1987, (18) Harris and Wynder 1988, (19) Adami et al. 1988, (20) Rohan and McMichael 1988, (21) Chu et al. 1989, (22) Toniolo et al. 1989, (23) Richardson et al. 1989, (24) Young 1989 (a = alcohol 18–35 yrs, b = alcohol after 35 yrs), (25) La Vecchia et al. 1989, (26) Nasca et al. 1990, (27) Sneyd et al. 1991, (28) Ferraroni et al. 1991, (29) Meara et al. 1989, (30) Longnecker et al. 1992 (a = recent alcohol, b = alcohol less than 30 yrs old), (31) Miller et al. 1987, (32) Hiatt et al. 1988a, (33) Howe et al. 1991, (34) Longnecker et al. 1988 (a = case-control studies, b = cohort studies).

↑ **More than gr/day indicated**

CC - Case Control Study

CO - Cohort Study

a weak association will be trivial. These hypotheses are investigated by observational epidemiological study (case-control studies or cohort studies) in which consumption of alcohol is measured according to amounts and sometimes type, sometimes temporal relationships with consumption, and related to risk using conventional methods.

The responses to questions on consumption are generally categorised according to daily amounts, without detailed reference to the type of alcohol or to when it was consumed. Since any biological hypothesis is so poorly specified a priori, many of the above possible associations have been investigated, which of course compromises the interpretation of any positive findings. Dickersin et al. (1987), for instance, has published an extensive study of published and unpublished clinical trials that show the existence of a publication bias of positive findings of importance both to meta-analysis and reviews of the epidemiological literature.

As far as can be established, in spite of much epidemiological attention and some publicity, public concern about the possibility of an association between alcohol and breast cancer, at least in Europe, is minimal.

The Scientific Consensus Concerning Possible Specific Associations Between Alcohol and Breast Cancer Risk

We begin with the main hypothesis that alcohol consumption itself causes an increased breast cancer risk. A current consensus probably does exist and is best argued by Steinberg and Goodwin (1991), in which the epidemiological literature is well reviewed and summarised.

The consensus would be that there is currently insufficient evidence to support a general causative relationship between alcohol and breast cancer risk. The studies that do find an association find only a weak positive association (with a relative risk of around 1.5), and this is not consistently found. With such a weak association and a relatively poor understanding of the aetiology of breast cancer, it is therefore impossible to exclude systematic confounding with some known or unknown risk factor. No particular specific relationship stands out, except the possibility that the association is strongest for large amounts of reported daily alcohol consumption and strongest for premenopausal breast cancer.

Confounding will be present when the consumption of alcohol is itself associated with exposure to some independent established or unknown risk factor. The most likely confounding factors are some aspects of diet, for which many quite well-established candidates exist and which are often poorly measured. Moreover, the nature of the consumption empirically found to be associated with breast cancer risk is not sufficiently consistent.

Epidemiological Evidence

The epidemiological studies we have reviewed are obviously not of an evenly high methodological quality. A very important source of variation is the definition and measurement of the amount and timing of alcohol intake; how difficult this is for the interpretation may be illustrated by the following definitions used in some of these studies: recent use, recent and past use, lifetime use, usual intake, frequency of drinking, current use, use 3 years ago, use in preceding year, use preceding 5 years, use more or less than 4 days per week, use per week, moderate use, infrequent use, use per day, use per month, and use with meals.

For the dose-response relationship (see Figure 1), we have translated the use into grams of pure alcohol per day whenever possible. One drink (wine, beer, or liquor) is described as containing 9–13 grams of ethanol; we chose to regard "one drink" as containing 10 g. Moderate use usually means 5–10 g/day. The numbers of "heavy drinkers" (more than 30 g/day) are usually very low, and their estimated relative risks are correspondingly rather volatile.

Many studies worked with questionnaires that asked about present use and/or the use in the past year. Some studies mentioned use before age 30 or 35 or specified duration of use as less or more than 30 years. The ratio of nondrinkers/drinkers differs considerably in the studies (sometimes 84% nondrinkers, which is certainly not average); nondrinkers are defined in several ways: using less than 10 g/week (Talamini et al. 1984), not having used alcohol in the last 5 years (Webster et al. 1983), or just "ex drinkers" (Sneyd et al. 1991).

In some studies alcohol use is differentiated into wine, beer, liquor, and total use. Some case-control studies have used hospital controls (cancer controls, noncancer controls), but the more recent ones usually used population controls that were often matched on important confounding variables. The use of screening programs has a possible weakness, because controls are possibly self-selected because they have volunteered in the programme (Harvey et al. 1987).

There are considerable differences in the extent and type of the questionnaires used to elicit alcohol histories. Some studies specify that the interviews were taken at home, by trained interviewers. There is the ubiquitous problem (for alcohol consumption particularly) of possible underreporting, which if associated with disease status in case-control studies will result in bias. In cohort studies this information is collected before the diagnosis but may have been gathered long ago, and not all studies have reported new interviews more recently. Sometimes information has been collected by telephone (Nasca et al. 1990).

Some studies were designed specifically for examining the question of an association between alcohol and breast cancer (Williams and Horm 1977, Rosenberg et al. 1990), but many studies were started long ago and were reanalysed subsequently when the question of an association between alcohol and breast cancer was suggested. In one instance the questionnaires had been collected in 1959 (Garfinkel et al. 1988).

Well-known risk factors for breast cancer were usually but not always taken into account (age, age at menarche and age menopause, marital status, age at first full-term pregnancy, family history of breast cancer, etc.), but there are more possible confounding variables: oestrogen use, SES, different population groups, tobacco use, body mass, and dietary factors. The published relative risks are not always corrected for the latter risk factors and not always adjusted for most known confounding factors.

One small study on male breast cancer and alcohol use (Casagrande et al. 1981) found no association with alcohol use, but an association with high body mass at the age of 30 years. Rohan and Cook (1989) has found no association between benign breast lesions and alcohol consumption. Lindegard (1987) found no association between the prevalence of breast cancer and alcohol-related diseases in a large homogeneous population study (commented upon by Graham [1987b]).

Two papers have presented overviews or "meta-analyses" of a number of individual studies: Longnecker et al. (1989) calculated dose-response curves from the data out of 16 published studies. They fitted mathematical models to the pooled data from the available literature, including 21 studies. Quality assessments were undertaken, and some of the analyses were weighted by the assessed quality of the studies. These analyses concluded that a small relative risk, which was dose related in a linear fashion, was consistent with the overall data. For case-control studies, the estimated risk increased linearly to 1.5 for 36 g/day or more. The results of cohort studies indicated a slightly higher risk of around 2.0 and a steeper linear relationship (see Figure 1). These authors interpret their findings as no proof of causality but strongly supportive of an association between alcohol consumption and breast cancer.

Howe et al. (1991) has performed a formal meta-analysis with original data from six dietary case-control studies (including two published studies—Rohan and McMichael [1988] and Toniolo et al. [1989]). The results from these studies are also represented in Figure 1. This study represents the strongest evidence for a causative association of alcohol with breast cancer, because it consists of the raw data from the majority of studies undertaken in the world in which an attempt at obtaining detailed dietary histories was made, and for which dietary adjustments could therefore be made.

These authors conclude that the adjusted relative risk for 40 g/day or more of alcohol is 1.7 (see Table 1) and unity for any lower consumption. However, the estimates for this particular cutoff of consumption level are entirely derived from the data and not from any prior hypothesis possibly suggested by other studies. Moreover, this group consisted of only 91 cases and 72 controls, from among 3500 in total, who were consuming 40 g or more daily. This is a relatively high level of consumption and is therefore likely to be among selected individuals; in addition, since this dose relationship differs from the unadjusted analyses of Longnecker et al. (1988), it is difficult to regard these analyses as strong evidence for a causative relationship.

The authors conclude that the observed association is not due to confounding by a number of diet-related factors. This is justified, however, by their analysis that statistical adjustments of the relative risk associated with alcohol show little evidence of confounding with individual measured dietary components. What is unclear is the extent to which a complex of dietary adjustment alters the strength of this association. From the tabulations, it appears that the relative risk associated with 40 g or more per day drops from around 1.74 to 1.69 after adjustment for all recorded dietary components, from which some evidence for confounding is apparent. The effect that dietary adjustments had on the estimated relative risk of around unity for consumption of less than 40 g/day remains unclear. This is an important unanswered question.

Table 1
Relative risk of breast cancer by daily alcohol intake
from Howe et al. (1991)

Alcohol g/day	Number of cases	Number of controls	Relative Risk	95% Confidence interval
0–	523	607	1.0	Reference
< 10–	479	642	0.9	0.8–1.1
< 20–	282	376	1.1	0.9–1.3
< 30–	138	210	1.0	0.7–1.3
< 40–	60	76	0.9	0.6–1.4
40+	91	72	1.7	1.2–2.4

Finally, cigarette smoking must be mentioned in the context of this review because of the possibility of a strong correlation between tobacco and alcohol exposure among women. The evidence that might implicate tobacco in the aetiology of breast cancer is extremely weak, however. MacMahon (1990), for instance, in a review of the epidemiology, estimates the relative risk of breast cancer among smokers to be around 1.14 of the risk among nonsmokers. His review examines the role of alcohol as a confounder in this association and argues firstly that alcohol exhibits a weak association with breast cancer, and secondly, that in those studies of the role of tobacco in which adjustment for alcohol is made, the relative risk associated with cigarettes is not consistently elevated. Hence, for this discussion, since tobacco is not apparently a risk factor for breast cancer, it cannot be an important confounder in the observed association of alcohol with breast cancer. Just conceivably tobacco could be a negative confounder if exposure to cigarettes reduced the risk of breast cancer (Baron 1984) and was associated strongly with alcohol consumption.

Examining Particular Associations

Nature of Consumption

Type of Alcohol

Some investigators have found that risk of breast cancer seemed to be associated with a specific type of drink, such as wine or beer, while others did not find such a specific association. Two studies were mainly concerned with use of wine. Most data on alcohol use are expressed as ethanol per unit of time. The data on specific drinks do not allow any clear conclusions about specific risks, in spite of many attempts to identify such a relationship.

For instance, data from the most positive large combined study (Howe et al. 1991) estimate the adjusted relative risk of breast cancer per 10 g alcohol/day by kind of beverage as 1.08 for beer, 1.06 for wine, and 1.13 for spirits. Only the figure of 1.07 per 10 g of total alcohol is significantly different from unity, because of the overall increased relative risk associated with more than 40 g/day of 1.7.

Quantity of Consumption

As mentioned previously, the definitions of alcohol use in the literature are rather variable. It is probably impossible for anyone to give exact quantitative data on the consumption of alcoholic beverages. In addition, there is probably much underreporting in general, as illustrated by Rathje and Murphy (1992), who, by comparing reported alcohol use with the contents of collected empty bottles in the garbage among several communities, found underreporting of around 60%. Friedenreich et al. (1990) report a study on recall bias in a nested case-control study in the National Breast Screening Study. Many authors mention the possibility of a recall bias, especially in case-control studies, where the cases might tend to be influenced by the recent diagnosis. Further, the use of alcoholic drinks is often dependent on social occasions such as parties or holidays, and on personal situations such as conflicts, depressions, or loneliness.

For several reasons it is difficult to form a conclusion about an association in a number of studies. For instance, Kato et al. (1989) used categories for drinking like "ever" and "occasional" and performed comparisons between daily versus occasional use. Zaridse et al. (1991) found (in Russia) a very high risk of breast cancer with consumption as low as less than 0.1 g/day, compared to nondrinking. Ewertz (1991) found an increasing risk of breast cancer with increasing use of alcohol in a subgroup of women, aged 50–59 years, and with lowest fat intake. With an intake of more than 24 g alcohol/day the relative risk was 18, but this subgroup contained only 14 cases and 2 controls.

Van't Veer et al. (1989) did a neat case control study, but the relatively low number of cases was divided over several subgroups (quantity of consumption, pre/postmenopausal, age at first consumption). Data on past drinking were obtained for only 120 cases. There is, however, a rather strong association with breast cancer in premenopausal women using more than 30 g/day compared with 1–4 g/day (not in postmenopausal women). In pre- and postmenopausal women, relative risk is not increased with consumption of less than 30 g/day.

The consensus does not reach far enough to cover a relationship between the consequences and a particular dose or range of doses for the reasons discussed above.

Age at Consumption

Four studies have found intake prior to age 25–30 to be associated with risk (Hiatt et al. 1988a, Harvey et al. 1987, Young 1989, Van't Veer et al. 1989), and one study found no association (La Vecchia et al. 1989).

In principle this might be important if the postulated biological mechanism for a causative hypothesis involves early- or late-stage carcinogenesis or particular constituents of alcoholic beverage associated with particular kinds of drink. Thus, effects on early-stage carcinogenesis exclusively would be expected to be detected according to measured alcohol consumption over a long period of time, possibly as much as 20 years (McPherson et al. 1986), before diagnosis. The extent to which such consumption predicts more recent consumption will determine the relevance of empirical associations of recent consumption with breast cancer. Thus, a finding of no association of recent consumption with breast cancer risk only excludes any possible association of distant use if such use reliably predicts recent use patterns. The associations found are far too weak to inform, however.

Nature of Breast Cancer

Willet et al. (1987b), Hiatt et al. (1988b), and Rohan and McMichael (1988) report from subgroup analyses that alcohol is associated with a stronger effect among (essentially) premenopausal women. These particular effect modifications are not themselves significant, but demonstrating such effects usually lacks power. If anything, a consistently stronger association is shown, however.

Nature of the Association

The possibility of confounding in the observed relationship between alcohol and breast cancer should first be examined. If any association is observed in an epidemiological study between the consumption of alcohol and breast cancer incidence, then broadly speaking such an association is deemed to be causative if and only if (1) chance is an unlikely explanation, (2) aspects of selection of the subjects in the study could not explain the association, and (3) confounding could not explain the finding.

All published studies report the extent to which chance is a plausible explanation for the observed association, and most make attempts to avoid selection bias. Hence, for this discussion it can be assumed that the literature consists of studies for which the role of chance is well quantified and the role of subject selection is minimal.

Confounding is present if a known or unknown risk factor for breast cancer is correlated among individuals with alcohol consumption. Whether such confounding can explain the association must therefore depend on the extent of the breast cancer risk associated with the confounding variable and the extent of the correlation with alcohol consumption.

The problem is, of course, that confounding can be with an unknown risk factor. In breast cancer this is particularly important, because its aetiology is relatively poorly understood in the sense that variation in known risk factors does not explain a large proportion of the variation in incidence of the disease. This implies that unknown potent risk factors remain, and hence the ability to analyze the true role of confounding is compromised.

Most known risk factors for breast cancer bestow a relative risk of around 3 or more. Clearly, in a complicated carcinogenic process, some exposures could be truly primary risk factors with a small relative risk, if for instance they only affected the probability of a particular cellular change in a multistage carcinogenic process. However, in epidemiological investigations of breast cancer, relative risks of less than 2 are most plausibly a consequence of confounding with a more potent risk factor.

Since this association is estimated to be almost universally around 1.5 at most, confounding must remain the strongest candidate for an explanation. These unproven yet plausible arguments in research interpretation are the main barriers to a complete consensus.

Thus, by examining the Bradford Hill (1971) criteria for a causal association, we find (and these arguments are strongly supported by Steinberg and Goodwin [1991]) that:

(1) There is a lack of consistency in the evidence; quite a number of studies do not find any association. There is, however, at least a suggestion of higher risk associated with more than moderate alcohol consumption.

(2) The associations found are not strong, with relative risks usually of the order of 1.5, and for individual higher-point estimates the

confidence limits are often rather wide and always include low relative risks close to unity.

(3) Dose-response gradients are observed in several studies, but the gradients are usually not monotonic, the maximum degree of risk being associated sometimes with intermediate levels of alcohol consumption. Some of the better studies seem to find an association only with quite extensive alcohol consumption. The one study that examined total alcohol exposure (La Vecchia et al. 1989) found no dose relationship. There is certainly no consistent pattern, which would be expected in a causal association. The key study by Howe et al. (1991) finds an effect only at very high levels of reported daily consumption.

(4) Temporal relationships between exposure and risk were examined in five studies. Four found intake prior to age 25–30 to be associated with risk (Hiatt et al. 1988a, Harvey et al. 1987, Young 1989, Toniolo et al. 1989), and one study found no association (LaVecchia et al. 1989).

(5) Alcohol use should make a contribution that is specific and unambiguously independent of other known risk factors; only a few studies (Schatzkin et al. 1987, Willet et al. 1987a, Rohan and McMichael 1988, La Vecchia et al. 1989, Rosenberg et al. 1990) adjusted for dietary fat intake, which has been regarded as a risk factor. Of course, the meta-analysis by Howe et al. (1991) did adjust for dietary factors, but reported no confounding and rather inconsistent alcohol daily dose relationships.

(6) Epidemiologic consistency was found in the low breast cancer incidence and low alcohol consumption in Mormon women (Lyon 1980), and in the findings of rising breast cancer incidence with increasing alcohol consumption in the United States (Smith 1989, Glass and Hoover 1988). International and national correlation studies (La Vecchia and Franceschi 1982, La Vecchia et al. 1988, Pochin 1976, Kono and Ikeda 1979, Wynder et al. 1990, Tuyns 1990, Henderson 1990) gave conflicting results, as did studies of breast cancer mortality and alcohol use (Breslow and Enstrom 1974, Pochin 1976, Kono and Ikeda 1979, Monson and Lyon 1975).

(7) Biologic plausibility is provided by, for instance, evidence that the primary metabolite of ethanol, acetaldehyde, does induce DNA replication and is mutagenic in cultured mammalian cells (Ristow and Obe 1978, Dellarco 1988). There is no evidence, however, that carcinogenic changes in mammary tissue have occurred as a consequence. Other evidence of promotional activity of ethanol or its metabolites is lacking.

The time span between menarche and first full-term pregnancy is known to be positively related to breast cancer risk, mediated possibly by exposure of the ductal system to repeated cycles of oestrogen and progesterone without progression to lactation (Drife 1981). It is conceivable that use of alcohol could increase the sensitivity of the breast to these exposures, either by delaying the metabolic degradation of these hormones by a hepatotoxic effect or by increasing the production of electrophilic compounds through induction of microsomal oxidases. There is no evidence to support either of these opposing mechanisms, nor is it likely that such an effect will be demonstrated since, if present, such an effect is likely to be small.

A similar result might be expected if alcohol consumption resulted in suppression of prolactin secretion by direct inhibition or through the stimulation of, for example, dopamine release. There is experimental evidence to support the suppression of prolactin by prolonged alcohol administration (Schrauzer et al. 1979). In man (male volunteers), alcohol was found to slightly increase prolactin levels in response to thyrotrophin-releasing hormone (TRH) but was followed by a phase in which TRH was without effect (Ylikahri et al. 1976). It is thus conceivable that chronic alcohol consumption leads to prolonged repression of the prolactic response, but there is no evidence in support of this.

(8) The association between alcohol consumption and cancer of the tongue, mouth, larynx, and oesophagus is rather strong, but in these cancers there is a very strong suggestion of a local carcinogenic effect. In the breast, the evidence for such an effect does not exist; moreover, breast cancer shares no risk factors with these cancers.

(9) Experimental evidence is not available and not likely to become available; it is difficult to postulate randomized controlled studies of alcohol intake.

Conclusions

A causative association of alcohol consumption and breast cancer certainly cannot be confirmed, but also cannot be finally excluded. However, all of the evidence would exclude a strong causative association. There is certainly the greatest possibility that the weak association found is an association only, a consequence of alcohol being related to a risk factor or factors that are as yet poorly understood or poorly measured.

Thus, efforts in research into the aetiology of breast cancer must concentrate on the identification of presently poorly understood risk factors that are most likely to explain this association. Of these, aspects of diet appear to be the most plausible, or some other life-style characteristic that is as yet unidentified. Tobacco is a most implausible confounding variable. Obviously, breast cancer is a major public health problem for which few practical interventions can offer any realistic hope of decreasing the burden of this disease.

New basic research into the biology of breast cancer aetiology clearly could ultimately suggest stronger hypotheses about the potential role of alcohol, which might then suggest more specific epidemiological hypotheses; inadequacies of adjustment for confounding will then be the object of particular attention.

The findings reviewed here do not depend on any particular piece of research, but rather the amalgamation of many studies. It is not clear to us that any hypothesis has received inadequate attention because of the biases of particular researchers, although it is fairly clear that alcohol, as a putative risk factor for serious disease, does attract more attention than might be appropriate, possibly because of its other social associations.

References

Adami HO, Lund E, Bergström R, Meirik O (1988). Cigarette smoking, alcohol consumption and risk of breast cancer in young women. Br J Cancer 58:823–27

Ames BN, Magaw R, Gold LS (1987) Ranking possible carcinogenic hazards. Science 236:271–80

Andrianopoulos G, Nelson RL (1987) Alcohol and breast cancer (letter). N Engl J Med 317:1286

Anonymous (1981) Two views of the causes of cancers (editorial). Nature 289:431–32

Anonymous (1985) Does alcohol cause breast cancer? (editorial). Lancet 1:1131–32

Anonymous (1988) Alcohol consumption and breast cancer. Nutr Rev 46:9–10

Anonymous (1990) Alcohol and cancer. (editorial). Lancet 335:634–35

Ballard-Barbash R, Schatzkin A, Taylor PR, Kahle LL (1990) Association of change in body mass with breast cancer. Cancer Res 50:2152–55

Baron JA (1984) Smoking and oestrogen related disease. Am J Epidemiol 119:9–22

Begg CB, Walker AM, Wessen B, Zelen M (1983) Alcohol consumption and breast cancer (letter). Lancet 1:2934

Beyers TE, Williamson DF (1991) Diet, alcohol, body size and the prevention of breast cancer. Dev Oncol 62:113–31

Blot WJ (1992) Alcohol and cancer. Cancer Res 52:2119–23

Boyd NF, McGuire V (1990) Evidence of association between plasma high-density lipoprotein cholesterol and risk factors for breast cancer. J Natl Cancer Inst 82:460–68

Breslow NE, Enstrom JE (1974) Geographic correlations between cancer mortality rates and alcohol-tobacco consumption in the United States. J Natl Cancer Inst 53:631–39

Byers T, Funch DP (1982) Alcohol and breast cancer. Lancet 1:799–800

Cairns J (1981) The origin of human cancers. Nature 289:353–57

Casagrande JT, Hanisch R, Pike MC, et al. (1981) A case-control study of male breast cancer. Cancer Res 48:1326–30

Chu SY, Lee NC, Wingo PA, Webster LA (1989) Alcohol consumption and the risk of breast cancer. Am J Epidemiol 130:867–77

Cohen M, Lippman M, Chabner B (1978) Role of pineal gland in aetiology and treatment of breast cancer. Lancet 2:814–16

Colditz GA (1990) The Nurses' Health Study: findings during 10 years of follow-up of a cohort of U.S. women. Curr Probl Obstet Gynecol Fertil 13:135–74

Dellarco VL (1988) A mutagenicity assessment of acetaldehyde. Mutat Res 195:1–20

Dickersin K, Chan S, Chalmers TC, et al. (1987) Publication bias and clinical trials. Contr Clin Trials 8:343–53

Drife JO (1981) Breast cancer, pregnancy and the pill. Br Med J 283:78

Drife JO (1991) Avoiding hormone-related risk factors. Dev Oncol 62:61–72

Driver HE, Swann PF (1987) Alcohol and human cancer. Anticancer Res 7:309–20

Epstein SS, Swartz JB (1981) Fallacies of lifestyle cancer theories. Nature 289:127–30

Ewertz M (1991) Alcohol consumption and breast cancer risk in Denmark. Cancer Causes Control 2:247–52

Ewertz M, Gillanders S, Meyer L, Zedeler K (1991) Survival of breast cancer patients in relation to factors which affect the risk of developing breast cancer. Int J Cancer 49:526–30

Feinstein AR (1988) Scientific standards in epidemiologic studies of the menace of daily life. Science 242:1257–63

Ferraroni M, Decarli A, Willett WC, Marubini E (1991) Alcohol and breast cancer risk: a case-control study from northern Italy. Int J Epidemiol 20:859–64

Fraenkel-Conrat H, Singer B (1988) Nucleoside adducts are formed by cooperative reaction of acetaldehyde and alcohols: possible mechanism for the role of ethanol in carcinogenesis. Proc Natl Acad Sci 85:3758–61

Friedenreich CM, Howe GR, Miller AB (1990) Recall bias in the association of diet and breast cancer (abstract). Am J Epidemiol 132:783

Friedenreich CM, Howe GR, Miller AB, Jain MG (1992) Cohort study of alcohol consumption and risk of breast cancer (abstract). Society for Epidemiological Research, 25th Annual Meeting, June 9–12, no 307

Galaver JS (1987) The determinants of estrogen levels in post menopausal women. Diss Abstracts Internat 47:4127b

Galaver JS, Rosenblum ER, Eagon PK, et al. (1987) Alcohol and breast cancer (letter). N Engl J Med 317:1286–17

Gapstur SM, Potter JD, Sellers TA, Folsom AR (1992) Interaction of alcohol consumption and estrogen use on risk of breast cancer in postmenopausal women (abstract). Society for Epidemiological Research, 25th Annual Meeting, June 9–12, no 110

Garfinkel L, Boffetta P, Stellman SD (1988) Alcohol and breast cancer: a cohort study. Prev Med 17:686–93

Garro AJ, Lieber CS (1990) Alcohol and cancer. Annu Rev Pharmacol Toxicol 30:219–23

Glass A, Hoover RN (1988) Changing incidence of heart cancer. J Natl Cancer Inst 80:1076–77

Graham S (1987a) Alcohol and breast cancer. N Engl J Med 316:1211–12

Graham S (1987b) Alcohol and breast cancer (letter). N Engl J Med 317:1289

Graham S (1988) Alcohol and breast cancer. Biomed Pharmacother 42:298

Graham S, Hellmann R, Marshall J, et al. (1991) Nutritional epidemiology of postmenopausal breast cancer in western New York. Am J Epidemiol 134:552–66

Harris JR, Lippman ME, Veronesi U, Willet W (1992) Breast cancer. N Engl J Med 327:319–28

Harris RE, Spritz N, Wynder EL (1988) Studies of breast cancer and alcohol consumption. Prev Med 17:676–82

Harris RE, Wynder EL (1988) Breast cancer and alcohol consumption. A study in weak associations. JAMA 259:2867–71

Harvey EB, Schairer C, Brinton LA, et al. (1987) Alcohol consumption and breast cancer. J Natl Cancer Inst 78:657–61

Henderson B (1990) Summary report of the sixth symposium on cancer registries and epidemiology in the Pacific Basin. J Natl Cancer Inst 82:1186–90

Herbert V, Jayatilleke E, Shaw S (1987) Alcohol and breast cancer (letter). N Engl J Med 317:1287–88

Hiatt RA, Bawol RD (1984) Alcoholic beverage consumption and breast cancer incidence. Am J Epidemiol 120:676–83

Hiatt RA, Klatsky AL, Armstrong MA (1988a) Alcohol consumption and the risk of breast cancer in a prepaid health plan. Cancer Res 48:2284–87

Hiatt RA, Klatsky AL, Armstrong MA (1988b). Alcohol and breast cancer. Prev Med 17:683–85

Hill AB (1971) Statistical evidence and inference. In Hill AB (ed), Principles of medical statistics. Oxford University Press, London, pp 309–23

Hocman G (1988) Prevention of cancer: restriction of nutritional energy intake (joules). Comp Biochem Physiol 91A:209–20

Holm LE, Callmer E, Hjalmar ML, et al. (1989) Dietary habits and prognostic factors in breast cancer. J Natl Cancer Inst 81:1218–23

Howe G, Rohan T, Decarli A, et al. (1991) The association between alcohol and breast cancer risk: evidence from the combined analysis of six dietary case-control studies. Int J Cancer 47:707–10

Hulker BS (1988) Hormones, alcohol and breast cancer risk. Prev Med 17:695–96

International Agency for Research on Cancer (1988) Alcohol drinking. IARC Monogr Eval Carcinog Risks Hum 44

Janerich D (1988) Hormones, alcohol and breast cancer risk. Prev Med 17:696–97

Kato I, Tominaga S, Terao Ch (1989) Alcohol consumption and cancers of hormone-related organs in females. Jpn J Clin Oncol 19:202–07

Kelsey J, Berkowitz GS (1988) Breast cancer epidemiology. Cancer Res 45:5615–23

Key TJA, Pike MC (1988) The role of oestrogen and progetogens in the epidemiology and prevention of breast cancer. Eur J Cancer Clin Oncol 24:29–43

Kono S, Ikeda M (1979) Correlation between cancer mortality and alcoholic beverage in Japan. Br J Cancer 40:449–55

Kritchevsky D (1990) Nutrition and breast cancer. Cancer 66:1321–25

La Vecchia C, Decarli A, Franceschi S, et al. (1985) Alcohol consumption and the risk of breast cancer in women. J Natl Cancer Inst 75:61–65

La Vecchia C, Franceschi S (1982) Alcohol and breast cancer (letter). Lancet 1:621

La Vecchia C, Harris RE, Wynder EL (1988) Comparative epidemiology of cancer between the United States and Italy. Cancer Res 48:7285–93

La Vecchia C, Negri E, Parazzini F, et al. (1989) Alcohol and breast cancer: update from an Italian case control study. Eur J Cancer Clin Oncol 25:1711–17

Lê MG, Moulton LH, Hill C, Kramar A (1986) Consumption of dairy produce and alcohol in a case-control study of breast cancer. J Natl Cancer Inst 77:633–36

Lieber CS, Seitz HK, Garro AJ, Worner TM (1979) Alcohol-related diseases and carcinogenesis. Cancer Res 39:2863–66

Lindegard B (1987) Alcohol and breast cancer (letter). N Engl J Med 317:1285

Longnecker MP, Berlin JA, Orza MJ, Chalmers TC (1988) A meta-analysis of alcohol consumption in relation to risk of breast cancer. JAMA 260:652–66

Longnecker MP, Berlin J, Orza M, Chalmers TC (1989) Meta-analysis of alcohol and risk of breast cancer (letter). JAMA 261:383

Longnecker MP, Newcomb PA, Mittendorf R, et al. (1992) Risk of breast cancer in relation to past and recent alcohol consumption (abstract). Society for Epidemiological Research, 25th Annual Meeting, June 9–12, no 309

Lowenfels AB (1990) Alcohol and breast cancer (letter). Lancet 335:1216

Lund E, Koster Jacobsen B (1990) Use of oral contraceptives in relation to dietary habits and alcohol consumption. Contraception 42:171–77

Lyon JL, Gardner JW, Klauber MR (1976) Alcohol and cancer. Lancet 1:1243

Lyon JL, Gardner JW, West DW (1980) Cancer incidence in Mormons in Utah during 1917–75. J Nat Cancer Inst 65:1055–61

MacMahon B (1990) Cigarette smoking and cancer of the breast. Wald N, Baron J (eds), In Smoking and hormone related disorders. Oxford Univ Press, Oxford, England

Mantel N (1988) An analysis of two recent epidemiologic reports in The New England Journal of Medicine associating breast cancer in women with moderate alcohol consumption. Prev Med 17:672–75

McPherson K, Coope P, Vessey M (1986) Early oral contraceptive use and breast cancer—theoretical effects of latency. Br J Epidemiol Community Health 40:289–94

McSween RNM (1982) Alcohol and cancer. Br Med Bull 38:31–33

Meara J, McPherson K, Roberts M, et al. (1989) Alcohol, cigarette smoking and breast cancer. Br J Cancer 60:70–73

Mendelson JH, Lukas SE, Mello NK, et al. (1988a) Acute alcohol effects on plasma estradiol levels in women. Psychopharmacology 94:464–67

Mendelson JH, Mello NK (1988b) Chronic alcohol effects on anterior pituitary and ovarian hormones in healthy women. J Pharmacol Exp Ther 245:407–12

Miller AB (1990) Diet and cancer, a review. Reviews in Oncology 3, Acta Oncol 29:87–95

Miller DR, Rosenberg L, Clarke AE, Shapiro S (1987) Breast cancer risk and alcohol beverage drinking. Am J Epidemiol 126:736

Monson RR, Lyon JL (1975) Proportional mortality among alcoholics. Cancer 36:1077–79

Nasca PC, Baptiste MS, Field NA, et al. (1990) An epidemiological case-control study of breast cancer and alcohol consumption. Int J Epidemiol 19:532–38

O'Connel DL, Hulka BS, Chambles LE, Wilkinson WE (1987) Cigarette smoking, alcohol consumption, and breast cancer risk. J Natl Cancer Inst 78:229–34

Paganini-Hill A, Ross RK (1983) Breast cancer and alcohol consumption. Lancet 2:626–27

Peto R (1980) Distorting the epidemiology of cancer: the need for a more balanced overview. Nature 284:297–300

Pochin EE (1976) Alcohol and cancer of breast and thyroid (letter). Lancet 1:1137

Rathje W, Murphy C (1992) Rubbish, the archeology of garbage. Harper Collins, London-Glasgow

Reynolds P, Camacho T, Kaplan GA (1988) Alcohol consumption and breast cancer: prospective evidence from the Alameda County Study (abstract). Am J Epidemiol 128:930

Richardson S, de Vincenzi I, Pujol H, Gerber M (1989) Alcohol consumption in a case-control study of breast cancer in southern France. Int J Cancer 44:84–89

Ristow H, Obe G (1978) Acetaldehyde induces cross-links in DNA and causes sister-chromatid exchanges in human cells. Mutat Res 58:115–19

Rohan TE, Cook MG (1989) Alcohol consumption and risk of benign proliferative epithelial disorders of the breast in women. Int J Cancer 43:631–36

Rohan TE, McMichael AJ (1988) Alcohol consumption and risk of breast cancer. Int J Cancer 41:695–99

Rookus MA, Chorus AMJ, Nijboer C, et al. (1992) The association between alcohol consumption and breast cancer risk (abstract). Society for Epidemiological Research, 25th Annual Meeting, June 9–12, no 278

Rose DP (1988) Hormones, alcohol and breast cancer risk. Prev Med 17:694–95

Rosenberg L (1989) Meta-analysis of alcohol and risk of breast cancer (letter). JAMA 261:383

Rosenberg L, Palmer JR, Miller DR, et al. (1990) A case-control study of alcoholic beverage consumption and breast cancer. Am J Epidemiol 131:6–14

Rosenberg L, Slone D, Shapiro S, et al. (1982) Breast cancer and alcoholic-beverage consumption. Lancet 1:267–71

Schatzkin A, Carter CL, Green SB, et al. (1989) Is alcohol consumption related to breast cancer? Results from the Framingham Heart Study. J Natl Cancer Inst 81:31–35

Schatzkin A, Greenwald P, Byar DP, Clifford CK (1989) The dietary fat-breast cancer hypothesis is alive. JAMA 261:3284–87

Schatzkin A, Hoover RN, Carter CL, et al. (1987) Alcohol and breast cancer (letter). N Engl J Med 317:1288

Schatzkin A, Jones DY, Hoover RN, et al. (1987) Alcohol consumption and breast cancer in the epidemiologic follow-up study of the first National Health and Nutrition Examination Survey. N Engl J Med 316:1169–73

Schottenfeld D (1979) Alcohol as a co-factor in the etiology of cancer. Cancer 43:1962–66

Schrauzer GN, McGuiness JE, Ishmael D, Bell LJ (1979) 1. Effects of long term exposure to alcohol on spontaneous mammary adencarcinoma and prolactin levels in C3H/St mice. J Stud Alcohol 40:240–46

Shah PN, Mhatre MC, Kothari LS (1984) Effect of melatonin on mammary carcinogenesis in intact and pinealectomized rats in varying photoperiods. Cancer Res 44:3403–7

Simon M, Carman W, Wolfe R, Schottenfeld D (1990) Alcohol consumption and the risk of breast cancer: a report from the Tecumseh Community Health Study (abstract). Am J Epidemiol 132:784

Simon MS, Carman W, Wolfe R, Schottenfeld D (1991) Alcohol consumption and the risk of breast cancer: a report from the Tecumseh Community Health Study. J Clin Epidemiol 44:755–61

Skegg DCG (1987) Alcohol, coffee, fat, and breast cancer. Br Med J 295:1011–12

Sluyser M (1987) Borrel en borstkanker. Tijdschr Kanker 11:107

Smith DI (1989) Relationship between alcohol consumption and breast cancer morbidity rates in Western Australia 1971–84. Drug Alcohol Depend 24:61–65

Smithline F, Sherman L, Kolodny HD (1975) Prolactin and breast carcinoma. N Engl J Med 784–91

Sneyd MJ, Paul Ch, Spears GFS, Skegg DCG (1991) Alcohol consumption and risk of breast cancer. Int J Cancer 48:812–15

Spitz MR, Fueger JJ, Hsu TC (1990) The synergistic role of alcohol in mutagen-induced chromosome damage (abstract). Am J Epidemiol 132:784

Stampfer MJ, Colditz GA, Willett WC (1988) Alcohol intake and risk of breast cancer. Compr Ther 14:8–15

Steinberg J, Goodwin PJ (1991) Alcohol and breast cancer risk (review). Breast Cancer Res Treat 19:221–31

Stellman SC, Garfinkel L (1986) Smoking habits and tar levels in a New American Cancer Society, prospective study of 1.2 million men and women. J Natl Cancer Inst 76:1057–63

Stevens RG, Hiatt RA (1987) Alcohol and breast cancer (letter). N Engl J Med 317:1287

Stoll BA (1991) Approaches and prospects. Develop Oncol 62:229–35

Talamini R, La Vecchia C, Decarli A, et al. (1984) Social factors, diet and breast cancer in a northern Italian population. Br J Cancer 49:723–29

Tamarkin L, Cohen M, Roselle D, et al. (1981) Melatonin inhibition and pinealectomy enhancement of 7,12-dimethylbenz(a)anthracene-induced mammary tumours in the rat. Cancer Res 41:4432–36

Toniolo P, Riboli E, Protta F, et al. (1989) Breast cancer and alcohol consumption: a case-control study in northern Italy. Cancer Res 49:5203–6

Trichopoulos D, Brown J, MacMahon B (1987) Urine estrogens and breast cancer risk factors among post-menopausal women. Int J Cancer 40:721–25

Turner TB, Bennet VL, Hernandez H (1985) The beneficial side of moderate alcohol use. Johns Hopkins Med J 148:53–63

Tuyns AJ (1979) Epidemiology of alcohol and cancer. Cancer Res 39:2840–43

Tuyns AJ (1990) Alcohol-related cancers in Mediterranean countries. Tumori 76:315–20

Tuyns AJ, Pequignot G, Abbatucci JS (1979) Oesophageal cancer and alcoholic consumption. Importance of the type of beverage. Int J Cancer 23:443–47

United Kingdom National Case-Control Study Group (1990) Oral contraceptive use and breast cancer risk in young women: subgroup analyses. Lancet 335:1507–9

Vandenbroucke JP (1987) Borstkanker en alcoholgebruik in perspectief. Ned Tijdschr Geneeskd 131:2007–9

Van Potter R (1945) The role of nutrition in cancer prevention. Science 101:105–9

Van't Veer P, Kok FJ, Hermus RJJ, Sturmans F (1989) Alcohol dose, frequency and age at first exposure in relation to the risk of breast cancer. Int J Epidemiol 18:511–17

Van't Veer P, van Leer EM, Rietdijk A, et al. (1991) Combination of dietary factors in relation to breast cancer occurrence. Int J Cancer 47:649–53

Wachter KW (1988) Disturbed by meta-analysis? Science 241:1407–8

Webster LA, Wingo PA, Layde P, Ory HW (1983) Alcohol consumption and risk of breast cancer. Lancet 2:724–26

Weiss P (1945) Biological research strategy and publication policy. Science 101:101–4

Wickramasinghe SN, Gardner B, Barden G (1986) Cytotoxic protein molecules generated as a consequence of ethanol metabolism in vitro and in vivo. Lancet 2:823–26

Wijngaarden BJ (1989) From the National Institutes of Health. JAMA 261:2481

Willet WC (1989) The search for the causes of breast and colon cancer. Nature 338:389–93

Willet WC, Stampfer MJ, Colditz GA (1989) Does alcohol consumption influence the risk of developing breast cancer? Two views. In DeVita VT, Hellman S, Rozenberg SA (eds), Important advances in oncology. Lippincott, Philadelphia, pp 267–81

Willet WC, Stampfer MJ, Colditz GA, et al. (1987a) Moderate alcohol consumption and the risk of breast cancer. N Engl J Med 316:1174–80

Willett WC, Stampfer MJ, Colditz GA, et al. (1987b) Alcohol and breast cancer (letter). N Engl J Med 317:1288–89

Williams RR (1976) Breast and thyroid cancer and malignant melanoma promoted by alcohol-induced pituitary secretion of prolactin, TSH, and MSH. Lancet 1:996–99

Williams RR, Horm JW (1977) Association of cancer sites with tobacco and alcohol consumption and socioeconomic status of patients: interview study from the Third National Cancer Survey. J Natl Cancer Inst 58:525–47

Witorsch RJ (1987) Alcohol and breast cancer (letter). N Engl J Med 317:1288

Wynder EL (1988a) American health foundation workshop on alcohol and breast cancer. Introductory remarks. Prev Med 17:667–69

Wynder EL (1988b) Hormones, alcohol and breast cancer risk. Prev Med 17:698–99

Wynder EL, Fujita Y, Harris RE, et al. (1990) Comparative epidemiology of cancer between the United States and Japan. Cancer 67:746–63

Wynder EL, Harris RE (1989) Does alcohol consumption influence the risk of developing breast cancer? Two views. In DeVita VT, Hellman S, Rozenberg SA (eds), Important advances in oncology. Lippincott, Philadelphia, pp 283–93

Ylikahri RH, Huttunen MO, Härkönen M (1976) Effect of alcohol on anterior-pituitary secretion of trophic hormones (letter). Lancet 1:1353

Young Th (1989) A case-control study of breast cancer and alcohol consumption habits. Cancer 64:552–58

Zaridze D, Lifanova Y, Maximovitch D, et al. (1991) Diet, alcohol consumption and reproductive factors in a case-control study of breast cancer in Moscow. Int J Cancer 48:493–501.

8

Alcohol and Pregnancy

M. Plant
Edinburgh University, United Kingdom

F.M. Sullivan
St. Thomas's Hospital, United Kingdom

C. Guerri
Valencia Foundation of Biomedical Investigations, Spain

E.L. Abel
C.S. Mott Center, Michigan, United States

Abstract

This report considers available evidence on the possible adverse effects of maternal and paternal alcohol consumption on pregnancy and on the development of the foetus and the child. Both human and clinical studies support the conclusion that chronic heavy maternal drinking, consistent with a diagnosis of "alcohol dependence" or "alcoholism" is an aetiological factor giving rise to "foetal alcohol syndrome" (FAS). Animal studies have shown the teratogenic actions of alcohol. Even so, in humans, whether an individual child will have FAS appears to be dependent on a constellation of factors in addition to alcohol, including low socioeconomic status, poverty, poor maternal health, diet, problematic past obstetric history, tobacco use, and illicit drug use. Current evidence is not consistent in showing a clear-cut relationship between adverse effects in pregnancy or individual pathognomonic effects on the foetus or child and lower levels of maternal alcohol consumption. There is some evidence of a threshold of drinking below which adverse effects cannot be detected. Current evidence is insufficient to define where this threshold lies, but it may be around 30–40 g/day. It should be noted that this is well above the levels defined as moderate drinking. It is also possible that some alcohol-related birth defects may be male-mediated, since in most cases fathers of FAS children are also heavy drinkers.

Introduction

Foetal alcohol syndrome (FAS), also known as alcohol embryopathy, is characterized by a cluster of anomalies occurring in children of alcohol-dependent women. First described in 1973 by Jones and Smith and their colleagues (Jones and Smith 1973, Jones et al. 1973), this syndrome was identified in children born to women with highly atypical drinking patterns. The descriptions of these women clearly shows that they fit the diagnosis of alcohol-dependent or "alcoholic."[1]

The pattern of anomalies in FAS consists of defects in the following categories (Rosett 1980):

(1)   pre- and/or postnatal growth deficiency, including intrauterine growth retardation, small-for-dates, failure to thrive,

---

[1]Note that the term "alcohol-dependent" is used throughout this report. This employs the terminology introduced by the World Health Organization in 1979. Even so, it is noted that many authors still use the term "alcoholism" (Edwards et al. 1977).

and continuing growth below the 10th percentile for gestational age;

(2) morphological anomalies, including a distinctive facial appearance; and

(3) central nervous system dysfunction, including cognitive disabilities, the most serious of which is mental retardation.

In addition to the pattern of anomalies defining FAS, each of the following individual features have also been associated with drinking during pregnancy:

- intrauterine and postnatal growth retardation;
- limb anomalies;
- cardiac anomalies (ventricular and atrial septal defects);
- urogenital anomalies (labial hypoplasia, hydronephrosis);
- ophthalmological problems (myopia, optic nerve hypoplasia, strabismus);
- otological problems (hearing deficits, serious otitis media);
- neurophysiological anomalies;
- neuroanatomical anomalies; and
- behavioural problems (fine and gross motor dysfunction, attention deficit disorder/hyperactivity, autism, sleep disorders, poor sucking reflex).

Not all of these individual features are associated with heavy maternal alcohol consumption during pregnancy, however, and one or more of them may be present in a child completely independent of any alcohol intake by the mother. This has led to difficulties in unambiguously attributing effects to alcohol intake, especially at lower levels of consumption, because the lower the alcohol consumption, the greater the influence of confounding factors.

Consensus in relation to FAS, in contrast to individual alcohol-related birth defects, is based on the fact that FAS has specific criteria and is present only in women who have a clearly identified drinking problem (Sokol and Abel 1992).

Despite the ambiguity relating to the impact of low alcohol intake, there is a widespread public misperception that FAS and physical anomalies are inevitable, even at low levels of consumption. This has led to a situation where women have become unduly alarmed about their own drinking behaviour, regardless of the amount, and have been advised on (Jones et al. 1974) or have themselves requested termination of pregnancy after consuming even small amounts of alcohol.

In contrast to this public misperception, there is general agreement among clinicians and research scientists that only alcohol-dependent women are at risk of giving birth to children with FAS. Even so, even in alcohol-dependent women it is certainly not inevitable that this damage will occur. In some studies, the prevalence among alcohol-dependent women has been as high as 26% (Seidenberg and Majewski 1978), and in others as low as 2% (Sokol et al. 1980). There are no particular patterns and levels of alcohol consumption that have been consistently shown to characterise this condition (Majewski 1981). It is not clear why this variation has been observed, but it strongly suggests that other factors interact with alcohol to cause this syndrome. While we know that consumption of alcohol has the potential for causing FAS and individual alcohol-related birth defects, the influence of these other factors means that we are currently unable to establish a realistic threshold. This problem is compounded by the fact that all such threshold estimates are presently based on unreliable self-reported data (Ernhart et al. 1988, Jacobson et al. 1991, Verkerk 1992). There is some evidence, however, that a threshold may exist below which adverse effects have not been detected (Sokol 1986). This threshold has not been consistently shown but lies below 30–40 g of alcohol daily. It should be noted that this level of drinking (210–280 g/week) is well above what would be regarded as moderate drinking in women. For example the United Kingdom "recommended limits" of weekly alcohol consumption for nonpregnant women is around 120 g or less.

Although studies in animals have clearly demonstrated alcohol-related effects for individual anomalies (for a review see Abel 1984), the same relationship is not as clearly evident in the epidemiological literature (Sokol et al. 1980, Little 1977, Little et al. 1976, Day et al. 1989, Hingson et al. 1982, Tennes and Blackard 1980, Marbury et al. 1983, Mills and Graubard 1987, Weiler et al. 1991). This may be due to the fact that few of the studies have large enough numbers of heavy drinkers included in the sample.

Another reason for inconsistency in the epidemiological data, as discussed above, is that the individual features of FAS may result from a variety of adverse influences in pregnancy interacting with alcohol. These influences can be summarized in relation to (1) parental characteristics, (2) foetal development, and (3) child development.

Parental Characteristics

Maternal Factors

Majewski (1981) postulated that the critical factor for alcohol-related embryonic damage is the degree of severity of maternal alcohol dependence. In animal models it has also been shown that the stage of maternal alcohol illness, as indicated mainly by the extent of liver damage, plays an important role in the frequency and severity of in-utero alcohol effects in the rat (Sanchis et al. 1987). However, the role of peak blood-alcohol level must also be taken into account (Bonthius et al. 1988).

Apart from the extreme of FAS, there is little consensus about the relationship between moderate maternal alcohol consumption and specific foetal anomalies. For example, reports linking urogenital anomalies and cleft palate with in-utero alcohol exposure are at variance with all other epidemiological studies in this area (Mills and Graubard 1987, Weiler et al. 1991).

Studies in animals clearly show that the presence of individual abnormalities, such as low birth weight, depend on the amount of alcohol consumed and the stage of pregnancy at which it occurs. Craniofacial malformations and gross central nervous system alterations, for example, result from ethanol exposure on gestation day 7 in mice, corresponding to the third week of human gestation (Sulik et al. 1981, Sulik 1984). Hydronephrosis and limb malformations occur in mice if the animals are exposed to ethanol on gestation day 9 (equivalent to the late fourth week of human gestation). Limb malformations (hemimelia, adactylia, syndactyly, and polydactyl) are induced by ethanol administration on days 9 to 11 of gestation in mice and rats (see the review by Blakley 1988).

One reason for the inconsistencies in the epidemiological literature is that there is much less precision in measuring the timing of alcohol exposure, and hence increased variability in outcome.

Socioeconomic Status and Ethnicity

In nearly every case where FAS has been found, the mother has been of lower as opposed to upper socioeconomic status (Abel and Sokol 1987). In many societies this variable is closely linked with ethnicity, which of itself can be a risk factor for alcohol-related adverse pregnancy outcome (Abel and Sokol 1987).

Nutritional Status

Poor nutritional status is closely linked with low socioeconomic status; this is particularly true in women. This risk factor is exacerbated by heavy alcohol consumption. Alcohol has a high caloric value, and excessive consumption can lead to unbalanced nutrition with deficiency in micronutrients and vitamins, which are essential for maintenance of a healthy pregnancy.

Access to and Use of Prenatal Care

An important factor in healthy pregnancy outcome is good prenatal care. Lack of prenatal care is associated with an increased risk of poor pregnancy outcome, such as perinatal mortality. Prospective studies on drinking and pregnancy are mainly conducted in groups of women who attend clinics to receive prenatal care. In these cases, the proportion of women giving birth to babies with FAS is relatively low. One of the reasons for this may be the somewhat chaotic lifestyle of female problem drinkers, which suggests that they will be less likely to attend regular prenatal checks (Abel and Sokol 1991). Therefore, most of the "at-risk" women are not included in these studies. These "at-risk" women showing a severe lack of prenatal care are often the subject of clinical reports on FAS, however; prospective studies are therefore likely to underestimate the incidence of FAS.

Past Obstetric History

If a female problem drinker has given birth to one child with FAS, there is a greatly increased risk of subsequent children also being affected if the problem drinking continues (Abel 1988). There is also some evidence that, even if the woman stops drinking prior to pregnancy, her offspring may be of lower birth weight than normal (Little et al. 1980). Other risk factors identified in relation to past obstetric history are history of spontaneous abortion and previous obstetric problems (Plant 1985).

Age and Parity

These two factors are closely linked. Maternal age may be a risk factor simply because the older the woman, the greater the likelihood of a longer drinking history. Regardless of alcohol intake, the greater the parity and the older the mother, the greater the likelihood that later children will be damaged (Sokol et al. 1986).

Concomitant Drug Use

There is a strong association between heavy drinking, heavy smoking, and heavy caffeine use. All of these factors affect birth weight. In certain areas, particularly in the United States, use of illicit drugs such as marijuana, cocaine, and heroin is also high. The concomitant use of drugs and alcohol raises the possibility of additive or synergistic effects on the embryo/foetus.

Metabolic Factors

There has been much controversy over the role of acetaldehyde in the aetiology of FAS. Acetaldehyde has teratogenic (O'Shea and

Kaufman 1979, Dreosti et al. 1981, Campbell and Fantel 1983) and mutagenic (Obe 1981) potential, and high levels may be associated with adverse pregnancy outcome (Veghelly et al. 1978a, Guerri and Sanchis 1985). However, the precise role of acetaldehyde in FAS is still uncertain (Schenker et al. 1990).

General Health

The general health of alcohol-dependent women or other problem drinkers is often poor. Immune deficiency is commonplace among alcohol-dependent people (Plant 1992), and liver damage is commonly associated with heavy drinking. Poorer women living in areas of high social deprivation are at increased risk for sexually transmitted diseases. In all of these cases the body's nutritional reserves will be depleted, and the risk of poor pregnancy outcome will be increased.

The Role of Animal Models

Animal studies on the effects of alcohol in pregnancy allow many of the confounding factors present in human studies to be adequately controlled. Alcohol reduces foetal growth and development in animals, and this reduction is related to dose and time of exposure during pregnancy (Abel 1982a). In relation to spontaneous abortion, the blood threshold level in nonhuman primates is about 200 mg/dl (Clarren et al. 1990). Reduced birthweight occurs with blood levels above 100 mg/dl (Abel 1982), but some studies have reported thresholds at 70 mg/dl.

Genetic factors may increase the susceptibility to alcohol-induced damage, mediated either through foetal (Christoffel and Salafsky 1975) or maternal genotype. With respect to the latter, there is a direct relationship between maternal alcohol levels and the incidence of teratogenesis (Chernoff 1980, Gilliam et al. 1989). Since the genetic variability of human alcohol-metabolizing enzymes is greater than in animals (Bosron and Li 1986), greater variability in alcohol-induced effects should be expected in humans.

Animal models have attempted to establish the teratogenic actions of alcohol by controlling potential confounding variables, such as malnutrition. There is a possibility that adverse effects may result from interaction between high alcohol intake and its associated nutritional problems, but evidence on this is not consistent. Harm has been observed in a variety of laboratory animals including rats, dogs, swine, sheep, ferrets, and monkeys (see the review by Blakley 1988). Intra- and interspecies differences in susceptibility to "in-utero" alcohol toxicity have been found in many studies. For example, rats are less susceptible than mice to the teratogenic effects of alcohol, and there are differences in the effects of alcohol on mice, depending on the strain. A recent study with different strains of mice showed that the maternal genotype plays an important role in foetal weight deficits and malformations (Gilliam and Irtenkauf 1990). Some of the mechanisms suggested as being responsible for alcohol-related birth defects have been reviewed by Schenker et al. (1990) and include toxicity of ethanol versus acetaldehyde, possible contribution of impaired nutrition, foetal hypoxia, the role of prostaglandins, and the effect of ethanol on cell growth and membrane lipids.

Paternal Factors

In nearly every case of FAS where information on the father is available or has been reported, the father has been described as a heavy drinker or alcohol-dependent (Abel 1991). This raises the interesting possibility that some of the features of FAS may be male-mediated. For instance, cardiovascular problems in the offspring, such as ventricular septal defect, have been associated with paternal consumption (Savitz et al. 1991). There are also reports of small but significant decreases in birth weight in children whose fathers consumed alcohol (Sokol et al. 1993, Little and Sing 1987). Studies in animals suggest that there are also changes in behaviour (Abel and Lee 1988, Abel and Tan 1988, Abel and Bilitzke 1990) and immune function (Berk et al. 1989, Hazlett et al. 1989) in the offspring of alcohol-consuming males.

The influence of paternal drinking on foetal development does not relate directly to the teratogenicity of ethanol but to the mutagenic properties of the drug (Badr and Badr 1975). In addition, where the male has an alcohol-related problem, other risk factors for the pregnant partner may come into play, such as the possibility of violence and increased stress due to inconsistent behaviour that are often associated with heavy alcohol use. Nevertheless, alcohol consumption by the father could interact with effects due to maternal consumption. Hence, careful analysis of all variables would be needed to document a separate paternal effect in humans.

Foetal Development

In clearly identified alcohol-dependent women, FAS is present in 2–26% of their babies (Abel and Sokol 1987). As noted in more detail above, the diagnosis of FAS should only be made if components of all of the following are present:

(1) pre- and postnatal growth deficiency, including intrauterine growth retardation, small-for-dates, failure to thrive, and continuing growth below the 10th percentile.

(2) physical anomalies, the most common being a specific cluster of facial features; and

(3) central nervous system dysfunctions, including cognitive disabilities, mental retardation, and hearing and visual disabilities.

At lower alcohol intake not resulting in FAS, the effect on intrauterine growth is less consistent. In contrast to studies on smoking in pregnancy, where reduced birth weight is observed in almost all studies, such an effect is only occasionally found in studies of "moderate" maternal alcohol consumption in pregnancy. Since a very large number of social, environmental, and nutritional factors are involved in decreased birth weight, it appears that the contribution from moderate alcohol intake is low.

From a diagnostic viewpoint, unusual facial features are among the most common characteristics. By themselves, these facial features tend to become less distinctive as the child enters adolescence (Majewski 1981), but in some cases they may indicate underlying brain damage.

Central nervous system deficits include microcephaly, mental retardation, attention deficit disorder/hyperactivity, fine and gross motor problems, and speech and language difficulties (Streissguth et al. 1990, Church and Gerkin 1988, Kyllerman et al. 1985).

The most serious problem of all is mental retardation (IQ below 70), which occurs in about 50% of the children with FAS (Abel 1982b). The remaining 50% of children have IQs ranging from 70 to normal. A recent study in which maternal IQ rather than educational level or occupation was taken into account showed that alcohol consumption no longer significantly affected IQ in alcohol-exposed children who do not have FAS (Greene et al. 1991a). The contribution of parental IQ has not received adequate attention in many studies. A failure to consider attention deficits and hyperactivity in the parents may likewise lead to false attribution of effects in the children to maternal alcohol intake.

Alterations of the central nervous system are among the most dramatic consequences of "in utero" alcohol exposure. Cognitive dif-

ficulties, hyperactivity, motor impairment, attention deficits, and behavioural problems are some of the problems commonly found in
children of women who were heavy drinkers during pregnancy
(Lemoine et al. 1968; Jones and Smith 1973, Streissguth et al. 1990).
Of particular importance is the fact that a high percentage of FAS
children have sensory-neural hearing impairment (Church 1987,
Church and Gerkin 1988), a finding that has also been replicated in
animal studies (Church and Holloway 1984). Abnormal visual system
development (Stromland 1987) and visual perceptual difficulties have
also been noted (Aronson et al. 1985).

Rats prenatally exposed to alcohol (PBAL = 130–180 mg/dl) exhibit numerous behavioural alterations, such as hyperactivity (Bond
1988, Shaywitz et al. 1979), inability to inhibit a response (Abel 1982a;
Riley and Meyer 1984), impaired feeding (Riley and Rockwood 1984),
learning disabilities (Barron et al. 1988) and deficits in spatial memory
processes (Gianoulakis 1990). Some of these behavioural disfunctions
appear to diminish with age, but others, such as hyperactivity and impaired learning, may persist into adulthood (Abel and Dintcheff 1986,
Plonsky and Riley 1983, Randall et al. 1986). The presence of these behavioural anomalies and their persistence in children with FAS and
alcohol-related birth defects has not been studied systematically.

Child Development

Not only is birth weight low in FAS children, there is consistent
failure of such children to thrive, regardless of postnatal environmental
conditions (Streissguth et al. 1985). As noted previously, the distinct
facial features resulting from tend to become less pronounced as the
child grows older.

For FAS children with IQs below 70, IQ tends to remain relatively stable, with little improvement being seen with age. For those
with a lesser degree of impairment, some improvement may occur
with adequate stimulation, but this has not been studied. Additional
attention to education may be of value in this group.

In a recent large multicentre study where current alcohol intakes
were recorded, an adverse effect on growth was noted in women drinking the equivalent of 120 g/week, yet no lasting impairment, either
mental or physical, was noted when the children were examined at
18 months (Du Florey et al. 1992). Except for facial anomalies, a similar result was reported for children up to 4 years and 10 months of
age (Greene et al. 1991b).

In animal studies, catch-up growth may be observed following exposure to low ethanol doses within 15 or 23 days of birth in rats (Abel and Dintcheff 1978) and monkeys (Scott and Fradkin 1984). Body and brain weight of rats exposed pre- and postnatally to alcohol did not reach the values in the controls even at adulthood (Guerri 1987). Intrauterine and postnatal growth retardation are characteristic of foetal ethanol exposure and are strong indicators of foetal injury (Day et al. 1989, Greene et al. 1991b, Middaugh and Boggan 1991).

Conclusions and Discussion

Available evidence supports the conclusion that alcohol-dependent women who drink heavily during pregnancy may produce offspring exhibiting features of FAS. Such women also have an increased risk of experiencing spontaneous abortions. FAS, as noted above, is based on a pattern of defects rather than on one or two features unique to the offspring of alcohol-dependent women. The aetiology of FAS appears to be complex, and in addition to alcohol is related to maternal life-style and health. Whereas chronic heavy drinking is a necessary component in the aetiology of alcohol-related birth defects, other factors will also be present. Even though most alcohol-dependent women do not give birth to FAS babies, this does not mean that heavy alcohol consumption does not pose a danger to the embryo/foetus. Heavy alcohol consumption is invariably associated with a variety of causal factors related to poor pregnancy outcome, including low socioeconomic status; poverty; poor diet and general health; heavy use of tobacco; illicit drug use; and previous poor obstetric history. The contribution of these factors to FAS needs to be clarified.

It has not been consistently shown that low to moderate levels of maternal alcohol consumption cause harm to the foetus or the child. Alcohol consumption levels and patterns of use are both critical. Studies in animals indicate that the critical variable associated with brain damage is peak alcohol concentration (Bonthuis et al. 1988), with the threshold for damage at around 200 mg/dl (Bonthuis et al. 1988). This threshold may be lower in humans, however.

In some countries it is common to consume wine daily as part of a meal; in other countries alcohol intake tends to be episodic and less frequent. These would produce quite different blood alcohol levels with regard to peak concentration and duration of alcohol exposure, and therefore the rates of children born with FAS would also be different.

Adequate definitions of alcohol consumption are a prerequisite to any future epidemiological studies if the results are to be meaningful to the public. For instance, one drink in the United Kingdom contains 8 g of alcohol, while in the United States it contains 13 g. Epidemiological studies on the effects of maternal alcohol consumption at lower levels need to cover a broad range of confounding variables; concentrating solely on alcohol to the exclusion of other factors will not clarify the issue. A wider spectrum of postnatal development must also be considered. One area that has yet to be examined is the risk of psychopathological behaviour resulting from prenatal alcohol exposure. Focus should also encompass paternal drinking as well as other risk factors that may affect pregnancy outcome. Further longitudinal epidemiological studies should be undertaken in affected children, and follow-up should extend well into school age to identify which effects are permanent and which are transient. It should be noted, however, that environmental factors could easily confound this issue.

Due to the many difficulties in controlling for confounding in epidemiological studies, we believe there is a continuing role for experimental studies in animals. Animal studies are also relevant if we wish to identify the mechanism(s) responsible for alcohol-related birth defects. The fact that so many mechanisms have been proposed indicates the difficulty of identifying alcohol's true role in harming the embryo/foetus.

In summary, although many mechanisms have been proposed to explain the teratogenic effects of alcohol, it is quite possible that more than one mechanism is involved in FAS and that different features of FAS may be manifestations of different pathophysiologies. Clarifying the pathogenesis is important for developing mechanism-based pharmacological interventions and for identifying individual risk factors for susceptibility to the deleterious effects of in-utero alcohol exposure.

The effects of low levels of maternal alcohol intake on behavioural development of the child are too dependent on studies of the limited population. Studies from Seattle, for instance, have shown adverse behavioural effects associated with moderate maternal alcohol consumption (Streissguth et al. 1981). Studies from a number of other sites (e.g., Cleveland [Greene et al. 1991a]) or other countries have not replicated these findings (Gusella and Fried 1984, Larsson et al. 1985, Forrest et al. 1991, 1992). This is one of the reasons why further epidemiological studies are needed. Regarding the fourth objective charged to this panel, we are not aware of instances where hypotheses have received insufficient attention due to the bias of particular researchers.

Acknowledgments: Dr. R. Sokol, Wayne State University (United States), is gratefully acknowledged for his contribution in critically reviewing the manuscript.

References

Abel EL (1982a) In utero alcohol exposure and developmental delay of response inhibition. Alcoholism 6:369–76

Abel EL (1982b) Consumption of alcohol during pregnancy: a review of effects on growth and development of offspring. Hum Biol 54:421–53

Abel EL (1984) Fetal alcohol syndrome: animal studies. CRC Press, Florida.

Abel EL (1988) Fetal alcohol syndrome in families. Neurotoxicol Teratol 10:1–2

Abel EL (1991) Fetal Alcohol Syndrome. Medical Economics Books, Oradell, New Jersey

Abel EL, Bilitzke, P (1990) Paternal alcohol exposure: paradoxical effect in mice and rats. Psychopharmacology 100:159–64

Abel EL, Dintcheff BA (1978) Effects of prenatal alcohol exposure on growth and development in rats. J Pharmacol Exp Ther 207:916–21

Abel EL, Dintcheff BA (1986) Effects of prenatal alcohol exposure on behavior of aged rats. Drug Alcohol Depend 16:321–30

Abel EL, Lee JA (1988) Paternal alcohol exposure effects offspring behavior but not body or organ weights in mice. Alcohol Clin Exp Res 12:349–55

Abel EL, Sokol RJ (1987) Incidence of fetal alcohol syndrome and economic impact of FAS-related anomalies. Drug Alcohol Depend 19:51–70

Abel EL, Sokol RJ (1991) A revised conservative estimate of the incidence of FAS and its economic impact Alc Clin Exp Res 15(3)514–24

Abel EL, Tan SE (1988) Effects of paternal alcohol consumption on pregnancy outcome in rats. Neurotoxicol Teratol 10:187–92

Aronson M, Kyllerman M, Sabel KG, et al. (1985) Children of alcoholic mothers: developmental, perceptual, and behavioral characteristics as compared to matched controls. Acta Paediatr Scand 74:27–35

Badr FM, Badr RS (1975) Induction of dominant lethal mutation in male mice by ethyl alcohol. Nature 253:134–36

Barron S, Gagnon WA, Mattson SN, et al. (1988) The effects of prenatal alcohol exposure on odour associative learning in rats. Neurotoxicol Teratol 10:333–39

Berk RS, Nowicki-Montgomery I, Hazlett LD, Abel EL (1989) Paternal alcohol consumption: effect on ocular response and serum antibody response to Pseudomonas aeruginosa infection in offspring. Alcohol Clin Exp Res 13:795–98

Blakley PM (1988) Experimental teratology of ethanol. In Kalter H (ed), Issues and Reviews in Teratology. Plenum Publishing Corp., pp 237–82

Bond NW (1988) Prenatal alcohol exposure and offspring hyperactivity: effects of physostigmine and neostigmine. Neurotoxicol Teratol 10:59–63

Bonthius DJ, Goodlett CR, West JR (1988) Blood alcohol concentration and severity of microencephaly in neonatal rats depend on the pattern of alcohol administration. Alcohol 5:209–14

Bosron WF, Li TK (1986) Genetic polymorphism of human liver alcohol and aldehyde dehydrogenases, and their relationship to alcohol metabolism and alcoholism. Hepatology 6:502–10

Campbell MA, Fantel AG (1983) Teratogenicity of acetaldehyde in vitro: relevance to the fetal alcohol syndrome. Life Sci 32:2641–47

Chernoff GF (1977) The fetal alcohol syndrome in mice: an animal model. Teratology 15:223–30

Chernoff GF (1980) The fetal alcohol syndrome in mice. Mater Variables Teratol 22:71–75

Christoffel KK, Salafsky I (1975) Fetal alcohol syndrome in dizygotic twins. J Pediatr 87:963–67

Church MW (1987) Chronic in utero alcohol exposure affects auditory function in rats and humans. Alcohol 4:231–39

Church MW, Gerkin KP (1988) Hearing disorders in children with fetal alcohol syndrome: Findings from case reports. Pediatrics 82:147–54

Church MW, Holloway JA (1984) Effects of parental ethanol exposure on the postnatal development of the brainstem auditory evoked potential in the rat. Alcohol Clin Exp Res 8:258–65

Clarren SK, Astley SJ, Bowden DM, et al. (1990) Neuroanatomic and neurochemical abnormalities in nonhuman primate infants exposed to weekly doses of ethanol during gestation. Alcohol Clin Exp Res 14:674–83

Clarren SK, Smith DW (1978) The fetal alcohol syndrome. N Eng J Med 298:1063–67

Day NL, Jasperse MS, Richardson G, et al. (1989) Prenatal exposure to alcohol. Effect on infant growth and morphologic characteristics. Pediatrics 84:536–641

Dreosti JE, Ballard FJ, Belling GB, et al. (1981) The effect of ethanol and acetaldehyde on DNA synthesis in growing cells and on fetal development in the rat. Alcohol Clin Exp Res 5:357–62

Du Florey C, Taylor T, Bolumar F, et al. (1992) A European concerted action: maternal alcohol consumption and its relation to the outcome of pregnancy and child development at 18 months. Int J Epidemiol 21(suppl 1)

Edwards G, Gross MM, Moser J, Room R (1977) Alcohol-Related Disabilities. World Health Organization, Geneva

Ernhart CB, Morrow-Tlucak M, Sokol RJ, Martier S (1988) Under-reporting of alcohol use in pregnancy. Alcohol Clin Exp Res 12:506–11

Forrest FM, Florey C du V, Taylor DJ, et al. (1991) Reported social alcohol consumption during pregnancy and infants' development at 18 months. Br Med J 303:22–26

Forrest F, Florey C du V, Taylor D (1992) Maternal alcohol consumption and child development. Int J of Epidemiol 21(suppl 4):17–23

Gianoulakis C (1990) Rats exposed prenatally to alcohol exhibit impairment in spatial navigation test. Behav Brain Res 36:217–28

Gilliam DM, Irtenkauf KT (1990) Maternal genetic effects on ethanol teratogenesis and dominance of relative embryonic resistance to malformations. Alcohol Clin Exp Res 14:539–45

Gilliam DM, Kotch LE, Dudek BC, Riley EP (1989) Thanol teratogenesis in mice selected for differences in alcohol sensitivity. Alcohol 5:513–19

Greene T, Ernhart CB, Ager J, et al. (1991a) Prenatal alcohol exposure and cognitive development in the preschool years. Neurotoxicol Teratol 13:57–68

Greene T, Ernhart CB, Sokol RJ, et al. (1991b) Prenatal alcohol exposure and preschool physical growth: a longitudinal analysis. Alcohol Clin Exp Res 15:905–13

Guerri C (1987) Synaptic membrane alterations in rats exposed to alcohol. Alcohol Alcohol Suppl 1:467–72

Guerri C, Sanchis R (1985) Acetaldehyde and alcohol levels in pregnant rats and their fetuses. Alcohol 2:267–70

Gusella JL, Fried PA (1984) Effects of maternal social drinking and smoking on offspring at 13 months. Neurobehav Toxicol Teratol 6:13–17

Hazlett LD, Barrett RP, Berk RS, Abel EL (1989) Maternal and paternal alcohol consumption increase offspring susceptibility to P. aeruginosa ocular infection. Ophthalmic Res 21:381–87

Hingson R, Alpert JJ, Day N, et al. (1982) Effects of maternal drinking and marijuana use on fetal growth and development. Pediatrics 70:539–46

Jacob T, Bremer DA (1986) Assortive mating among men and women alcoholics. J Stud Alcohol 47:219–22

Jacobson SW, Jacobson JL, Sokol RJ, et al. (1991) Maternal recall of alcohol, cocaine and marijuana use during pregnancy. Neurotoxicol Teratol 13:535–40

Jones KL, Smith DW (1973) Recognition of the fetal alcohol syndrome in early infancy. Lancet 2:999–1001

Jones KL, Smith DW (1974) Offspring of chronic alcohol women. Lancet 2:349

Jones KL, Smith DW, Streissguth AP, Myrianthopoulos MC (1974) Outcome in offspring of chronic alcoholic women. Lancet 1:1076–78

Jones KL, Smith DW, Ulleland CN, Streissguth AP (1973) Pattern of malformation in offspring of chronic alcoholic mothers. Lancet 1:1267–71

Kyllerman M, Arouson M, Sokol KG, et al. (1985) Children of alcoholic mothers. Growth and motor performance compared to matched controls. Acta Paediatr Scand 74(1)20–26

Larsson G, Bohlin A-B, Tunnell R (1985) Prospective study of children exposed to variable amounts of alcohol in utero. Arch Dis Child 60:316–21

Lemoine P, Hurries H, Borteyru JP, Menuet JC (1968) Les enfants de parents alcooliques. Anomalies observées. A propos de 127 cas. Quest Med 21:476–92

Little RE (1977) Moderate alcohol use during pregnancy and decreased infant birth weight. Am J Public Health 67:1154–56

Little RE, Schultz FA, Mandall W (1976) Drinking during pregnancy. J Stud Alcohol 37(2)375–79

Little RE, Sing CF (1987) Father's drinking and infant birth weight: report of an association. Teratology 36:59–65

Little RE, Streissguth AP, Barr HM, Herman CS (1980) Decreased birth weight in infants of alcoholic women who abstain during pregnancy. J Pediatr 96:974–77

Majewski F (1981) Alcohol embryopathy: some facts and speculations about pathogenesis. Neurobehav Toxicol Teratol 3:129–44

Marbury MC, Linn S, Monson R, et al. (1983) The association of alcohol consumption with outcome of pregnancy. Am J Public Health 73:1165–68

Middaugh LD, Boggan WO (1991) Postnatal growth deficits in prenatal ethanol-exposed mice: characteristics and critical periods. Alcohol Clin Exp Res 15:919–26

Mills JL, Graubard BI (1987) Is moderate drinking during pregnancy associated with an increased risk for malformations? Pediatrics 80:309–24

O'Shea KS, Kaufman MH (1979) The teratogenic effect of acetaldehyde: implications for the study of the fetal alcohol syndrome. J Anat 128:65–76

Obe G (1981) Acetaldehyde not ethanol is mutagenic. In Kappas A (ed), Progress in environmental mutagenesis and carcinogenesis. Elsevier/North-Holland, Amsterdam, pp 19–23

Plant MA (1992) Alcohol, AIDS and sex. In Sherr L (ed), Heterosexual AIDS. Harwood, Reading (in press)

Plant MA, Plant ML (1992) Risk-takers: alcohol, drugs, sex and youth. Tavistock/Routledge, London, pp 76–87

Plant ML (1985) Women, drinking and pregnancy. Tavistock, London

Plonsky M, Riley EP (1983) Head-dipping behaviors in rats exposed to alcohol prenatally as a function of age at testing. Neurobehav Toxicol Teratol 5:309–14

Randall CL, Becker HC, Middaugh LD (1986) Effect of prenatal ethanol exposure on activity and shuttle avoidance behavior in adult C57 mice. Alcohol Drug Res 6:351–60

Riley EP, Meyer LS (1984) Considerations for the design, implementation, and interpretation of animal models of fetal alcohol effects. Neurobehav Toxicol Teratol 6:97–101

Riley EP, Rockwood GA (1984) Alterations in suckling behavior in preweaning rats exposed to alcohol prenatally. Pharmacol Biochem Behav 10:255–59

Rosett ML (1980) A clinical perspective of the fetal alcohol syndrome (editorial). Alcohol Clin Exp Res 4:119–22

Sanchis R, Sancho-Tello M, Chirivella M, Guerri C (1987) The role of maternal alcohol damage on ethanol teratogenicity in the rat. Teratology 36:100–208

Savitz DA, Schwingl PJ, Keele MA (1991) Influence of paternal age, smoking, and alcohol consumption on congenital anomalies. Teratology 44:429–40

Schenker S, Becker HC, Randall CL, et al. (1990) Fetal alcohol syndrome: current status of pathogenesis. Alcohol Clin Exp Res 14:635–47

Scott WJ, Fradkin R (1984) The effects of prenatal ethanol in cynomolgus monkeys maca fascicularis. Teratology 29:49–56

Seidenberg J, Majewski F (1978) Zur Haufigkeit der Alkoholembryopathis in den verschiedenen Phasen der mutterlichen Alkoholkrankheit (On the frequency of alcohol embryopathy in the different phases of maternal alcoholism). Suchtgefahren, Hamburg 24:63–75

Shaywitz BA, Griffieth GG, Warshaw JB (1979) Hyperactivity and cognistive defects in developing rat pups born to alcoholic mothers: an expanded fetal alcohol syndrome (FAS). Neurobehav Toxicol 1:113–22

Sokol RJ, Abel EL (1992) Risk factors for alcohol-related birth defects: threshold, susceptibility and prevention. In Sonderegger TB (ed), Perinatal substance abuse. Johns Hopkins University Press, Baltimore

Sokol RJ, Ager J, Martier S, et al. (1986) Significant determinants of susceptibility to alcohol teratogenicity. Ann N Y Acad Sci 477:87–102

Sokol RJ, Martier SS, Ager JW, et al. (1993) Paternal drinking may affect intrauterine growth. Society of Perinatal Obstetricians Abstracts (submitted)

Sokol RJ, Miller SI, Reed G (1980) Alcohol abuse during pregnancy: an epidemiologic study. Alcohol Clin Exp Res 4:135–45

Streissguth AP, Barr EM, Sampson PD (1990) Moderate prenatal alcohol exposure: effects on child IQ and learning problems at age 7½ years. Alcohol Clin Exp Res 14:662–69

Streissguth AP, Clarren SJ, Jones KL (1985) Natural history of the fetal alcohol syndrome: a 10-year follow-up of eleven patients. Lancet 2:85–91

Streissguth AP, Martin DC, Martin JC, Barr HM (1981) The Seattle longitudinal prospective study on alcohol and pregnancy. Neurobehav Toxicol Teratol 3:223–33

Stromland K (1987) Ocular involvement in the fetal alcohol syndrome. Surv Opthalmol 31:277–84

Sulik KK (1984) Critical periods for alcohol teratogenesis in mice, with special reference to the gastrulation stage of embryogenesis. In Mechanisms of alcohol damage in utero, Ciba Foundation Symposium 105. Pitman, London, pp 124–41

Sulik KK, Johnston MC, Webb MA (1981) Fetal alcohol syndrome: embryogenesis in a mouse model. Science 214:936–38

Tennes K, Blackard C (1980) Maternal alcohol consumption, birth weight, and minor physical anomalies. Am J Obstet Gynecol 138:774–80

Veghelly PV, Osztovics M, Kardos G, et al. (1978a) The foetal alcohol syndrome: symptoms and pathogenesis. Acta Pediatr Hung 19:171–89

Veghelly PV, Osztovics M, Szaszovszky E (1978b) Maternal alcohol consumption and birth weight. Br Med J 2:1365–66

Verkerk PH (1992) The impact of alcohol misclassification on the relationship between alcohol and pregnancy outcome. Int J of Epidemiol 21(4 Suppl I):33–37

Waterson EJ, Murray-Lyon IM (1990) Preventing alcohol related birth damage: a review. Soc Sci Med 30(3)349–64

Weiler MW, Lammer EJ, Rosenberg L, Mitchell AA (1991) Maternal alcohol use in relation to selected birth defects. Am J Epidemiol 134:691–98

9

Alcohol and Overweight

I. Macdonald
University of London, United Kingdom

G. Debry
University of Nancy, France

K. Westerterp
University of Limburg, The Netherlands

Abstract

From an epidemiological standpoint, a relationship between moderate alcohol intake and body weight is difficult to establish, and the results of surveys are conflicting. The surveys are difficult to interpret because of many uncontrolled variables such as personality patterns and life-styles, level of education, physical activity, and tobacco consumption. There is a negative relationship between smoking and body weight, and a positive association between smoking and alcohol intake.

Under normal living conditions, studies on moderate alcohol consumption in men have shown no effect on energy balance and body weight over intervals of up to 4 weeks. Investigations have failed to identify a mechanism for increased metabolism or energy deposition after alcohol ingestion but do suggest that at moderate levels alcohol is efficiently used as a fuel by the liver; it still remains a mystery, however, as to what happens to the energy from alcohol in the body.

Alcohol tends to supplement rather than displace macronutrient energy, although there are some alterations in the dietary pattern. Individuals who consume alcohol but who are not alcoholic appear to add the energy from alcohol to their normal energy intake rather than replace food with alcohol. Further research is clearly needed to provide evidence of how the energy from ingested alcohol disappears.

Introduction

There is a common perception among the general public that alcohol consumption leads to overweight and even obesity, and this is exemplified by the so-called "beer belly." But is the excess abdominal adipose tissue associated with beer consumption due to energy from the alcohol, other sources of energy in beer, or the frequent association between beer consumption and overnutrition? On the other hand, the excess spirit drinker may be perceived as being thin, but is this thinness due to the alcohol or to the general malnutrition often associated with those whose preferred form of nourishment is spirits?

Alcohol constitutes approximately 4–6% of the energy intake in the Western diet. It is obvious that alcohol intake is not equally distributed over the population; however, the majority of people in a "drinking" population will be moderate drinkers. Here the focus is on the effect of alcohol consumption on energy balance in the group of moderate drinkers—that is, subjects with an average consumption of 15–45 g/day of alcohol, or those individuals who consume alcohol but are not alcoholic.

It is curious that the role of alcohol intake is not emphasized (except by Roe [1979]) in scientific and related books on alcohol and obesity.

Epidemiology

From an epidemiological point of view, a relationship between moderate alcohol intake and body weight is difficult to establish, and the results of surveys are conflicting. The surveys are difficult to interpret because of the many uncontrolled variables such as personality patterns and life-style (Chalmers et al. 1990), socioeconomic status (Lapidus et al. 1989, Wheeler 1990), level of education (Williamson et al. 1987, Rissanen et al. 1991), physical activity (Shephard et al. 1969, Gyntelberg and Meyer 1974, Williamson et al. 1987, Kromhout et al. 1988, Shah et al. 1989, Hellerstedt et al. 1990, Rissanen et al. 1991), and tobacco consumption (Higgins and Kjelsberg 1967, Shephard et al. 1969, Gyntelberg and Meyer 1974, Dyer et al. 1977, Cooke et al. 1982, Kozarevic et al. 1982, Baeke et al. 1983, Gordon and Kanell 1983, Fisher and Gordon 1985, Friedman and Kimbal 1986, Gordon and Doyle 1986, Williamson et al. 1987, Kromhout et al. 1988, Hellerstedt et al. 1990, Rissanen et al. 1991, Wannamethee and Shaper 1992).

The results of many surveys conflict in that the correlation between moderate alcohol consumption and body mass index (BMI) has been reported to be positive, negative, or nonexistent. These contrary findings may be due to the fact that all the confounding factors are not taken into account.

Many surveys that evaluate the relationship between alcohol and blood pressure and/or blood lipids measured body weight, but most, unfortunately, do not indicate the relationship, if any, between body weight and alcohol consumption.

Analysis of the Surveys

Between 1968 and 1992, 46 surveys were published: 41 were cross-sectional, three were combined cross-sectional and prospective, one was a case control study, and one was a prospective study. Most of the surveys were carried out in North America and Europe with some in Australia, New Zealand, and Japan.

The most frequent measurements of adiposity were based on height and weight, with skin fold measurements sometimes carried out. Several methods were used to assess alcohol and food intakes such as 24-hour recall, frequency checklists, diet histories, and diet diaries; these data were collected by mail or by interview. Many statistical methods were employed, but because of the diversity of these methods not all data have the same validity.

Results

Most of the surveys (see Table 1) did not account for smoking habits, and this omission is very important since the influence of smoking on body weight is more powerful than that of alcohol. There is an inverse relationship between smoking and body weight (U.S. Department of Health and Human Services 1988) and a positive association between smoking and alcohol intake (see the review by Hellerstedt et al. 1990); therefore, only the surveys that have taken smoking into account should be considered.

Smoking can also explain why the effect of alcohol is often different between men and women (see the discussion of this topic below). Some reports found that in women, smoking reduces any body weight increase that may be due to alcohol consumption (Higgins and Kjelsberg 1967, Cooke et al. 1982, Fischer and Gordon 1985, Friedmann and Kimbal 1986, Schatzkin et al. 1987, Willett et al. 1987, Williamson et al. 1987, Stampfler et al. 1988, Colditz et al. 1991, Rissanen et al. 1991), while others found the opposite effect (Tofler et al. 1969, Gyntelberg and Meyer 1974, Lang et al. 1987, Trevisan et al. 1987). Similarly, in men the effects of smoking are unclear. It may reduce any body weight increase due to alcohol (Higgins and Kjelsberg 1967, Cooke et al. 1982, Williamson et al. 1987, Rissanen et al. 1991, Wannamethee and Shaper 1992) or weakly increase the weight (Tofler et al. 1969, Gyntelberg and Meyer 1974, Dyer et al. 1977, Friedmann and Kimbal 1986, Lang et al. 1987, Trevisan et al. 1987, Colditz et al. 1991).

It is interesting that the results of several European and Australian surveys (Tofler et al. 1969, Gytelberg and Meyer 1974, Lang et al. 1987, Trevisan et al. 1987) showing a positive association between smoking, alcohol consumption, and body weight in women are different from those of many North American surveys.

A further complication is that the alcohol and smoking effects may depend on the race of the individual and the nature of the alcoholic drink. In one survey (Klatsky et al. 1977), the correlation between

Table 1
Reported correlations between alcohol intake and body weight

Men	Women	Men and women
	Positive	
Gyntelberg 1974	Trevisan 1987	Abdushelishvili 1976
Klatsky 1977	Lang 1987	Shephard 1969
Barboriak 1978		Tofler 1969
Kromhout 1983		
Colditz 1991		
Rissanen 1991		
Wannamethee 1992		
	Negative	
Henze 1977	Higgins 1967	Bebb 1971
	Klatsky 1977	Roe 1978
	Schatzkin 1987	Jones 1982
	Willett 1987	Gruchow 1985
	Stampfer 1988	Shah 1989
	Colditz 1991	
	No Correlation	
D'Alonzo 1969	Colditz 1991	Klatzky 1977
Myrhed 1974		Jacobsen 1987
Dyer 1977		Remig 1990
Kozarevic 1982		
Milon 1982		
Hillers 1985		
Kornhuber 1985		
Gordon 1986		
Sawata 1986		
Camargo 1987		

alcohol consumption and body weight is positive for white men but not for black men. The body weights of black and white female abstainers were heavier than those of drinkers, with no relationship in Oriental subjects between alcohol consumption and body weight.

The nature of the alcoholic drink may be of importance. One survey (Jacobsen and Thelle 1987) found that in men and in women (when the highest BMI quartile is excluded) there is a positive association between the use of spirits and BMI, while negative correlations were found for beer (men) and wine (women). A high alcohol consumption, particularly of spirits, has been reported to contribute to an elevated waist/hip ratio, with its possible cardiovascular complications (Bjorntorp et al. 1989).

Therefore, it is not possible to draw any firm conclusions from epidemiological studies on the relationship between moderate alcohol consumption and body weight.

Physiological and Metabolic Aspects

In contrast to the survey-type of study, another approach is the intervention study, ideally with a crossover design, in which the effects of alcohol consumption are studied in subjects with and without the addition of moderate alcohol to the diet.

Alcohol Consumption, Energy Balance, and Body Weight

Valimaki et al. (1988) measured the body weight in 10 healthy nonalcoholic men aged 30–43 years during a 3-week baseline period with no alcohol consumption, then 3 weeks with 30 g alcohol/day, again 3 weeks with no alcohol and finally 3 weeks with 60 g alcohol/day. The subjects consumed their "own" normal diets and were requested to maintain their habitual dietary and exercise patterns during the trial. The mean body weight did not change during the entire period, despite the fact that with the extra alcohol energy consumed a minimal weight gain of 1.5 kg would have been expected, had the alcohol been converted to body fat.

Contaldo et al. (1989) measured the energy intake, body weight, and resting energy expenditure in 10 healthy men aged 30–47 years before and during a 2-week period with and without the exchange of dietary energy with 75 g alcohol/day. Before the intervention the subjects were asked to keep a diary of their intake over 7 days and were asked not to drink alcohol and to maintain a stable weight over a run-in period of 10 days. The body weight and resting metabolic rate showed no significant changes during the two periods of isocaloric diets with or without alcohol.

In studying the effect of wine versus alcohols, McDonald and Margen (1976) measured the body weight in six healthy men aged 22–29 years during four consecutive 18-day intervals in a metabolic ward. The subjects were supplied with a standard liquid diet and, respectively, 1 l of wine with 9.3% alcohol/day, 1 l of 9.3% pure ethanol in water/day, or 1 l water/day, in randomized order, each over an 18-day interval. There was a universal loss of weight during the wine and alcohol administration, resulting in an overall mean weight loss of 1.0 kg.

Crouse and Grundy (1984) studied twelve men aged 22–62 years and in the weight range from normal to obese in a metabolic ward for 10 weeks. In the first 2 weeks the men adjusted to a liquid diet, followed by a 4-week "control" period. Eight of the subjects who were not unduly overweight continued with this diet with the addition of 90 g alcohol/day. This resulted in a mean weight loss of 0.85 kg (range –0.1 to –1.9 kg). In four overweight subjects, 90 g alcohol/day was added to the "control" diet, with half of the alcohol energy replacing dietary energy, and it was found that there was a mean weight gain of 1.03 kg (range +0.2 to +1.8 kg).

It seems therefore that in men, under normal living conditions, moderate alcohol consumption had no measurable effect on energy balance and body weight over intervals of up to 4 weeks. Under strictly controlled conditions in a metabolic ward, even 4 weeks of heavy drinking resulted in a slightly negative energy balance, as indicated by a tendency to lose weight in normal-weight subjects, while overweight subjects, partly substituting the same amount of alcohol with dietary energy, tended to gain weight.

The effect of alcohol consumption on energy balance, if any, may thus be a function of the subject's status with respect to weight.

Alcohol Consumption and Energy Expenditure

It has been suggested that during alcohol ingestion ethanol becomes the major fuel of hepatic metabolism, without any mechanism of storage or feedback control (i.e., the energy is wasted) (Pirola and Lieber 1972, 1976). More recently, it has been suggested that ethanol consumption damages the mitochrondia, resulting in an alteration in energy use through uncoupling of oxidation with phosphorylation (Lieber 1991).

There are few studies on the implications of alcohol consumption for energy metabolism and on resting metabolic rate (Perman 1962, Rosenberg and Durnin 1978, Weststraete et al. 1990), and these all showed an increased energy expenditure after alcohol consumption. However, the increased energy expenditure only partly offsets the alcohol energy at lower levels of alcohol intake and did not substantially offset the large energy surplus seen at higher levels of consumption; one reason for this may be that the observation period was too short.

In a recent study eight young men were studied on two occasions over 2 consecutive days in a metabolic chamber when, on the first day, they received foods in amounts calculated to cover their expected energy expenditure. On the second day they received three 32-g portions of ethanol diluted with water, one portion of which was consumed with each of their three main meals. The energy provided by the alcohol was equivalent to 25% of the subject's predicted 24-hour energy expenditure. During one of the sessions, food was kept constant on the second day, while on the other the addition of alcohol was compensated for by an equivalent decrease in energy from food. On both occasions when alcohol was consumed there was an increase in energy expenditure equivalent to about one-fourth of the energy content of the ethanol. These studies showed that ethanol exerts a lipid-sparing rather than a carbohydrate-sparing effect, which results in a shift in macronutrient intake that, in theory, favours the development of overweight (Suter et al. 1992).

Alcohol ingestion induces a significant increase in metabolic rate during the 90 minutes after ingestion, and this increase is similar to or slightly lower than the thermic effects of fats or carbohydrates (Perman 1962, Rosenberg and Durnin 1978, Weststrate et al. 1990). To the contrary, two studies have reported no increase in metabolic rate after alcohol intake (Barnes et al. 1965, Stock and Stuart 1974).

Another possibility is that alcohol might increase the metabolic rate during the digestion of a meal (DIT). One recent study reported that alcohol slightly increased the DIT (Weststrate et al. 1990), another found no significant effect (Rosenberg and Durnin 1978), and a third found that whisky taken with a meal produced a 22% increase in DIT compared with 13% after a meal with no whisky (Stock and Stuart 1974). More recently it has been hypothesized that the ingested alcohol enters an unregulated "futile" cycle in which it is broken down to a compound with the release of energy and that the compound is immediately resynthesised with further loss of energy (Lands and Zakhari 1991).

Physiological and Metabolic Studies

When measuring the effects of alcohol consumption on energy balance and body mass, the limits of analytical precision have to be considered. Body mass can be measured with a precision of 1 g, but constancy of body mass is no guarantee for energy balance, since the body's composition can change while body mass remains the same. Reinus et al. (1989) reported a weight loss of 700 g in one week in subjects receiving a high alcohol dose, while energy balance remained unchanged. It would seem that an intervention interval of 30–90 days at a moderate alcohol intake of 45–15 g, respectively, would be necessary to assess the effect of alcohol on body weight.

Thus, what happens to the energy from alcohol remains a metabolic mystery. Detailed biochemical studies have failed to identify a mechanism for an increased fat deposition after alcohol ingestion (Frayn et al. 1990). Most studies suggest that at moderate levels alcohol is efficiently used as a fuel by the liver (Mitchell and Herlong 1986).

Animal studies have shown alcohol to reduce body weight gain. Rats prefer dilute alcohol solutions over water (Richter 1941), and when alcohol solutions are offered, rats consume a significant proportion of their daily intake as alcohol while reducing normal food intake. Total daily energy intake remains the same during the period on a diet containing alcohol. Despite the constancy of energy intake, body weight goes down in this situation (Rothwell and Stock 1984, Larue-Achagiotis et al. 1990).

Clinical Observations

The majority of observational studies show that alcohol, though usually providing additional energy to the diet, is not associated with greater levels of overweight (Bebb et al. 1971, Jones et al. 1982, Fisher and Gordon 1985, Hillers and Massey 1985, Camargo et al. 1987, Le Marchand et al. 1989). The results of various experimental studies agree with these findings (Pirola and Lieber 1972, McDonald and Margen 1976, Crouse and Grundy 1984). In another study, after controlling for smoking, age, total daily calorie intake, physical activity, race, education, and height, it was reported that alcohol caused only a slight increase in BMI (Williamson et al. 1987).

There have been reports as well that alcohol consumers weigh less than nondrinkers at similar or higher energy intakes (Camargo et al. 1987, Hellerstedt et al. 1990), and that postmenopausal female nondrinkers had a higher BMI than drinkers, and among the drinkers there was a negative association between BMI and the amount consumed (Kaye et al. 1990).

In a recent analysis of data from two large cohort studies it was found that increasing alcohol intake does not lead to increased BMI in men and actually reduces BMI in women (Colditz et al. 1991).

Based on the above studies, it seems that no support can be given to recommending that alcohol consumption be reduced in order to maintain or reduce body weight. On the other hand, the Dutch Zutphen Study found that obese middle-aged men have a lower energy intake but a higher alcohol intake than their lean counterparts (Kromhout 1983) and that alcohol intake was directly related to BMI (Kromhout et al. 1988).

Sex Differences in Alcohol Intake and Body Weight

Most human studies have involved men, and in many of those that included women no differences in alcohol consumption and body weight between the sexes were noted. There are some reports, however, that suggest that the sex response may not be the same. There seems to be an inverse relationship between alcohol consumption and BMI in women but not in men (Gruchow et al. 1985, Fischer and Gordon 1985, Jones et al. 1982, Williamson et al. 1987).

A more recent study of data from 89,538 women showed a clear inverse relationship between alcohol consumption and BMI but not among 48,493 men, even after adjustment for smoking (Colditz et al. 1991). As mentioned earlier, these differences between men and women may be due to different life-styles, variations that may not have been controlled for in all reported studies.

Dietary Changes Associated With Alcohol Intake

Though alcohol tends to supplement rather than displace macronutrient energy, some alterations in the dietary pattern do occur. In one study (Colditz et al. 1991) the strongest relation between alcohol consumption and intake of specific nutrients was observed for carbohydrates. Intake of carbohydrates decreased from an average of 153 g/day in abstainers to 131 g/day in women consuming 25–50 g ethanol/day. In men carbohydrate intake fell from 231 g/day in abstainers to 213 g/day in those consuming 25–50g ethanol/day. In both groups the sucrose intake decreased significantly with increasing alcohol intake. This reduced sucrose intake seemed to be due to fewer servings of added sugar to foods or beverages. A definite inverse relationship between sugar consumption and alcohol consumption has also been reported (Kubler 1990).

In addition to carbohydrates, the consumption of vitamins, calcium, fruits, and raw vegetables was greater among abstainers, while consumption of fat (particularly polyunsaturated fats), meat, pickled vegetables, and dried fish was greater among drinkers (Le Marchand et al. 1989). In contrast to this, data from Ireland suggests an inverse relationship between the energy derived from alcohol and that derived from dietary fat (Gibney et al. 1989).

Alcohol Calories and Distribution of Body Fat

Since body fat distribution (rather than total fat or obesity) may be an independent risk factor for cardiovascular disease, hypertension, and diabetes, a study was carried out on 40,980 postmenopausal women to determine whether a correlation between alcohol consumption and waist/hip ratio (WHR) exists. It was found that WHR was obviously strongly related to BMI but was significantly and negatively associated with alcohol consumption, with the lowest WHR present in women who drank 2–7.4g ethanol/day (Kaye et al. 1990). In Swedish women, however, alcohol consumption was positively associated with WHR (Lapidus et al. 1989), and no relation was found between WHR and alcohol consumption in a sample of Mexican and non-Hispanic women (Haffner et al. 1986).

In a study of 1936 men aged 21–80 years a positive association was found between alcohol intake and WHR that remained significant after adjustment for BMI, age, and smoking (Troisi et al. 1990). In a later study of 765 men, the same group found that alcohol was only weakly and positively associated with WHR (Troisi et al. 1991).

Thus, in view of the possible significance of WHR as a predictor of cardiovascular disease, further investigation of body fat distribution associated with alcohol consumption seems to be needed.

The Fate of Ingested Alcohol Calories

Individuals who consume alcohol but who are not alcoholic appear to add the energy from alcohol to their normal energy intake rather than replace food with alcohol. This means that they consume more total energy than individuals who do not drink (Fisher and Gordon 1985, Gruchow et al. 1985). Thus it seems as if energy derived from alcohol does not replace that derived from other nutrients but is supplemental (Jones et al. 1982). It has also been reported that on drinking days the mean total calorie intake is higher than on days when no drinking occurred (Bebb et al. 1971).

In a study of the data from 48,493 men, the total energy consumption was 7576 kJ/day in abstainers and 9822 kJ/day in those whose alcohol intake was greater than 50 g/day, and the energy intake varied little with alcohol intake (Colditz et al. 1991). This, however, was not so in women.

Since there seems to be little support for the view that the energy in ethanol per se can or is used to any extent by the metabolism of the body, what is the explanation? Every gram of alcohol burned in the laboratory releases 28 kJ, yet it seems that the body uses alcohol less efficiently.

Alcohol increases the basal metabolic rate, and this increased basal expenditure may partially offset the energy of the alcohol ingested at lower levels of alcohol intake, but it does not substantially offset the large energy surplus seen at higher levels of consumption (Camargo et al. 1987).

Thus the energy contributed by alcohol does not appear to enter into overall energy regulation in that the fuel from alcohol is additional to overall intakes and does not replace other energy sources, at least in men. Further research in this area is clearly needed to provide evidence of how the energy from ingested alcohol disappears.

Plans for Further Research

As ethanol is rarely consumed per se, it is not surprising that the evidence for the role of alcohol in overweight is confusing. Therefore, it is necessary to use ethanol only in any studies that are carried out.

In man it would be useful to learn more about the effect of ethanol on metabolic rate using the double-labeled water technique, both acute and sub-chronic.

There seems to be a consensus view that alcohol energy is not handled according to the laws of thermodynamics. This does not seem to attract much interest from biochemists and others, but it could be of value to initiate animal studies that address the apparent problem of the "lost calories." Perhaps studies at the cellular or molecular level that look at cell pumps, futile cycles, etc. after ethanol consumption, or perhaps some studies on the effect of ethanol consumption on such hormones as those from the thyroid. (The apparent sex difference reported in the literature in response to ethanol should also encourage some endocrine studies).

Though in theory epidemiological surveys would be the best way to determine whether moderate chronic alcohol consumption can modify body weight, there are too many variables that cannot be controlled, so it may be necessary to carry out detailed metabolic studies in the controlled surroundings of a metabolic ward where the exact food and ethanol intake can be monitored. These studies would need to cover a period of months rather than weeks because, in addition to a control period, the changes in body weight are likely to be small. During such an investigation it would be possible to make frequent biochemical and metabolic measurements that might provide a lead as to whether energy derived from ethanol is additive to the energy derived from other nutrients or is in some way "lost" by the body.

References

Abdushelishvili G (1976) The peculiarities of obesity frequency in the Georgian Republic. Proceedings fo the 10th International Congress of Nutrition, Kyoto, Japan. Victory-sha Press, pp 263–64

Baecke JAH, Buremma J, Fritjers JER, et al. (1983) Obesity in young Dutch adults II. Daily life-style and body mass index. Int J Obes 7:13–24

Barboriak JJ, Rooney CB, Leitschuh TH, Anderson AJ (1978) Alcohol and nutrient intake of elderly men. J Am Diet Assoc 72:493–95

Barnes EW, Cooke NJ, King AJ, et al. (1965) Observations on the metabolism of alcohol in man. Br J Nutr 19:485–89

Bebb HT, Houser HB, Witschi JC, et al. (1971) Calorie and nutrient contribution of alcoholic beverages to the usual diets of 155 adults. Am J Clin Nutr 1971 24:1042–52

Bjorntorp P, Seidell J, Petterson P (1989) Alcohol consumption and adipose tissue distribution. Int J Obes 13(suppl):Abstr 70

Camargo CA, Vranizan KM, Dreon DM, et al. (1987) Alcohol, calorie intake and adiposity in overweight men. J Am Coll Nutr 6:271–78

Chalmers DK, Bowyer CA, Olenick NL (1990) Problem drinking and obesity: a comparison in personality patterns and life styles. Int J Addict 25:803–17

Colditz GA, Giovannuci E, Rimm EB, et al. (1991) Alcohol intake in relation to diet and obesity in men and women. Am J Clin Nutr 54:49–55

Contaldo F, d'Arrigo E, Caradente V, et al. (1989) Short term effects of moderate alcohol consumption on lipid metabolism and energy balance in normal men. Metabolism 38:166–71

Cooke KM, Frost GW, Thornell IR, et al. (1982) Alcohol consumption and blood pressure. Survey of the relationship at a health screening clinic. Med J Aust 1:65–69

Crouse JR, Grundy SM (1984) Effects of alcohol on plasma lipoproteins and cholesterol and triglyceride metabolism in man. J Lipid Res 25:486–96

D'Alonzo CA, Pell S (1969) Cardiovascular disease among problem drinkers. J Occup Med 10:865–72

Dyer AR, Stamler J, Paul O, et al. (1977) Alcohol consumption, cardiovascular risk factors and mortality in two Chicago epidemiologic studies. Circulation 56:1067–74

Fisher M, Gordon T (1985) The relation of drinking and smoking habits to diet: the Lipid Clinics Prevalence Study. Am J Clin Nutr 41:623–30

Frayn KN, Coppack SW, Walsh PE, et al. (1990) Metabolic responses of forearm and adipose tissue to acute ethanol ingestion. Metabolism 39:958–66

Friedman LA, Kimbal AW (1986) Coronary heart disease mortality and alcohol consumption in Framingham. Am J Epidemiol 124:481–89

Gibney MJ, Moloney M, Shelley E (1989) The Kilkenny Health Project: food and nutrient intakes in randomly selected healthy adults. Br J Nutr 61:129–37

Gordon T, Doyle JT (1986) Alcohol consumption and its relation to smoking, weight, blood pressure and blood lipids. The Albany Study. Arch Intern Med 146:262–65

Gordon T, Kanell WB (1983) Drinking and its relation to smoking, BP, blood lipids and uric acid. Arch Intern Med 143:1366–74

Gruchow HW, Sobocinski KA, Barboriak JJ, et al. (1985) Alcohol consumption, nutrient intake and relative body weight among U.S. adults. Am J Clin Nutr 42:289–95

Gyntelberg F, Meyer J (1974) Relationship between blood pressure and physical fitness, smoking and alcohol consumption in Copenhagen males aged 40–59. Acta Med Scand 195:375–80

Haffner SM, Stern MP, Hazuda HP, et al. (1986) Upper and centralized adiposity in Mexican Americans and non-Hispanic whites: relationship to body mass index and other behavioral and demographic variables. Int J Obes 10:493–502

Hellerstedt WL, Jeffrey RW, Murray DM (1990) The association between alcohol intake and adiposity in the general population. Am J Epidemiol 132:594–611

Henze K, Bucci A, Signoretti P, et al. (1977) Alcohol intake and coronary risk factors in a population in Rome. Nutr Metab vol 21 (suppl 1):157–59

Higgins MW, Kjelsberg M (1967) Characteristics of smokers and non-smokers in Tecumseh, Michigan II. Am J Epidemiol 86:60–77

Hillers VN, Massey LK (1985) Interrelationships of moderate and high alcohol consumption with diet and health status. Am J Clin Nutr 41:356–62

Jacobsen BK, Thelle DS (1987) The Tromso Heart Study: the relationship between food habits and the body mass index. J Chron Dis 40:795–800

Jones BR, Barett-Connor E, Criqui MH, et al. (1982) A community study of calorie and nutrient intake in drinkers and non-drinkers of alcohol. Am J Clin Nutr 35:135–41

Kaye SA, Folsom AR, Prineas RJ, et al. (1990) The association of body fat distribution with lifestyle and reproductive factors in a population study of postmenopausal women. Int J Obes 14:583–91

Klatsky AL, Friedman GD, Siegelaub AB, et al. (1977) Alcohol consumption among white, black or Oriental men and women. Am J Epidemiol 195:311–23

Kornhuber HH, Lisson G, Suschka-Suuermann L (1985) Alcohol and obesity: a new look at high blood pressure and stroke. Eur Arch Psychiatry Neurol Sci 234:357–62

Kozarevic D, Demirovic J, Gordon T, et al. (1982) Drinking habits and coronary heart disease: the Yugoslavia Cardiovascular Disease Study. Am J Epidemiol 116:748–58

Kromhout D (1983) Energy and macronutrient intake in lean and obese middle-aged men (The Zutphen Study). Am J Clin Nutr 37:295–99

Kromhout D, Saris WH, Horst CH (1988) Energy intake, energy expenditure and smoking in relation to body fatness. The Zutphen Study. Am J Clin Nutr 47:668–74

Kubler W (1990) Zum Verbrauch von Zucker in der Bundesrepublik Deutschland. Z Ernahrungswiss 29(suppl):3–10

Lands WEM, Zakhari S (1991) The case of the missing calories. Am J Clin Nutr 54:47–48

Lang T, Degoulet P, Aime F, et al. (1987) Relationship between alcohol consumption and hypertension prevalence and control in a French population. J Chronic Dis 40:713–20

Lapidus L, Bengtsson C, Hällström T, Björntorp P (1989) Obesity. Adipose tissue distribution and health in women. Appetite 12:25–35

Larue-Achagiotis C, Poussard AM, Louis-Sylvestre J (1990) Alcohol drinking, food and fluid intakes and body weight gain in rats. Physiol Behav 47:545–48

Le Marchand L, Kolonel LN, Hankin JH, et al. (1989) Relationship of alcohol consumption to diet: a population-based study in Hawaii. Am J Clin Nutr 49:567–72

Lieber CS (1991) Perspectives: do alcohol calories count? Am J Clin Nutr 54:976–82

McDonald JT, Margen S (1976) Wine versus ethanol in human nutrition. I. Nitrogen and calorie balance. Am J Clin Nutr 29:1093–1103

Milon H, Froment A, Gaspard P, et al. (1982) Alcohol consumption and blood pressure in French epidemiological study. Eur Heart J 3 October (suppl. c):59–64

Mitchell MC, Herlong HF (1986) Alcohol and nutrition: caloric value, bioenergetics and relationship to liver damage. Ann Rev Nutr 6:457–74

Myrhed M (1974) Alcohol consumption in relation to factors associated with ischaemic heart disease. Acta Med Scand 567(suppl):9–93

Perman ES (1962) Increase in oxygen uptake after small ethanol doses in man. Acta Physiol Scand 55:207–9

Pirola RC, Lieber CS (1972) Energy cost of the metabolism of drugs, including ethanol. Pharmacol 7:185–96

Pirola RC, Lieber CS (1976) Energy wastage in alcoholism and drug abuse: possible role of hepatic microsomal enzymes. Am J Clin Nutr 29:90–93

Reinus JF, Heymsfield SB, Wisking R, et al. (1989) Ethanol: relative fuel value and metabolic effects in vivo. Metabolism 38:125–35

Remig VM, Mitchell MC, Johnson WA (1990) Alcohol, energy and nutrient intake of healthy elders. J Am Diet Assoc 90 (suppl):Abstr A74

Richter CP (1941) Alcohol as a food. Q J Stud Alcohol 1:650–62

Rissanen AM, Heliovaara M, Knekt P, et al. (1991) Determinants of weight gain and overweight in adult Finns. Eur J Clin Nutr 45:419–30

Roe DA (1978) Physical rehabilitation and employment of AFCD recipients (final report). Report DLMA-51-36-75-01-1. New York State College of Agriculture and Life Sciences, Ithaca NY

Roe DA (1979) Alcohol consumption and body weight. In Roe, DA (ed), Alcohol and the Diet. Avi Publishing Co., Westport, Connecticut, pp 89–95

Rosenberg K, Durnin JVGA (1978) The effect of alcohol on resting metabolic rate. Br J Nutr 40:293–98

Rothwell NJ, Stock MJ (1984) Influence of alcohol and sucrose consumption on energy balance and brown fat activity in the rat. Metabolism 33:768–71

Sawata S, Sato R, Hidaka H, et al. (1986) Relationship between alcohol consumption, body weight, family history of hypertension and blood pressure in young adults. Clin Exp Hypertens [A] A8:21–35

Schatzkin A, Jones DY, Hoover RN, et al. (1987) Alcohol consumption and breast cancer in the epidemiologic follow-up study of the First National Health and Nutrition Examination Survey. N Engl J Med 316:1169–73

Shah M, Jeffrey RW, Haan RJ, et al. (1989) Relationship between sociodemographic and behaviour variable and body mass index in a population with high-normal blood pressure: hypertension prevention trial. Eur J Clin Nutr 43:583–96

Shepard RJ, Jones G, Ishii K, et al. (1969) Factors affecting body density and thickness of subcutaneous fat. Am J Clin Nutr 1175–89

Stampfer MJ, Colditz GA, Willett WC, et al. (1988) A prospective study of a moderate alcohol consumption and the risk of coronary disease and stroke in women. N Engl J Med 319:267–73

Stock MJ, Stuart JA (1974) Thermic effects of ethanol in the rat and man. Nutr Metab 17:297–305

Suter PM, Schutz Y, Jequier E (1992) The effect of ethanol on fat storage in healthy subjects. N Engl J Med 326:983–87

Tofler AB, Sake BM, Rollo KA, et al. (1969) Electrocardiogram of the social drinker in Perth, Western Australia. Br Heart J 31:306–13

Trevisan M, Krogh V, Farinaro E (1987) Alcohol consumption, drinking pattern and blood pressure: analysis of data from the Italian National Research Council Study. Int J Epidemiol 16:520–27

Troisi RJ, Heinold JW, Vokonas PS, et al. (1991) Cigarette smoking, dietary intake, and physical activity: effects on body fat distribution—The Normative Aging Study. Am J Clin Nutr 53:1104–11

Troisi R, Weiss ST, Segal MR, et al. (1990) The relationship of body fat distribution to blood pressure in normotensive men: the normative aging study. Int J Obes 14:515–25

U.S. Department of Health and Human Services (1988) The health consequences of smoking: nicotine addiction. Surgeon General Report, DHHS Publ No (CDC) 88-84-8406, U.S. General Printing Office, Washington, D.C.

Valimaki M, Taskinen M-R, Ylikahri R, et al. (1988) Comparison of the effects of two different doses of alcohol on serum lipoproteins, HDL subfractions and apolipoproteins A-1 and A-2: a controlled study. Eur J Clin Invest 18:472–80

Wannamethee G, Shaper AG (1992) Blood lipids: the relationship with alcohol intake, smoking and body weight. J Epidemiol Community Health 46:197–202

Weststrate JA, Wunnik P, Deurenberg J, et al. (1990) Alcohol and acute effects on resting metabolic rate and diet-induced thermogenesis. Br J Nutr 64:413–25

Wheeler EF (1990) The effect of alcohol abuse on energy and nutrient intakes. Eur J Gastroenterol Hepatol 2:395–98

Willett WC, Stampfer MJ, Colditz GA, et al. (1987) Moderate alcohol consumption and the risk of breast cancer. N Engl J Med 316:1174–80

Williamson DF, Forman MR, Binkin NJ, et al. (1987) Alcohol and body weight in United States adults. Am J Public Health 77:1324–30

10

Genetics and Alcohol

P. Couzigou
University of Bordeaux

H. Begleiter
State University of New York, United States

K. Kiianmaa
Alko Ltd., Finland

D.P. Agarwal
University of Hamburg, Germany

Abstract

(1)   *What is the consensus of the body of research addressing the question of whether there is a genetic explanation for alcoholism or a genetic predisposition toward alcoholism?*

Animal studies initially established that heredity influences the level of voluntary alcohol consumption as well as sensitivity to different components of alcohol intoxication. Experiments in humans then supported the hypothesis that genetic factors influence style of drinking and the probability of developing alcoholism. Most notable are studies examining the degree of concordance for alcohol drinking in monozygotic and dizygotic twins and studies of adopted children with or without alcoholics as biological parents.

(2)   *What is the direction and quality of the evidence found in twin and adoption studies, pedigree and family analysis, population and ethnic comparisons, and breeding experiments with animals?*

Relative to other biomedical questions, evidence for a genetic influence in alcoholism is firm. Emphasis in the field has thus moved on to more specific questions. Studies with humans have examined how the genetic influence differs in different forms of alcoholism (or at different extremes along a continuum) and between men and women. Similarly, animal studies are beginning to ask more specific questions about alcohol drinking, e.g., questions relating to the increase in drinking caused by deprivation, the decrease caused by satiety, and the changes caused by reinforcement and learning. Some of the clearest results relate to low drinking. Both animal and human work has shown that genetics not only predisposes some individuals to heavier drinking but also works in the other direction, preventing some individuals from drinking large amounts and protecting them from alcoholism.

(3)   *Are there new technologies or strategies to determine whether there is a specific genetic predetermination factor that promotes alcoholism?*

Selectively bred animal lines have been examined to find the behavioral, neurological, and enzymatic factors that may cause a specific predetermination to heavy drinking. Similar factors are being examined in high-risk humans (e.g., those with an alcoholic relative) and in different human populations. These studies can be expected to continue in the future, aided by improved techniques for precise measurement of the factors. Studies of alcohol drinking behavior in animal lines developed for other alcohol-related characteristics are now beginning to be done. A new direction would be the selective breeding of animal lines to test for specific components of alcohol drinking (e.g., for high or low increases after forced abstinence) or to try to match specific human drinking patterns (e.g., binge drinking or the characteristics of human type II alcoholics).

Family studies with the collection of information by direct interviews would be of major importance. Such family studies could explore the genetics of each specific aspect of alcohol consumption (initial sensitivity, alcoholism, end-organ damage). The linkage map of the human genome, in progress now, will be of tremendous importance to localize, using family data, the part of the genome implicated in the specific genetic factor studied. Research on the polymorphism for contributive genes in alcohol and acetaldehyde metabolism, neuromediators, and enzymes implicated in end-organ metabolism would be useful. Identifying individuals at genetic risk of alcoholism and/or alcohol-related diseases would be possible using the knowledge of a specific genetic predetermination and the results of longitudinal studies. In longitudinal studies, the choice of criteria that could be easily used a second time for identifying a high-risk population, avoiding for example reaction to alcohol absorption, would be relevant.

(4) *If genetic factors promote alcoholism, would it be possible to identify individuals at risk and thus allow them to adapt their life-styles accordingly?*

Research has already made it possible to identify individuals, especially in Oriental populations, with a particularly low risk for alcoholism, and it seems likely that in the future, markers will be found for a high risk for alcoholism. The markers could be genotypic or phenotypic. A single "alcoholism gene," however, is unlikely to be identified. Current evidence in animals and humans instead points toward polygenic control, probably with several genes having substantial influence but a very large number of other genes having some effect. Although the influences are generally imagined as additive, more complex interactions are possible.

The ethical problems raised by the likely discovery of such markers are already being considered. Educational strategies need to be determined to allow identified high-risk subjects to change their life-styles most effectively.

(5) *How long might it take to determine a specific genetic profile for alcoholism, assuming there is such a profile?*

The answer depends on the degree of accuracy required. Even today we can, to a limited extent, identify people with an increased risk for alcoholism simply from the presence of alcoholism among their relatives. This knowledge probably has already helped direct some individuals away from danger, and can be seen as a benefit already accruing from earlier research in the field.

Existing markers can improve the accuracy for identifying high-risk people. Most likely, in future years, many markers will be discovered, each one contributing slightly to the improvement of identification. Even in the next few years, we may well have a set of markers related to some particular form of alcoholism that is sufficiently accurate to warrant general practical use. Complete determination of the entire genetic profile contribution to alcoholism, however, may not be possible.

(6)   *What new research should be undertaken?*

Animal models should be used for physiopathological studies investigating the relationships between preference, tolerance, dependence, and withdrawal. For such studies transgenic models, especially in the mouse, would be worthwhile. Animal and human studies of low alcohol consumption should be extended. Also of interest are racial and interethnic studies of initial sensitivity and alcohol metabolism. Family studies and longitudinal studies are needed on alcohol behavior, alcohol abuse, alcohol dependence, alcoholism, and alcohol-related diseases. These studies must relate to the study of putative markers and the linkage map of the human genome.

Research goals should also be extended. In addition to markers for alcoholism, efforts should be made to discover markers for genetically determined susceptibility to various form of alcohol-induced organ damage independent of consumption differences and markers for high degrees of functional impairment from alcohol intoxication. Furthermore, genetic research should be used not only to aid in identifying problems but also in the search for ways to correct and cure them. Animal models with a specific genetic component related to alcohol— e.g., heavy drinking caused by especially high reinforcement from alcohol—could be used to search for treatments that would be effective in humans with a similar feature.

Introduction

Genes have long been suspected to play a role in the etiology of alcoholism. Ancient Greek scholars such as Aristotle and Plutarch observed that "alcoholism runs in families." Well-conducted studies (Cotton 1979, Guze et al. 1986) have confirmed this observation. Cotton's review of familial alcoholism studies estimated that one of three alcoholics will have at least one parent who is also alcoholic. Males more frequently than females present alcoholic symptoms.

"Familial" does not necessarily imply "hereditary." Segregation analysis of alcoholism in families pointed to the existence of a genetic factor but did not succeed in determinating the transmission modalities (Gilligan et al. 1987, Aston and Hill 1990). A single gene is unlikely to account wholly for the transmission of such a complex disorder as alcoholism. More probably, different genes will be shown to affect different aspects of alcoholism and alcohol-related diseases. To try to disentangle genetic and environmental interactions, several twin and adoption studies have been conducted. Additionally, experiments using animal models have delineated the genetic transmission of alcohol-relevant traits.

Twin Studies

Twin studies are one way to assess the relative strength of genetic and environmental components of alcohol problems. Since monozygotic (MZ) twins are genetically identical and dizygotic (DZ) twins share only part of their genes, a greater concordance between MZ than DZ twins is expected if a trait is under strong genetic control. An estimate of heritability can be calculated from the exact difference between MZ and DZ concordances. Heritability estimates can range from zero to one; zero implies no genetic source of variation for an observed characteristic whereas a value of one implies that all of the variation is genetic. Partanen et al. (1966) interviewed 902 pairs of male twins and reported that the heritability estimates for the amount and frequency of alcohol drinking were 0.36 and 0.39, respectively. Heritability estimates of about 0.3 and 0.6 for amount and frequency of alcohol consumption were obtained by other investigators (reviewed in Marshall and Murray 1989), and other studies reported similar trends.

The data on alcohol dependence and alcoholism reported in twin studies also point to the existence of a genetic factor (reviewed in Merikangas 1990). Only Murray et al. (1983) failed to find significant differences in concordance rates for alcohol dependence in MZ and DZ twins. At least one twin presented with a psychiatric illness, so there may have been confounding with other forms of psychopathology. In the study by Pickens et al. (1991), heritability of alcoholism appeared to be stronger for males than for females and varied with DSM III diagnosis; the proportion of genetic influence was higher for alcohol dependence. A recent and especially well designed twin study by Kendler et al. (1992) supported the hypothesis that genetic factors play a major role in the aetiology of alcoholism in women. The probandwise concordance for alcoholism was consistently higher in MZ than in DZ twins. Multifactorial threshold models suggested that the heritability of liability to alcoholism in women is in the range of 0.5 to 0.6.

Twin studies are a powerful tool to estimate heritability, but they do not completely exclude environmental effects. Living together increases the similarity of alcohol consumption patterns in twin pairs (Gedda and Brenci 1983). Cohabitation and frequent social contacts between twins were greater in MZ than in DZ twins; when these influences were factored out, however, there still remained a much higher concordance of alcohol drinking habits in MZ twins (Kaprio et al. 1987, Clifford et al. 1984b). In another twin study Heath et al. (1989) examined the influence of marital status and social contact in twins in modifying the effects of inheritance of alcoholism. Social contact did not modify the concordance rate, but marital status significantly decreased the genetic influence on alcohol drinking habits. The greater proximity of MZ than DZ twins is one possible explanation of the higher concordance rates in MZ pairs for chronic infectious diseases such as tuberculosis and leprosy.

One way to avoid such bias is to study pairs of twins where each was reared in a different family. Kaprio (1984) compared MZ and DZ twins separated before age 11 with matched pairs reared together. The intrapair correlation in monthly alcohol use was greater for twins reared together; the concordance rate, however, was higher in MZ twins, both those reared together and those who were separated, suggesting a genetic effect. Alcohol-related hospitalisation concordance is greater for twins living within a limited geographic area; twin analyses, however, confirmed significant genetic variation in alcohol-related disorders (Romanov et al. 1991). Another study investigated factors associated with adolescent alcohol use (Heath and Martin 1988). Among males, age of initiation of drinking was uninfluenced by genetic factors but was strongly influenced by shared environment. Among females, a moderate genetic influence and little effect on shared environment were found. In contrast, current alcohol consumption by adult twins was strongly influenced in both sexes by genetic factors.

Another recent twin study (McGue et al. 1992) found a modest genetic influence on alcohol problems in women and in late-onset men;

genetic influences were substantial only in the aetiology of early-onset male alcoholism. Opposite-sex dizygotic twin data revealed significant cross-sex transmission. Alcohol problems were greatest among male cotwins of female probands (McGue et al. 1992). Finnish twin cohort studies confirm that genetic factors are important contributors to social patterns of alcohol use and abuse. They also indicate the complexity of the genetics of these traits (Kaprio et al. 1991). Follow-up analyses of absolute changes in alcohol use revealed heritable influences on the disposition to alter behavior (Kaprio et al. 1992).

Taken together, the data from these studies confirm the significant importance of genetic factors in determining individual differences in alcohol use and abuse. In males, genetic differences are important in youth, but environmental factors increasingly influence drinking habits with age. In females, although genetic factors determine alcohol consumption profiles, the influence of both genetic and environmental variance increases considerably with age.

Adoption Studies

Adoption studies allow genetic and environmental factors to be assessed independently. They began with a study by Roe (1944), who found no difference in alcohol abuse in a small sample of foster children with or without a parental history of drinking problems. The sample size was small, however, and it was not clear that the biological parent would today be classified as alcoholic; also, many adoptees had not entered the age of alcoholism risk at the time they were studied.

Interest in the study of adopted children of alcoholics was revived in the 1970s. Schuckit et al. (1972) observed that half-siblings of alcoholic probands who had an alcoholic biological parent but were raised by nonalcoholics more frequently became alcoholics than did those whose biological parents were moderate drinkers. This emphasizes the role of some heritable factor, more especially as alcoholism in the surrogates did not increase the risk in the children. Subsequent extensive studies were conducted in Denmark, Sweden, and the United States (Goodwin et al. 1973, 1974, 1977, Bohman 1978, Cadoret and Gath 1978, Goodwin 1985, 1986), which showed that the sons of alcoholics had a nearly fourfold higher alcoholism rate than did adoptees whose biological parents were nonalcoholic, whether raised by nonalcoholic foster parents or by their own biological parents. Adopted sons of alcoholics were more likely to be alcoholic at a relatively early stage than were their peers. There are no significant differences among adopted daughters of alcoholics, but the sample size was small. Sons of alcoholics were similar to sons of nonalcoholics regarding susceptibility to non-alcohol-related psychiatric disturbances when both groups were raised by nonalcoholic adoptive parents. Further extended analysis of large-scale adoption studies from Sweden (Bohman et al. 1981, Cloninger et al. 1981) provided substantial data on at least two types of genetically influenced alcoholism: type I and type II.

Type I alcoholism is the more common type and occurs in both men and women. It is also called "milieu-limited alcoholism" because its acquisition requires both genetic predisposition and environmental provocation. If only one of these factors is present the risk of alcohol abuse is lower than it is among the general population, but if both are present the risk is doubled. Type I alcohol abuse starts after age 25. It is associated with mild alcohol abuse in either biological parent and is usually not severe (i.e., it is milder than type II alcoholism). Type I alcoholics typically show infrequent encounters with the legal system.

Type II alcoholism is less common than type I (about 25% of all male alcoholics in the general population are type II) and is limited to males. It is particularly heritable, with the risk of developing alcohol abuse nine times greater in predisposed sons than in the general population. Environmental factors seem to play only a minor role. The time of onset of type II alcohol abuse is early adolescence. It is associated with a father who is a severe alcoholic but it is not associated with alcohol abuse in the biological mother. Type II alcoholism is typically severe and is difficult to treat. It is often accompanied by serious encounters with the law. The personality profile of a type II alcoholic is characterized by impulsivity and excitability (high novelty seeking), brash and uninhibited behavior (low harm avoidance), and distant social relations (low reward dependence). Although type II men become severe alcoholics, type II women exhibit instead life-long somatization problems such as irritable bowel syndrome.

It is widely believed that there is a major gene effect in type II alcoholism. A twin study (Pickens et al. 1991) also found evidence for differential genetic heritability of alcoholism subtypes, but there has been criticism of the data on which the classification is based (Littrell 1988, Searles 1988). Recent research does not support this alcoholic typology (Schuckit and Irwin 1989), and simple division into familial and nonfamilial cases can be as useful as Cloninger classification (Buydens-Branchey et al. 1989, Marshall and Murray 1991). However, failure to find differences in drinking behavior as a function of familial risk for alcoholism does not favor such simple classification (Alterman et al. 1989). Alcoholism is a heterogeneous disorder with numerous phenotypes. Phenotypic heterogeneity not only arises from various gene-environment interactions, but may also occur because of comorbidity with such other disorders as antisocial personality and/or other psychiatric disorders. Phenotype definitions are evolving (Schuckit 1991); for example, Hill (1992) recently suggested a type III alcoholism.

Further analysis of a U.S. study found a tendency for adopted children to misuse drugs and for alcoholism in the adoptive parents to somewhat raise the risk of alcoholism in their adopted children (Cadoret et al. 1985). The findings for a genetic factor in female alcoholism are more equivocal than for male alcoholism. A recent analyses from Sweden, however, points to such a factor (Dinwiddie and Cloninger 1989).

The twin and adoption studies on alcoholism to date are not perfect. Biases can be introduced by the practices of adoption agencies that match the adoptees to the adopting parents, and by differences between persons who place their children for adoption and those who do not. Some of the studies used cohorts that spanned several decades, and some used nonstandard definitions of alcoholism. The lack of agreement on a valid definition of alcoholism is a major difficulty, because definitions of alcoholism have evolved markedly over the years and are still evolving (Keller and Doria 1991). These limits on twin and adoption studies can decrease the perceived role of genetic influences on the genesis of alcohol abuse and alcoholism (Murray et al. 1983, Peele 1986, Fillmore 1988, Searle 1988). The evidence to date for a genetic role, however, is compelling. Evidence of a genetic contribution also may be found in animal models showing that alcohol-related behaviors may be transmitted to offspring.

Animal Studies

In studies of animals presented with a choice of water or ethanol solution, some animals prefer the ethanol solution over water. Inbred strains of mice play an important role in studies on the heritability of ethanol consumption. Inbred strains represent populations of genetically identical individuals that have been produced by more than 20 generations of mating of closely related animals, such as siblings (Belknap 1980). Theoretically this has resulted in random fixation of homozygous genes. When ethanol intake in several inbred strains of mice was compared, C57B1 mice voluntarily consumed high amounts of ethanol whereas C3H/2, A/2, BALB/c, and DBA/2N strains preferred water (McClearn and Rodgers 1959; Rodgers and McClearn 1962; Yoshimoto and Komura 1987). Demonstration of significant strain differences is itself presumptive evidence of a genetic involvement in ethanol preference. Studies of inbred rat strains have also shown differences in ethanol preference (Brewster 1968, Satinder 1970) and provide further evidence of a genetic factor in ethanol preference.

These early studies stimulated the use of selective breeding to study the genetics of ethanol drinking. Selected individuals are mated to produce offspring of desired phenotype—an ancient technique man has used to breed, for instance, dogs and domestic cattle. This technique has also been used to develop animals that will voluntarily drink large amounts of ethanol. Although cattle breeders mostly are interested in selection in one direction, in basic research selection is usually performed bidirectionally, i.e., selecting for high and low extremes. This was done with rats almost 30 years ago by Eriksson (1968, 1969, 1971) in the Alko Research Laboratories in Helsinki and resulted in the establishment of the AA (Alko, alcohol) line that voluntarily consumes high amounts of ethanol and the ANA (Alko, non-alcohol) line that chooses water to the virtual exclusion of ethanol. Similar programs were started elsewhere, leading to the UCHA and UCHB rat lines at the University of Chile (Mardones 1960, 1972) and to the P and NP lines as well as the HAD and LAD lines at Indiana University (Li et al. 1981, 1987, Lumeng et al. 1986). The results of these selection programs clearly indicate that genetic factors influence the drinking of ethanol by animals.

Animal Models in Studies of Ethanol Abuse

Because animal studies have demonstrated that what occurs in humans can also be found in animals, an animal model would be useful for studying a genetically transmitted trait, since it makes possible the study of both genetic and environmental influences by manipulating both the genotype and the environment. The development of animal models of ethanol abuse, however, raises questions of the criteria for such a model. Some authors (cf. Lester and Freed 1973, Cicero 1980, Li et al. 1987) have suggested the criteria that an animal model of alcoholism ideally has to meet: (1) the animal must self-administer ethanol in pharmacologically significant amounts, (2) tolerance to ethanol should be demonstrable following a period of continuous consumption, and (3) dependence on ethanol should develop after a period of continuous consumption.

Although these criteria include some features characteristic of some human alcoholics, human alcoholism is a complex, heterogeneous disorder. These criteria also emphasize the chronic effects of ethanol, such as tolerance and dependence, and assume that they contribute to the abuse of ethanol. Our knowledge of the mechanisms that are primary in the development of ethanol abuse and alcoholism are, however, sparse. We do not know what mechanisms are related to ethanol sensitivity and development of tolerance and dependence on ethanol in the initiation and the maintenance of excessive ethanol intake. Therefore animal models of ethanol abuse should focus on the different biological factors that may contribute to the problem. An animal model makes it possible to separate, for genetic analysis and pharmacological investigations, different variables such as ethanol-seeking behavior and voluntary ethanol consumption, sensitivity, tolerance, and dependence.

Selected animal lines are useful in studies of the mechanisms of ethanol abuse and the effects of ethanol. Since the lines are produced by selectively breeding animals from a heterogeneous base population for a specific ethanol-related trait, the selected lines should theoretically differ from each other only in the trait on which selection has been applied and in traits that are related to the selected trait; selected lines are therefore a valuable tool for searching for the existence of genetic correlation between the selected trait and a specific biochemical, neurochemical or behavioral trait and to test hypotheses regarding underlying causes of ethanol abuse (Deitrich and Spuhler 1984, Crabbe et al. 1985, Schuckit et al. 1985, Crabbe et al. 1985, 1990b, Dietrich 1990).

The early studies used selected lines differing in voluntary ethanol consumption to investigate ethanol abuse. It soon became evident, however, that many characteristics related to the effects of ethanol, such as sensitivity to ethanol, capacity to develop tolerance, likelihood of developing physical dependence, and withdrawal severity after chronic ethanol administration, may also contribute to the development of ethanol abuse. Consequently, several sets of selected lines based on different ethanol-related traits have been developed to produce animal models for testing specific hypotheses concerning the bases for genetic differences and the specific biological mechanisms of ethanol abuse and ethanol's actions. The lines and related work are discussed elsewhere (McClearn 1981, Deitrich and Spuhler 1984, Li et al. 1987, Crabbe 1989, Kiianmaa et al. 1989, Phillips et al. 1989, Sinclair et al. 1989, Deitrich and Pawlowski 1990); lines will only be listed here.

Voluntary Ethanol Consumption

UCHA and UCHB rats are the oldest lines selected for differential voluntary ethanol intake. They were developed by J. Mardones in Santiago, Chile (Mardones 1960, 1972).

AA (Alko, alcohol) and ANA (Alko, nonalcohol) rats have been selectively outbred for their voluntary intake of 10% ethanol solution in a free-choice situation (Eriksson 1968, 1969, 1971, Sinclair et al. 1989).

P (preferring) and NP (nonpreferring) rats are inbred lines. They also differ in their preference for 10% ethanol solution (Li et al. 1981, 1987).

HAD (high alcohol drinking) and LAD (low alcohol drinking) rats resulted from replicating the development work of the P and NP lines through outbreeding (Lumeng et al. 1986).

SP (Sardinia preferring) and SNP (Sardinia nonpreferring) rats differ in their preference for 10% ethanol solution. The lines were recently developed in Cagliari, Italy (Fadda et al. 1989).

Sensitivity to Ethanol

LS (long-sleep) and SS (short-sleep) mice have been selectively outbred at the Institute for Behavioral Genetics in Boulder, Colorado for the duration of ethanol-induced loss of righting reflex "sleep time" (McClearn and Kakihana 1981, Phillips et al. 1989, Deitrich 1990).

Fast and slow mice differ in the stimulatory effects of ethanol (2 g/kg) in an open field apparatus (Crabbe et al. 1987b, 1990a, Phillips et al. 1989, 1991).

Hot and cold mice have been produced by selecting the hypothermic effect of an acute dose of ethanol (3 g/kg) (Crabbe et al. 1987a, 1990a, Phillips et al. 1989). Both fast/slow and hot/cold mice are also outbred lines.

AT (alcohol tolerant) and ANT (alcohol nontolerant) rats are outbred lines selected for differential ethanol-induced (2 g/kg) impairment of motor performance on the tilting plane (Eriksson and Rusi 1981, Eriksson 1990).

HAS (high alcohol sensitive) and LAS (low alcohol sensitive) rats have been selectively outbred for the duration of ethanol-induced (3 g/kg) loss of righting reflex in a test similar to that used in the breeding of LS and SS mice (Spuhler et al. 1990).

Ethanol Withdrawal

SEW (severe ethanol withdrawal) and MEW (mild ethanol withdrawal) mice have been selectively outbred for the severe ethanol withdrawal syndrome (McClearn et al. 1982, Phillips et al. 1989). Physical dependence is produced by administration of an ethanol-containing liquid diet for 9 days, and withdrawal severity is scored on a battery of tests.

WSP (withdrawal seizure prone) and WSR (withdrawal seizure resistant) mice have been selected for severe and mild signs of withdrawal induced by handling after 3 days of chronic inhalation of ethanol vapor (Crabbe et al. 1985, Crabbe 1989, Phillips et al. 1989). WSP and WSR mice are also outbred lines.

The Benefits of Animal Models

Animals can be used to search for predisposition markers. This is not, however, efficient. Markers may have only an accidental relationship to a factor affecting alcohol drinking, or the factor may be altered in several ways. For instance, the low drinking of ANA rats and among Orientals is caused apparently by a genetic alteration that reduces ALDH activity, but preliminary results suggest a differential cause in rats compared with humans. In other words, the animal models are better for discovering critical, essential factors resulting in overt differences than for revealing factors that are accidental, incidental, or indirectly involved (e.g., a predisposition marker). Animal lines especially can be used to search for the "primary sites" where genetics first produce an influence.

Animal lines point the way to treatments for alcoholism related to genetic predisposition, and then provide a basis for testing them.

Reinforcement

The amount of an addictive agent (e.g., alcohol) that an animal consumes is determined by the reinforcing effects (i.e., encourages intake) of the agent on the one hand and by the adversive effects (i.e., discourages intake) on the other. Like the effects of other addictive agents, the ethanol effect is biphasic: a low dose is reinforcing and a high dose is adversive. The AA and P rat lines, developed for high alcohol consumption, get more reinforcement from alcohol than do ANA, NP, and non-selected Wistar rats. Furthermore, P rats get reinforcement from alcohol directly into the brain.

Learned Behavioral Disorder

Alcoholism in humans is thought to be a learned behavioral disorder. Some individuals receive so much reinforcement so often from alcohol that the responses involved in getting and drinking alcohol come to dominate all of their behavior and cannot be controlled by normal social incentives and pressures. Culture, society, peer pressure, and alcohol laws influence how often a person gets reinforcement from alcohol. Genetics may also influence this by helping to direct some individuals toward gangs and groups that drink larger amounts of alcoholic beverages. The amount of reinforcement per drinking experience, however, almost certainly is under strong genetic control. This is illustrated by animal studies and can be studied best with animal models.

Blocking Reinforcement

Blocking alcohol reinforcement in the brain should be a useful addition to alcoholism treatment. Punishment of alcohol drinking, however, is not the same as blocking reinforcement. A large body of animal studies, supported amply by work with alcoholics, illustrates that punishment is not an effective method for treating alcoholism. What is needed instead is a pharmacological method for blocking reinforcement from alcohol in the brain. This could then be used to extinguish alcohol drinking or prevent the progressive development of alcoholism.

Particularly useful animal genetics research will discover a pharmacological means to block genetic reinforcement, and research will then test whether the drug is reducing alcohol drinking by affecting reinforcement or by some other means.

Alcohol Resistance

Some animals have a genetically determined greater susceptibility to motor impairment. Work in humans also suggests that genetics influences severity of intoxication. It seems likely that individuals who are more sensitive to alcohol-induced motor impairment or less able to counteract alcohol's effects are responsible for many accidents involving alcohol. It might be possible to find drugs or other means to raise the alcohol resistance of overly sensitive individuals to average levels. Animal lines genetically developed for low resistance to alcohol-induced motor impairment should be useful.

Relapse and Binge Intoxication Predisposition

Most animals including humans increase alcohol drinking temporarily after a period of forced abstinence, often leading to severe intoxication, accidents, alcohol poisoning, and perhaps adverse medical consequences. This alcohol deprivation effect also promotes relapse. There is increasing evidence that the time course for the alcohol deprivation effect and its magnitude are influenced by genetics. Important new work would be the development of lines differing in alcohol deprivation effects and of drug treatments for suppressing the alcohol deprivation effect or, more specifically, for suppressing excessively large alcohol deprivation effects.

Satiety

It has been claimed that a major difference between alcoholics and social drinkers is that social drinkers have better alcohol satiety systems that usually help them stop imbibing after only a couple of drinks. In accord, we have initial findings in rats that such a satiety system does exist and some evidence to suggest that it might be affected by genetics. Important new work would be the study of genetic factors that affect satiety and the development of drugs to enhance the system and overcome any genetically determined deficit.

Genetic Heterogeneity: Biological Markers

The extensive heterogeneous nature of alcoholism explains the difficulties in determining the genetic part of the disorder. One valuable approach would be to assess the manner in which alcohol consumption, alcohol dependence, and alcohol-related problems are transmitted within families, assuming that all three are not transmitted together. It will be easier to then identify the different genes that confer susceptibility.

The transmissible component in alcoholism undoubtedly involves multiple genes whose expression can be quite specific (e.g., disposition to end-organ injury) or much less specific (e.g., development of personality traits that predispose to alcoholism). Moreover, the ultimate phenotype can be greatly affected by environmental factors.

Although alcoholism is a genetically influenced disorder, it is in many respects different from other disorders that follow a more traditional Mendelian mode of inheritance. In contrast to a number of disorders such as cystic fibrosis, Huntington's disease, and sickle cell anemia, the development of alcoholism in some individuals depends on the presence of genetically influenced predisposition factors that interact with environmentally determined precipitating factors. It is the interaction between predisposing and precipitating factors that results in alcoholism. The search for potential causative genes is complicated because alcoholism is a common and complex non-Mendelian disorder with a number of features characteristic of complex diseases:

(1) Alcoholism is a clinically heterogeneous disorder with variable age of onset.

(2) The disorder may not be caused by any one single gene, but may develop from the additive effects of multiple genes (polygenetic inheritance).

(3) Single mutations at different genetic loci may result in clinically indistinguishable disease states (genetic heterogeneity).

(4) Not every individual who inherits the genes will develop the disorder (reduced penetrance).

(5) The disorder may reflect the complex interactions between alleles at several loci (epistatic effects).

(6) A substantial number of individuals without a disease genotype manifest alcoholism resulting from nongenetic causes (phenocopies).

It would appear that the quest for uncovering genes in alcoholism is a seemingly intractable problem. However, the presence of genetic factors predisposing individuals to develop alcoholism offers an unique opportunity to assess potential biological factors associated with alcoholism. Because of solid evidence that implicates genetic factors in the development of alcoholism, the study of offspring of alcoholic patients from high-density families should provide an important sample of individuals at high risk for the development of alcoholism. Such a sample of individuals would be ideal for studying antecedent biological factors that predispose some individuals to develop alcoholism.

The search for predisposing biological markers associated with genetic factors in alcoholism must be conducted in accordance with a specific set of criteria. First, it should be demonstrated that in the general population, the trait (marker) can be reliably measured and is stable over time, is genetically transmitted, and has a low base rate and that individuals at risk can be identified with a significant degree of accuracy and reliability. Second, studies in patients should demonstrate that the "abnormal trait" is prevalent in the patient population, is present during symptom remission and is not just a state marker, occurs among first-degree relatives of the proband at a rate higher than that of the normal population, and segregates with the illness in affected relatives of the proband.

Some of the most widely studied biological markers include the P300 event-related potential, the A1 allele of the D2 dopamine (DA) receptor, monoamine oxidase activity in platelets, and adenylate cyclase activity. Although these trait markers may identify individuals at risk of developing alcoholism, other trait markers may denote protection. The best example of the latter is the protective effect of ALDH2*2 (aldehyde dehydrogenase 2 deficiency), which will be discussed later.

The P300 Event-Related Potential

Although EEG measures the spontaneous electrical activity of the brain, event-related potential (ERP) measures, by computer averaging, the specific brain wave response to external sensory stimuli. One component of ERP is a positive wave observed at about 300 msec (the P300) after a sensory stimulus that requires an individual to attend to and interpret its contextual meaning. The stimulus is anticipated but occurs as a rare event. The size of the P300 is believed to correlate with the individual's ability to selectively recognize and properly interpret subtle stimuli in the environment. Thus, P300 measures the sensory, perceptual, and cognitive responses of the individual. Early on, P300 was found to be reduced in abstinent alcoholics and was thought to be a consequence of alcohol abuse (Begleiter et al. 1980). However, Begleiter et al. (1984) reported that preadolescent sons of alcoholic fathers manifested a reduced P300 amplitude before any exposure to alcohol compared with controls with nonalcoholic fathers. Reduced P300 voltages in ERP were found in sons of alcoholics by using either a visuospatial "evoke" paradigm or an auditory "oddball" paradigm. Additionally, at least three separate research groups have replicated the finding of reduced P300 voltages in high-risk subjects without the administration of alcohol. Because abnormal P300 has been reported by various laboratories under different experimental conditions, this electrophysiological marker seems to be generalizable. Of note, the young sons of alcoholics tested by Begleiter met the criteria for the male-limited, type II alcoholism as delineated by Cloninger. To date, no follow-up studies have been done to compare the development of alcoholism in these sons of alcoholics showing and not showing the decreased P300 amplitude. At this time, the only measure that meets all of the criteria necessary to be a bona fide phenotypic biologic marker is in fact ERP (i.e., specific criteria 1a.b.c.d–2a.b.c.d). In addition, ERP measures are currently the only ones demonstrated experimentally and statistically to discriminate reliably between high-risk and low-risk subjects.

The A1 Allele of the D2 Dopamine Receptor

Publicity has been given to an article by Blum and his colleagues (1990) on the association of the A1 allele of D2 dopamine receptor gene with alcoholism. From brain samples of 35 severe alcoholics and 35 nonalcoholics, DNA was digested with the Taq1 restriction enzyme and probed with a clone that contained the entire 3' coding exon, the polyadenylation signal, and about 16.4 kilobase of noncoding 3' sequence of human D2 dopamine receptor gene. These investigators found that 69% of the alcoholics in contrast to 20% of the nonalcoholics carried the A1 allele, a highly significant difference. Their data were criticized, however, because the frequency of the A1 allele in their sample of alcoholics was similar to frequencies obtained in other population studies, whereas the frequency of the A1 allele in their nonalcoholic controls was inordinately low.

Three additional studies were performed in attempts to replicate the original report. Two of the studies seemed to confirm the original observation, but that by Bolos et al. (1990) produced negative results. The latter study was criticized because it investigated only alcoholic subjects with less severe alcoholism, since by design medically ill alcoholics were excluded. Further studies by Blum et al. (1991) and Parsian et al. (1991) confirmed a significant association between severe alcoholism and the A1 allele. Analyses carried out by Bolos et al. and Parsian et al. revealed no linkage between A1 allele polymorphism and alcoholism in more than 19 nuclear families with multigenerational pedigrees of alcoholics. As concluded by Conneally (1991) in his commentary, "It appears that the association between alcoholism and the A1 allele of the D2 dopamine receptor locus may be real. It is clearly not due to linkage with a gene for alcoholism, but could be a cause of the progression of the disease in individuals genetically predisposed to alcoholism." More recent studies suggest that the A1 allele could aggravate susceptibility to the medical complications of alcoholism (Cook et al. 1992, Karp 1992). How the A1 allele affects D1 binding has yet to be adequately investigated.

Monoamine Oxidase Activity in Platelets

Monoamine oxidase (MAO) catalyzes the oxidation of monamine neurotransmitters, e.g., norepinephrine, dopamine, and 5-HT, and it exists in two isoforms: MAO A and B. Both MAO isoenzymes are present in the central nervous system, but MAO B is also found in circulation platelets. The cDNAs for MAO A and B have been cloned and the genes have been localized to the X chromosome. The activity of MAO B in platelets is under strong genetic control and has been reported repeatedly to be lower in alcoholic patients (Schuckit et al. 1982), with lower activity in type II alcoholics than in type I (Von Knorring et al. 1991). The low MAO B platelet activity in alcoholics is due to a decrease in the amount of enzyme rather than the Km for substrate, and it persists with abstinence. Thus, it is not simply caused by the toxic effect of ethanol. It is unknown how low platelet MAO relates to central nervous system MAO activities. Likewise, it is unknown whether low MAO activities in platelets or in the central nervous sytem play a mechanistic role in the aberrant alcohol-seeking behavior found in alcoholics. The major problem with platelet MAO activity is that it is complicated by a wide range of normal MAO activities and a great overlap between populations with high and low risk for alcoholism. Thus, the interpretation of platelet MAO activities remains a difficult problem.

Lymphocyte and Platelet Adenylate Cyclase Activities

Another enzyme activity that is decreased in alcoholics is adenylate cyclase. In peripheral lymphocytes obtained from alcoholic subjects, both the basal and the adenosine agonist-stimulated rates of cAMP production were reduced by as much as 74% (Diamond 1987). Similarly, the accumulation of cAMP in platelets exposed to cesium fluoride, prostaglandin E or nonhydrolyzable analogs of GTP was impaired in cells obtained from alcoholics relative to those from nonalcoholics (Tabakoff et al. 1988). These abnormalities in alcoholics persisted even after weeks of abstinence, suggesting that the decreased adenylate cyclase activity in lymphocytes and platelets is more of a trait marker (one that identifies vulnerability to developing alcoholism) than a state marker (one that reflects the extent of alcohol abuse). Since the activity of adenylate cyclase is reduced when stimulated by a battery of receptor ligands and nonhydrolyzable GTP analogs, the molecular basis for the defect most likely results in an abnormality in the Gs guanine nucleotide-binding proteins that couple receptor binding by ligand to adenylate cyclase activation. So far, decreased adenylate cyclase activity in lymphocytes and platelets as a trait marker of alcoholism has not been extensively replicated. Very recently, lymphocyte adenylate cyclase activity has been studied in familial alcoholism. The marker, which is independent of the level of alcohol consumption, occurred in about 40% of the offspring of multigenerational alcoholics. Segregation was consistent with a major locus dominant gene (Palmour et al. 1992).

Associations between other markers and alcoholism have been tested (Hill et al. 1975, reviewed in Merikangas 1990 and Eskay and Linnoila 1991). No association between acetylation phenotype and alcoholism was discovered (Guthrie et al. 1989). Linkage may exist between alcoholism and esterase D (Tanna et al. 1988). An association has been described between alcoholism and A1 A2 BO and MNS polymorphisms (Hill et al. 1988, Clemente et al. 1992). A specific variant of the human brain protein PC 1 Duarte has an increased frequency in populations of alcoholics (Comings 1977). Protein III, which plays a critical role in the functioning of nerve cells, may exist in a genetically defined variant form in individuals at heightened risk for alcohol dependence (Perdahl 1984). A defect in serotonin metabolism is one hypothesis for alcoholism, and tests of tryptophan oxygenase (Comings 1992) and tryptophan pyrrolase (Comings et al. 1991) should be done. A pilot study suggests phospholipase D activity in lymphocyte as a potential marker in adult men at risk for becoming alcoholics (Mueller et al. 1988, Eskay and Linnoila 1991).

Another approach is to determine high-risk populations. Subjective responses to alcohol were investigated (Moss et al. 1989, Schuckit 1991). Differences between subjects with positive and negative family histories were observed after an alcohol challenge by measurement of body sway and endocrinological changes (prolactin, cortisol and adrenocorticotropin hormone). Less intense reaction to alcohol was found in sons of alcoholic fathers (Schuckit 1991). A longitudinal study demonstrated that a decreased reaction at age 20 appears to be a major predictor of alcoholism by age 30 (Schuckit 1992). Various indices of sober and alcohol-intoxicated cardiovascular reactivity may serve as markers for familial risk of alcoholism (Peterson et al. 1992). A review of neuropsychological factors that predispose to alcoholism found apparent inconsistencies in the findings regarding the cognitive abilities of subjects at high risk and low risk for alcoholism (Hesselbrock et al. 1991). A recent and extensive review of children of alcoholics was recently published (Sher 1991).

In conclusion, the identification of valid and reliable genetic markers of risk of developing alcoholism has begun in earnest, and is critical to the search for the genes that influence the development of alcohol dependence. Several putative markers have been evaluated in cross-sectional studies. The value of any potential marker, however, will be significantly increased by testing its predictive power in longitudinal studies. Moreover, we need to assess the relationship of all of the putative markers in several different populations of individuals at risk of developing alcoholism. Although the current epidemiological data indicate that males are at higher risk than females to develop alcoholism, similar studies of females must be done. It is also important to determine whether similar putative markers exist in females and to assess the predictive value of such markers for the development of alcoholism or other psychiatric conditions.

The identification of genetic trait markers correlated with a predisposition to develop alcoholism not only will be critical for identifying potential genes but will be equally important in elucidating the etiological factors involved in the development of alcoholism. A better understanding of the causes of alcoholism will result in the development of more rational and effective treatment procedures and the implementation of efficacious primary prevention initiatives.

Alcohol and Acetaldehyde Metabolism: Initial Sensitivity

Normal twins have been used to examine genetic influences on the absorption, breakdown, and elimination of a single challenge dose of alcohol. Short-term environmental factors influence alcohol metabolism, particularly in the absorption phase, but the repeatable variance in peak blood alcohol concentration and rate of elimination is due mainly to genetic factors (Kopun and Propping 1977, Martin et al. 1985; reviewed in Marshall and Murray 1989).

Alcohol dehydrogenase (ADH alcohol:NAD oxidoreductase, EC 1.1.1.1.) oxidises ethanol to acetaldehyde via hydrogen transfer from the substrate to the cofactor *nicotinamide adenin* dinucleotide (NAD), resulting in conversion to its reduced form, NADH. Polymorphisms have been reported at two of the five loci encoding ADH subunits (ADH2 and ADH3). The variant enzyme form produced at the polymorphic ADH2 locus is commonly known as "atypical" ADH, which contains a variant β2 subunit instead of the usual β1 subunit. It exhibits a much higher catalytic activity than the normal enzyme at a relatively high physiological pH (pH 8.8), and migrates more cathodically in starch gel electrophoresis. About 5-10% of the English, 9-14% of the German, and 20% of the Swiss population possess the atypical ADH, whereas the variant enzyme occurs in about 85% of the Japanese, Chinese, and other Oriental populations. Differences in the kinetic properties of the polymorphic forms of ADH isozymes may contribute to interethnic differences in the in vivo rate of ethanol metabolism. Any genetically determined variation in the ethanol metabolism rate could also influence steady-state blood acetaldehyde levels.

Individuals who are ADH2/2 homozygotes eliminate alcohol more rapidly (about 30% faster) than do heterozygotes. Some individuals homozygous for ADH2/2 with normal ALDH2 have a greater degree of flushing than do heterozygotes or Caucasians homozygous for ADH 2/1. Presence of the ADH 2/3 allele is associated with faster alcohol elimination (May et al. 1992). Preliminary results on ADH3 polymorphism are not in favor of an effect of ADH3 genotype on ethanol metabolism (Couzigou et al. 1990).

Oxidation of acetaldehyde in human liver and other organs is catalyzed by the NAD-dependent aldehyde dehydrogenase (ALDH). At least four isozymes of ALDH coded by different gene loci have been detected in human organs and tissues that differ in their electrophoretic mobility, isoelectric point, kinetic properties, subcellular and tissue distribution, and chromosomal assignment. A widely prevalent genetic polymorphism has been observed for ALDH2 isozyme. In about 50% of the Japanese and Chinese, liver lacks an ALDH2 isozyme activity band. Phenotype distribution studies indicate that a significant percentage of Orientals of Mongoloid origin have this isozyme abnormality, whereas none of the Caucasian or Negroid populations investigated so far exhibit this polymorphism. About 40% of South American Indian tribes (Mapuche, Atacamenos, Shuara) exhibit the ALDH2 deficiency phenotype, but only a very small percentage of North American Indians (Sioux, Navajo, mestizos) have this deficient phenotype (Goedde et al. 1986). Protein structural studies revealed that a point mutation is responsible for the inactivation of ALDH2 isozyme in Orientals; glutamic acid at the 14th position from the C terminus (487th position from the amino terminus) is substituted with lysine in the deficient isozyme (Hempel et al. 1984).

Alcohol flushers exhibit rapid facial flushing, elevation of skin temperature, and increase in pulse rate when they drink less than 0.5 mL of ethanol/kg body weight. Incidence of alcohol flushing in Orientals is correlated with lack of the mitochondrial aldehyde dehydrogenase ALDH2 activity and is confirmed by a genotyping aldehyde dehydrogenase study (Shibuya et al. 1989). Inherited defects in the cytosolic ALDH isozyme (ALDH1) in Caucasian subjects who reported alcohol-related flushing have also been described (Peters et al.

1990). Accordingly, "Caucasian flushing" is possibly due to the synthesis of proteins with reduced and/or altered enzyme activity.

Behavioral and physiological responses to alcohol are in part inherited (reviewed in Marshall and Murray 1989, Heath and Martin 1992). Electroencephalogram patterns after alcohol ingestion became more dissimilar between DZ twins than MZ twins (Propping 1977). Genetic factors contribute to the response of heart rate and body sway to a challenge of alcohol (Cobb et al. 1984). A study of psychomotor performance and subjective intoxication in twin pairs not selected for risk of alcoholism after intake of alcohol (0.75 g/kg body weight) showed a significant difference in alcohol-specific reactivity such as body sway and other psychomotor performance (Martin et al. 1985). Multivariate genetic analysis of these studies (Heath and Martin 1992) has further helped identify two genetic factors. The first factor had high loadings on drinking history, subjective intoxication, and body sway. The second factor had high loadings on blood alcohol curve and on tests of psychomotor coordination but low loading on drinking history and subjective ratings. In females only, body sway also loaded on this second, BAC-sensitive factor as well as on the first, drinking-history-sensitive factor. Inherited differences in reactivity or sensitivity to a standard dose of alcohol, noted in the sons of alcoholics, were hypothesised to account for their increased propensity to alcoholism (Schuckit 1988).

Acute Reactions to Acetaldehyde

In humans, the effects of ethanol per se are influenced by its sympathomimetic activity and by its metabolites, acetaldehyde and acetate (Truitt and Walsh 1973, Kupari et al. 1983). In some individuals, ingestion of moderate amounts of alcohol exerts the so-called alcohol sensitivity symptoms (facial flushing, increase in heart rate, enhancement of left ventricular function, hot feeling in stomach, palpitation, tachycardia, muscle weakness, etc.). Wolff (1972, 1973) reported significant differences between Caucasians, with 5% of subjects showing a flush response to alcohol, and Mongoloids and American Indians, over 80% of whom showed flushing reactions. It is evident from all of the published studies that compared with Caucasians, a greater percentage of Orientals (Mongoloid ancestry) and American Indians show adverse reactions to alcohol.

ALDH2 isozyme-deficient subjects show a significantly higher blood acetaldehyde level than do nonflushers with a normal ALDH2 isozyme profile. Thus, the initial vasomotor flushing after alcohol ingestion in Orientals might be due to their inability to metabolize acetaldehyde quickly and effectively in the absence of the mitochondrial ALDH2 isozyme with a low Km for acetaldehyde (reviewed by Goedde and Agarwal 1992).

The Role of Alcohol Sensitivity in Alcohol Drinking Habits

An interesting correlation exists between flushing response and alcohol drinking habits of Orientals. In one study, Asian Americans living in Hawaii were questioned about their use of alcoholic beverages and the postdrink physical consequences they experienced (Wilson et al. 1978). Comparison between groups showed that (1) a larger proportion of Orientals than Caucasians reported no use of alcohol, (2) Caucasians reported heavier alcohol use, (3) a smaller percentage of Orientals reported ever using alcohol and the overall amount they consumed was a little smaller, and (4) a large proportion of Orientals who drank alcohol experienced facial flushing and associated sensitivity symptoms after drinking alcohol.

Suwaki and Ohara (1985) conducted a comprehensive survey of drinking patterns (drinking frequency and drinking quantity) and alcohol-related problems, including alcohol-induced facial flushing, in a large number of middle-aged Japanese men. Of the 2035 individuals questioned, 1646 drank alcohol regularly and 389 reported not drinking at all. Of those who consumed alcohol, about 61% reported that they flushed after ingesting alcohol and 48% did not experience any flushing response. Flushers drank a small amount of alcohol compared with nonflushers, who frequently drank a fairly large amount of alcohol and suffered from alcohol-related problems.

In a large study of Koreans and Chinese in Taiwan (Park et al. 1984), subjects who showed fast flushing consumed substantially less alcohol than did those who exhibited no flushing or slow flushing. The Chinese in Hawaii and Taiwan resembled each other closely regarding flushing response and alcohol use. Accordingly, only fast flushing appears to have a substantial influence on alcohol use as observed in Japanese in Hawaii, in homeland Koreans and to some extent in Taiwanese (Johnson et al. 1984, Park et al. 1984). Reed and Hanna (1986) reported between-race and within-race variation in cardiovascular responses to alcohol consumption. The alcohol response data show similarities between Japanese and Chinese and marked differences between either of these and Europeans. The mean usual alcohol consumption (g/week) was found to be 40.8, 73.0, and 135.8 for the Chinese, Japanese, and Europeans, respectively. A relationship has been observed between subtypes of alcohol-induced flushing and DSM III alcohol abuse (Higushi et al. 1992b).

ALDH2 Abnormality, Alcohol Sensitivity, and Alcohol Consumption

Individuals who experience an initial adverse reaction to alcohol by virtue of their genetically controlled deficiency of ALDH2 may be discouraged from alcohol abuse. Harada et al. (1985) determined the frequency of ALDH2 isozyme deficiency in two Japanese districts in the regions of Sendai and Gifu, which differed significantly in their per capita alcohol consumption. The role of ALDH2 isozyme deficiency in affecting alcohol drinking habits was further supported by Japanese studies (Ohmori et al. 1986, Higushi et al. 1992a). Men who had inactive ALDH2 drank significantly less alcohol than did those with active ALDH2, and a similar but less noticeable efffect was detected in women. Two types of flushing responses have been noted. The great majority of subjects who reported that they always flushed were shown to have inactive ALDH2, whereas infrequent flushing and absence of flushing were associated with active ALDH2. A recent study of Asian-American men corroborated the association between the presence of an ALDH2-2 allele, increased pulse rate, and alcohol-induced flushing. In this study, flushers reported experiencing significantly more positive feelings of intoxication than did nonflushers, despite equivalent blood alcohol concentrations. The alcohol sensitivity reaction that many Asian flushers experience may contribute to their lower tendency to drink excessively, even though their response to alcohol is not predominantly negative (Wall et al. 1992).

ADH and ALDH Polymorphism and Alcoholism

Few data are available on ADH polymorphism and alcoholism. The ADH2-2 allele was more common in a nonalcoholic control group than in alcoholics (Thomasson et al. 1991). In the same study, the ADH3-1 allele was also more prevalent in the nonalcoholics than in the alcoholics. However, no association between ADH3 phenotype and alcoholism was found (Fleury et al. 1990). An association between ADH RFLP polymorphism and alcoholism was recently described (Ward et al. 1992).

A significantly low incidence of ALDH2 isozyme deficiency was observed in a group of alcoholics compared with psychiatric patients, drug-dependent patients, and healthy controls in a Japanese psychiatric hospital (Harada et al. 1982, Goedde 1983). In 175 alcoholics, only about 2% were found to have the isozyme deficiency, whereas in drug-dependent patients, schizophrenics, and healthy controls, more than 40% had the deficiency. In a subsequent study of alcoholics and healthy controls from the Kanto area in Japan, a similar distribution of isozyme deficiency was observed (Harada et al. 1985). Of 247 alcoholics, only 5.4% were deficient in ALDH2 isozyme, whereas about 42% of the 61 healthy controls were ALDH2 deficient. Nearly identical findings were observed in other psychiatric clinics in Japan and Taiwan (Ohmori et al. 1986). Thus, the higher the prevalence of ALDH2 isozyme deficiency in racial or ethnic groups, the lower the prevalence of alcohol-related problems.

Interestingly, Sioux and Navajo tribes and a mestizo group showed a very low percentage of isozyme deficiency, wherease Indians from Chile and Ecuador were deficient to an extent comparable to Japanese and Chinese (Goedde et al. 1986). Although no deficiency of ALDH2 isozyme at autopsy in the livers of American Indians of northern New Mexico was observed (Rex et al. 1985, Bosron et al. 1988), 14% of 51 Oklahoma Indians were deficient (Zeiner et al. 1984). This study also showed that ALDH2 isozyme-deficient Indians drank significantly less alcohol than did nondeficient Indians, and a family history of alcoholism was significantly lower in deficient subjects than in Indians without the isozyme deficiency.

In a study of Chinese males living in Taiwan, the frequency of the ALDH2-2 allele was 30% in a nonalcoholic control group and 6% in a group of alcoholic individuals (Thomasson et al. 1991).

Genetics and Alcoholic Liver Disease

Although there is a relationship between alcohol consumption and alcoholic liver disease, at both the aggregate and the individual level, fewer than one-third of alcoholics or heavy drinkers develop serious alcohol-related liver damage. Autopsy series or studies based on liver biopsy have shown that the incidence of cirrhosis in heavy drinkers is under 30% (Leevy 1968, Von Olderhausen 1970, Bhathal et al. 1975). Additionally, under a well-controlled experimental situation, only about 30% of baboons given high doses of ethanol developed cirrhosis (Lieber et al. 1975).

Whatever the explanation, alcohol is necessary but not sufficient to induce alcoholic cirrhosis. Associated factors, genetic and environmental, influence hepatic vulnerability to alcohol. One twin study (Hrubec and Omenn 1981) specifically addressed the existence of a genetic factor in alcoholic cirrhosis. Among 15,924 twin pairs, the prevalence between individual twin subjects was 2.96% for alcoholism and 1.42% for alcoholic cirrhosis. The respective concordance rates were 26.3 (MZ twins) versus 11.9 (DZ twins) for alcoholism and 14.6 (MZ) versus 5.4 (DZ) for alcoholic cirrhosis. The greater concordance in MZ twins for alcoholic cirrhosis could not be explained by the difference in alcoholism concordance between MZ and DZ twins. There is a gender difference in alcoholic liver disease, with women more susceptible to alcohol-induced hepatic disease than men (reviewed in Van Thiel 1991). These results suggest a genetic predisposition to alcohol-induced liver injury and prompted the research for candidate genes and genetic markers.

Many investigators have analyzed the distribution of HLA phenotypes in patients suffering from alcoholism with and without organ damage. A number of studies (reviewed by Devor and Cloninger 1989) showed that alcoholic cirrhosis is significantly associated with HLA B8, B13, B15, B40, CW3, DR2, DR4, and DRW9. A protective role has also been reported for HLA B8, B12, and B13. Accelerated development of alcoholic cirrhosis has been observed in patients with HLA B8 (Saunders et al. 1982). These associations must be viewed with caution. Statistically significant associations with HLA antigens may occur by chance if a large number of antigens are screened with a sufficient sample size (Gilligan and Cloninger 1989, Poupon et al. 1991). A meta-analysis of race and degree of liver disease showed that none of the HLA phenotypes was significantly more common in the patient categories studied than in controls (Gluud 1992).

Phenotypes of immunoglobulin allotypes were associated with alcoholic cirrhosis (Schmidt et al. 1987), but this finding has not been replicated (Poupon et al. 1991). Data recently were published on HLA class III alleles, with the C4B-Q0 allele reported to be associated with cirrhosis. The C4B-Q0 allele would be linked to the development of cirrhosis whatever the etiology (Pasta et al. 1992).

Conflicting results have been reported about the association between polymorphism of type I collagen and increased risk of alcoholic cirrhosis (Weiner et al. 1988, Day et al. 1990, Christa et al. 1992). This polymorphism is plausible and merits further exploration.

Alcohol dehydrogenase class I is polymorphic at the ADH2 and ADH3 loci, and the difference in the kinetic properties of the corresponding enzymes may explain different susceptibility to alcoholic liver disease. The ADH2-2 allele is not associated with increased risk of alcoholic cirrhosis (Shibuya and Yoshida 1988b, Tanaka et al. 1990), and the same observation was made for the ADH2-3 allele (Couzigou et al. 1990b). For ADH3, conflicting results are described for alleles and an association with alcoholic cirrhosis: an increased risk with the ADH3-1 allele (Day et al. 1991) or the ADH3-2 allele (Tanaka et al. 1990) but an absence of significant risk with the ADH3 polymorphism in a genotyping study (Couzigou et al. 1990, Wermuth et al. 1991) and a phenotyping study (Ricciardi et al. 1983, Poupon et al. 1992).

Mitochondrial aldehyde dehydrogenase ALDH2 is polymorphic in Oriental populations, and the mutant dominant ALDH2-2 allele has a protective role against alcoholism. ALDH2-2 is also protective against alcoholic liver disease (Shibuya and Yoshida 1988b). Heterozygosity for mutant ALDH2 also seems to predispose to more severe liver damage, the estimated daily intake of ethanol being lower among individuals with the ALDH2 genotype. ALDH2-2-deficient individuals also had a higher prevalence of alcoholic hepatitis (Enomoto et al. 1991).

Association of glutathione S transferase I polymorphism and alcoholic cirrhosis has been described in a Japanese population (Harada et al. 1987) but failed to be replicated in Caucasians (Groppi et al. 1991). Preliminary results do not support an association between apoprotein E polymorphism and alcoholic cirrhosis (Iron et al. 1992).

The alpha I antitrypsin gene has been studied as a potential "candidate gene" in predisposition to alcoholic cirrhosis, without significant results (Morin et al. 1975, Brind et al. 1991). Associations between alcoholic cirrhosis and other genetic markers such as colour blindness and blood groups have been described but have not been confirmed (reviewed in Saunders and Williams 1983).

Genetics and Other End-Organ Alcohol-Related Disease

Only a minority of alcoholics develop chronic pancreatitis. The reasons for individual susceptibility to this disease are unknown. Only one twin study has tried to assess the genetic component of this susceptibility, but no twin pairs concordant for pancreatitis were found (Hrubec and Omenn 1981). A genetic predisposition for alcoholic pancreatitis was suggested by reports of an increased incidence of various HLA antigens as well as blood groups (reviewed in Haber et al. 1991). A statistically significant association may occur by chance in view of the number of HLA antigens tested. No significant differences were found in alpha I antitrypsin phenotypes between alcoholics with or without pancreatitis (Haber et al. 1991). A trend is observed in preliminary data for an association between ADH3 polymorphism and alcoholic pancreatitis, but confirmation on a more important sample is required (Couzigou et al. 1990b, Day et al. 1991).

One study (Hrubec et al. 1981) addressed the concordance of alcoholic psychosis between alcoholic twins. The concordance rate for alcoholism was 26.3 (MZ) versus 5.4 (DZ) and for alcoholic psychosis was 21.1 (MZ) versus 6.0 (DZ). The greater concordance in MZ twins for alcoholic psychosis could not be explained by the difference in concordance for alcoholism between MZ and DZ twins. These results suggest a genetic predisposition to alcoholic psychosis.

A biochemical basis for differences in susceptibility to Wernicke-Korsakoff (WE) syndrome is sustained by a difference in Km for thiamine for erythrocyte and fibroblast transketolase between alcoholics with and without WE syndrome (Blass and Gibson 1977). Evidence for an association between WE syndrome and an apparent genetic variant of transketolase, however, is indirect and conflicting and requires further exploration (Nixon et al. 1990, Eskay and Linnoila 1991).

Another organ adversely affected by alcohol abuse is the cardiovascular system. Myrhed (1974) conducted a study of twins in Scandinavia that suggested a genetic influence on alcohol-induced hypertension.

Glutathione S transferase I polymorphism has been shown to be associated with carcinoma of the lung (linked with tobacco). No association has been found between oesophageal carcinoma (linked with alcohol and tobacco) and lack of glutathione S transferase I (Coutelle et al. 1992).

Genetic polymorphism has been described for other enzymes implicated in ethanol metabolism, such as cytochrome P450IIE1 (Hayashi et al. 1991), fatty acid ethyl ester synthase (Devor [in Crabb and Lands 1992]), gastric ADH (Baraona et al. 1991), and in the metabolism of organs injured by chronic alcohol intake. This gives some support for the eventual discovery of a genetic factor in other end-organ alcohol-related disease, and future studies addressing this hypothesis would be worthy.

Suggested Future Studies

Certain technologies and strategies will be especially helpful to determine prospectively whether there is a specific genetic predetermination to alcoholism. In animal models, development of specific mouse genetic models for different aspects of alcohol drinking and behavior would be worthwhile (far more is known about the mouse genome than the rat genome). Animal models of alcoholism do not exist, but animal models are of importance for answering questions related to alcoholism, now that transgenic models are being developed using gene insertion or deletion. A mechanistic approach seems more relevant than a molecular approach for searching out genes responsible for alcoholism. Animal models of ethanol abuse should be focused on the different genetic factors that contribute to alcohol abuse. An animal model makes it possible to separate different variables—such as voluntary ethanol consumption, sensitivity, tolerance, dependence, and withdrawal—for genetic analysis and pharmacological investigation. New work should thus study genetic factors of voluntary ethanol consumption to solve where the genetic factors come in. The studies should clarify whether there are genetic differences in the satiety and deprivation effects of alcohol and in reinforcement from alcohol. This could be done by developing animal models designed to answer specific questions, e.g., developing animal lines showing high versus low deprivation effects and animal lines differing in the amount drunk in one bout. Genetic studies should also be aimed at clarifying how ethanol sensitivity and tolerance contribute to ethanol consumption.

Family studies with the collection of information by direct interviews would be of major importance. These family studies could investigate specific aspects of genetics and alcoholism (e.g., initial sensitivity, alcoholism, and end-organ damage). Genetic factors influence alcoholism risk, but the current debate centers on the strength of that influence and the extent to which it is moderated by age, sex, diagnostic subtype, and psychiatric comorbidity. New knowledge is needed to improve understanding in these areas, especially regarding phenotype and subtype of alcoholism.

Regarding genetics markers, genotypic and phenotypic markers should be studied, because probably a number of genes are involved but with small additive effects. A linkage map of the human genome, now in progress, will be of tremendous importance in localising, with the use of family data, that part of the genome implicated in the genetic factor studied. Longitudinal studies are necessary to determine high-risk populations. Research on polymorphisms as contributive genetic factors in alcoholism and acetaldehyde metabolism, on neuromediators, and on enzymes implicated in end-organ metabolism would be worthwhile. Identification of individuals at genetic risk of alcoholism and/or alcohol-related diseases should be possible using knowledge of a specific genetic predetermination and the results of longitudinal studies.

In longitudinal studies, the choice of criteria that can easily be used a second time for identification of high-risk populations, e.g., reactions to alcohol absorption, would be relevant and useful in exploring related ethical problems. Educational strategies should be developed to allow high-risk subjects to adapt their life-styles. From a curative and therapeutic point of view, animal studies could contribute to the development of treatments related to genetic aspects of alcohol abuse.

It is not possible to predict how long it will take to establish a genetic profile of alcoholism and alcohol-related disease. Indeed, such a genetic profile may not be specific for alcoholism. It is possible that the genes involved in the predisposition to alcoholism may also be useful in identifying individuals predisposed to other disorders of behavioral dysregulation. It is hoped that in the next decade such a genotypic profile can be developed.

What new research should be undertaken? Animal models can be used for physiopathological studies (relationships between preference, tolerance, dependence, drinking and tolerance, tolerance-dependence and withdrawal). For such studies transgenic models, especially of the mouse, would be worthwhile. Animal and human studies involving low levels of alcohol drinking should be undertaken. Also of interest would be racial and interethnic studies about initial sensitivity and alcohol metabolism. Family studies and longitudinal studies are necessary to understand the impact of alcohol on behavior, including alcohol abuse, alcohol dependence, and alcohol-related diseases. Such studies should relate to the study of putative markers and the linkage map of the human genome.

Acknowledgments: Prof. M. Joernvall, Karolinska Institute (S) is gratefully acknowledged for his contribution in critically reviewing the manuscript.

References

Agarwal DP, Goedde HW (1989) Human aldehyde dehydrogenases: their role in alcoholism. Alcohol 6:517–23

Agarwal DP, Goedde HW (1990) Alcohol metabolism, alcohol intolerance and alcoholism. Springer-Verlag, Berlin, Heidelberg

Agarwal DP, Goedde HW (1991) The role of alcohol metabolizing enzymes in alcohol sensitivity, alcohol drinking habits, and incidence of alcoholism in Orientals. In Palmer TN (ed), The molecular pathology of alcoholism. Oxford University Press, Oxford, pp 211–37

Agarwal DP, Goedde HW (1992) Medico-biological and genetic studies on alcoholism. Role of metabolic variation and ethnicity on drinking habits, alcohol abuse and alcohol-related mortality. Clin Investig 70:465–77

Akabane J, Nakanishi S, Kohei H, et al. (1964) Studies on the sympathomimetic action of acetaldehyde. Jpn J Pharmacol 14:295–307

Allan AM, Harris RA (1989) Sensitivity to ethanol and modulation of chloride channels does not cosegregate with pentobarbital sensitivity in HS mice. Alcohol Clin Exp Res 13:428–34

Alterman AI, Searles JS, Hall JG (1989) Failure to find differences in drinking behaviour as a function of familial risk for alcoholism: a replication. J Abnorm Psychol 98:50–53

Ambroziak W, Pietruszko R (1987) Human aldehyde dehydrogenase metabolism of putrescine and histamine. Alcohol Clin Exp Res 11:528–32

Aston CE, Hill SY (1990) Segregation analysis of alcoholism in families ascertained through a pair of male alcoholics. Am J Hum Genet 46:879–87

Baraona E, DiPova C, Tabasco J, Lieber CS (1987) Transport of acetaldehyde in red blood cells. Alcohol Alcohol Suppl 1:203–6

Baraona E, Yokoyama A, Ishii H, et al. (1991) Lack of alcohol dehydrogenase isoenzyme activities in the stomach of Japanese subjects. Life Sci 49:1929–34

Baribeau JC, Eier M, Braun CMJ (1987) Neurophysiological assessment of selective attention in males at risk for alcoholism. In Johnson Jr R, Rohrbaugh JW, Parasuraman R (eds), Current trends event-related potential research (EEG Suppl 40). Elsevier Science Publishers BV (Biomedical Division), pp 651–56

Begleiter H, Porjesz B, Tenner M (1980) Neuroradiological and neurophysiologic evidence of brain deficits in chronic alcoholics. Acta Psychiatr Scand 62:3–13

Begleiter H, Porjesz B, Chou CL (1981) Auditory brainstem potentials in chronic alcoholics. Science 211:1064–66

Begleiter H, Porjesz B, Bihari B (1987) Auditory brainstem potentials in sons of alcoholic fathers. Alcohol Clin Exp Res 11:477–83

Begleiter H, Porjesz B, Bihari B, Kissin B (1984) Event-related brain potentials in boys at risk for alcoholism. Science 225:1493–96

Belknap JK (1980) Genetic factors in the effects of alcohol: neurosensitivity, functional tolerance and physical dependence. In Rigter H, Crabbe JC (eds), Alcohol tolerance and dependence. Elsevier, Amsterdam, pp 157–80

Bhathal PS, Wilkinson P, Clifton S, et al. (1975) The spectrum of liver disease in alcoholism. Aust N Z J Med 5:49–57

Blass JM, Gibson GE (1977) Abnormality of a thiamine requiring enzyme in patients with Wernicke-Korsakoff syndrome. N Engl J Med 297:1367–70

Blum K, Noble EP, Sheridan PJ, et al. (1990) Allelic association of human dopamine D2 receptor gene in alcoholism. JAMA 263:2055–60

Blum K, Noble EP, Sheridan PJ, et al. (1991) Association of the A1 allele of the D2 dopamine receptor gene with severe alcoholism. Alcohol 8:409–16

Bohman M (1978) Some genetic aspects of alcoholism and criminality: a population of adoptees. Arch Gen Psychiatry 5:269–76

Bohman M, Sigvardsson S, Cloninger CR (1981) Maternal inheritance of alcohol abuse. Arch Gen Psychiatry 38:965–69

Bolos AM, Dean M, Lucas-Derse S, et al. (1990) Population and pedigree studies reveal a lack of association between the dopamine D2 receptor gene and alcoholism. JAMA 264:3156–60

Brewster DJ (1968) Genetic analysis of ethanol preference in rats selected for emotional reactivity. J Hered 59:283–86

Brian LC, Wang ZW, Raymond RC, et al. (1992) Alcoholism and the D2 receptor gene. Alcohol Clin Exp Res 16:806–9

Brind AM, MacIntosh I, Day CP, et al. (1991) Alpha-I-antitrypsin genotype—a risk factor for alcoholic cirrhosis. J Hepatol 13(suppl 2):234

Buydens-Branchey L, Branchey MH, Noumair D, Lieber CS (1989) Age of alcoholism onset. Arch Gen Psychiatry 46:231–36

Cadoret RJ, Cain C, Grove WM (1980) Development of alcoholism in adoptees raised apart from alcoholic biologic relatives. Arch Gen Psychiatry 37:561–63

Cadoret R, Gath A (1978) Inheritance of alcoholism in adoptees. Br J Psychiatry 132:252–58

Cadoret RJ, O'Gorman TW, Troughton E, Haywood E (1985) Alcoholism and antisocial personality: interrelationships, genetic and environmental factors. Arch Gen Psychiatry 42:161–67

Campbell KB, Lowick BM (1987) Ethanol and event-related potentials: the influence of distractor stimuli. Alcohol 4:257–63

Carr LG, Mellencamp RJ, Crabb DW, et al. (1991) Polymorphism of the rat liver mitochondrial aldehyde dehydrogenase cDNA. Alcohol Clin Exp Res 15:753–56

Cederlof R, Friberg L, Lundman T (1977) The interactions of smoking, environment and heredity and their implication for a disease aetiology. Acta Med Scand Suppl 612:1–128

Christa L, Zarski JP, Nalpas B, et al. (1992) Nested PCR on cellular DNA in plasma to investigate the collagen type I A2 polymorphic restriction sites in alcoholic patients. J Hepatol 16:515–16

Cicero TJ (1980) Animal models of alcoholism? In Eriksson K, Sinclair JD, Kiianmaa K (eds), Animal models in alcohol research. Academic Press, London, pp 99–117.

Clemente IC, Fananas L, Moral P, Sanchez-Turet M (1992) A study of association of alcoholism with A1 A2 BO and MNSs polymorphisms. Genetics and alcohol related diseases, ISBRA Satellite Symposium, Bordeaux, France, June 18–19

Clifford CA, Fulker DW, Gurling HMD, Murray RM (1981) Preliminary findings from a twin study of alcohol use. In Gedda L, Parisi P, Nance WE (eds), Twin research 3. Part C. Epidemiological and clinical studies. Alan R. Liss, Inc., New York, pp 47–52

Clifford CA, Fulker DW, Murray RM (1984a) Genetic and environmental influences on drinking patterns in twins. In Krasner N, Madden JS, Walker RJ (eds), Alcohol related problems. Wiley, New York, pp 115–26

Clifford CA, Hopper JL, Fulker DW, Murray RM (1984b) A genetic and environmental analysis of a twin family study of alcohol use, anxiety and depression. Genet Epidemiol 1:63–79

Cloninger CR (1987) Neurogenetic adaptive mechanisms in alcoholism. Science 236:410–16

Cloninger CR, Bohman M, Sigvardsson S (1981) Inheritance of alcohol abuse. Arch Gen Psychiatry 38:861–68

Cobb MJ, Blizard RA, Fulker DW, Murray RM (1984) Preliminary findings from a study of the effects of a challenge dose of alcohol in male twins. Acta Genet Med Gemellol 33:451–56

Cohen HL, Porjesz B, Begleiter H (1991) EEG: characteristics in males at risk for alcoholism. Alcohol Clin Exp Res 15:858–61

Cohen HL, Porjesz B, Begleiter H (1992a) Ethanol induced alterations in EEG activity in adult males. Neuropsychopharmacology (in press)

Cohen HL, Porjesz B, Begleiter H (1992b) The effects of ethanol on EEG activity in males at risk for alcoholism. Electroencephalogr Clin Neurophysiol (in press)

Comings DE (1977) PC 1 Duarte, a common polymorphism of a human brain protein and its relationship to depressive disease and multiple sclerosis. Nature 277:28–32

Comings DE (1992) Serotonin and alcoholism as a spectrum disorder. Alcohol Alcohol 27(suppl):1–10

Comings DE, Muhleman D, Dietz Jr GW, Donlon T (1991) Human tryptophan oxygenase localised to 4q31: possible implication for alcoholism and other behavioral disorders. Genomics 9:301–8

Conneally PM (1991) Association between the D2 dopamine receptor gene and alcoholism: a continuing controversy. Arch Gen Psychiatry 48:757–59

Conterio F, Chiarelli B (1962) Study of the inheritance of some daily life habits. Heredity 17:347–59

Cook BL, Wang ZW, Crowe RC, et al. (1992) Alcoholism and the D2 receptor gene. Alcohol Clin Exp Res 16:806–9

Cotton NS (1979) The familial incidence of alcoholism: a review. J Stud Alcohol 40:89–116

Coutelle C, Dumas F, Fleury B, et al. (1992) Glutathione S tranferase μ (GST1) gene deletion and cancer in alcoholic patients. Function of glutathione in gut and liver. Basel Liver Week, Basel, Switzerland, October 21. Falk Foundation, Freiburg, Germany

Couzigou P, Fleury B, Groppi A, et al. and the French Group for Research on Alcohol and Liver (1990a) Genotyping of alcohol dehydrogenase class I polymorphism in French patients with alcoholic cirrhosis. Alcohol Alcohol 25:623–26

Couzigou P, Fleury B, Groppi A, et al. (1990b) Role of alcohol dehydrogenase polymorphism in ethanol metabolism and alcohol-related diseases. In Weiner H, Flynn TG, Crabb DW (eds), Enzymology and molecular biology of carbonyl metabolism 3. Plenum Press, New York, pp 263–70

Crabb DW, Edenbergh JH, Bosron WF, Li TK (1989) Genotypes for aldehyde dehydrogenase deficiency and alcohol sensitivity. J Clin Investig 83:314–16

Crabb DW, Lands W (1992) Highlights of the RSA Symposium on Enzymes of Alcohol Metabolism. Alcohol Clin Exp Res 16:870–74

Crabbe JC (1989) Genetic animal models in the study of alcoholism. Alcohol Clin Exp Res 13:120–27

Crabbe JC, Feller DJ, Phillips TJ (1990a) Selective breeding for two measures of sensitivity to ethanol. In Deitrich RA, Pawlowski AA (eds), Initial Sensitivity to Alcohol. NIAAA Research Monograph 20, U.S. Government Printing Office, Rockville, Maryland, pp 123–50

Crabbe JC, Kosobud A, Tam BR, et al. (1987a) Genetic selection of mouse lines sensitive (cold) and resistant (hot) to acute ethanol hypothermia. Alcohol Drug Res 7:163–74

Crabbe JC, Kosobud A, Young ER, et al. (1985a) Bidirectional selection for susceptibility to ethanol withdrawal seizures in Mus musculus. Behav Genet 15:521–36

Crabbe JC, McSwigan JD, Belknap JK (1985b) The role of genetics in substance abuse. In Galizio M, Maisto SA (eds), Determinants of substance abuse. Plenum Publishing Corp., New York, pp 13–64

Crabbe JC, Phillips TJ, Kosobud A, Belknap JK (1990b) Estimation of genetic correlation of experiments using selectively bred and inbred animals. Alcohol Clin Exp Res 14:141–51

Crabbe JC, Young ER, Deutsch CM, et al. (1987b) Mice genetically selected for differences in open field activity after ethanol. Pharmacol Biochem Behav 27:577–81

Day CP, Bashir R, James OFW, et al. (1991) Investigation of the role of polymorphism at the alcohol and aldehyde dehydrogenase loci in genetic predisposition to alcohol related end organ damage. Hepatology 14:798–801

Day CP, Bashir R, Sykes B, et al. (1990) Investigation of the role of five "candidate genes" in genetic susceptibility to alcoholic cirrhosis. Hepatology 12:925

De Fiebre MC, Romm E, Collins JT, et al. (1991) Responses to cholinergic agonists of rats selectively bred for differential sensitivity to ethanol. Alcohol Clin Exp Res 15:270–76

Deitrich RA (1990) Selective breeding of mice and rats for initial sensitivity to ethanol: contributions to understanding of ethanol's action. In Deitrich RA, Pawlowski AA (eds), Initial sensitivity to alcohol. NIAAA Research Monograph 20, U.S. Government Printing Office, Rockville, Maryland, pp 7–59

Deitrich RA, Spuhler K (1984) Genetics of alcoholism and alcohol actions. In Smart K, Sellers EM (eds), Research advances in alcohol and drug problems. Plenum Publishing Corp., New York, vol 8, pp 47–98

Devor EJ, Cloninger CR (1989) Genetics of alcoholism. Annu Rev Genet 23:19–36

Diamond IB, Wrubel B, Estrin W, Gordon A (1987) A. Basal and adenosine-receptor-stimulated levels of cAMP are reduced in lymphocytes from alcoholic patients. Proc Natl Acad Sci U S A 84:1413–16

Dinwiddie SH, Cloninger CR (1989) Family and adoption studies of alcoholism. In Goedde HW, Agarwal DP (eds), Alcoholism biochemical and genetic aspects. Pergamon Press, New York, pp 259–76

Ehlers CL, Schuckit MA (1990) EEG fast frequency activity in the sons (a/b) of alcoholics. Biol Psychiatry 24:631–41

Elmasian R, Neville H, Woods D, et al. (1982) Event-related potentials are different in individuals at right risk for developing alcoholism. Proc Nat Acad Sci 79:7900–7903

Emmerson RY, Dustman RE, Shearer DE, Chamberlin HM (1987) Visually evoked and event related potentials in young abstinent alcoholics. Alcohol 4:241–48

Enomoto N, Takase S, Takada N, Takada A (1991) Alcoholic liver disease in heterozygotes of mutant and normal aldehyde dehydrogenase-2 genes. Hepatology 13:1071–75

Eriksson CJP (1990) Finnish selective breeding studies for initial sensitivity to ethanol: update 1988 on the AT and ANT rat lines. In Deitrich RA, Pawlowski AA (eds), Initial sensitivity to alcohol. NIAAA Research Monograph 20, U.S. Government Printing Office, Rockville, Maryland, pp 61–86

Eriksson K (1968) Genetic selection for voluntary alcohol consumption in the albino rat. Science 159:739–41

Eriksson K (1969) Factors affecting voluntary alcohol consumption in the albino rat. Ann Zool Fenn 6:227–65

Eriksson K (1971) Rat strains specifically selected for their voluntary alcohol consumption. Ann Med Exp Biol Fenn 49:67–72

Eriksson K, Rusi M (1981) Finnish selection studies on alcohol-related behaviors: general outline. In McClearn GE, Deitrich RA, Erwin G (eds), Development of animal models as pharmacogenetic tools. NIAAA Research Monograph 6, U.S. Government Printing Office, Rockville, Maryland, pp 87–117

Eskay R, Linnoila M (1991) Potential biochemical markers for the predisposition toward alcoholism. In Galanter M (ed), Recent developments in alcoholism. Vol 9: children of alcoholics. Plenum Press, New York, pp 41–51

Fadda F, Mosca E, Colombo G, Gessa GL (1989) Effect of spontaneous ingestion of ethanol on brain dopamine metabolism. Life Sci 44:281–87

Fillmore KM (1988a) alcohol use across the life course: a critical review of 70 years of international longitudinal research. Addiction Research Foundation, Toronto, pp 75–87

Fillmore KM (1988b) The 1980s dominant theory of alcohol problems—genetic predisposition to alcoholism: where is it leading us? Drugs and Society 2:69–87

Fleury B, Couzigou P, Coutelle C, et al. and the French Group for Research on Alcohol and Liver (1990) Comparative: genetic polymorphism of alcohol dehydrogenase ADH in alcoholics and controls in France. Alcohol Clin Exp Res 14:288

Fuller JL (1985) The genetics of alcohol consumption in animals. Soc Biol 32:210–21

Fuller JL, McClearn GE, Wilson JR, Crowe L (1985) Genetics and human encounter with alcohol. Soc Biol 32:327

Gabrielli WF, Mednick SA, Volavka J, et al. (1982) Electroencephalograms in children of alcoholic fathers. Psychophysiology 19:494–507

Gedda L, Brenci G (1983) Twins living apart test: progress report. Acta Genet Med Gemellol 32:17–22

George SR, Roldan L, Lui A, Naranjo CA (1991) Endogenous opioids are involved in the genetically determined high preference for ethanol consumption. Alcohol Clin Exp Res 15:668–72

Gill K, Amit Z (1989) Serotonin uptake blockers and voluntary consumption: a review of recent studies. In Galanter M (ed), Recent developments in alcoholism. Plenum Press, New York, vol 7, pp 225–50

Gilligan SB, Cloninger CR (1989) The genetics of alcoholism. In Crow KE, Batt Rd (eds), Human metabolism of alcohol. CRC Press, Boca Raton, Florida, vol 1, pp 171–86

Gilligan SB, Reich T, Cloninger CR (1987) Etiologic heterogeneity in alcoholism. Genet Epidemiol 4:395–414

Gluud C (1992) HLA antigens in alcoholics and in alcoholic liver disease. Genetics and alcohol related diseases, ISBRA Satellite Symposium, Bordeaux, France, June 18–19

Goedde HW, Agarwal DP (eds) (1987) Genetics and alcoholism. Proc Clin Biol Res, Liss, New York, vol 241

Goedde HW, Agarwal DP, Fritze G (1992) Distribution of ADH2 and ALDH2 genotypes in different populations. Hum Genet 88:344–46

Goedde HW, Agarwal DP, Harada S (1986) Aldehyde dehydrogenase polymorphism in North American, South American and Mexican Indians. Am J Hum Genet 38:395–99

Goedde HW, Harada S, Agarwal DP (1979) Racial differences in alcohol sensitivity: a new hypothesis. Hum Genet 51:331–34

Goedde HW, Singh S, Agarwal DP (1989) Genotyping of mitochondrial aldehyde dehydrogenase in blood samples using allele-specific oligonucleotides. Hum Genet 81:305–7

Goodwin DW (1985) Alcoholism and genetics. The sins of the fathers. Arch Gen Psychiatry 42:171–78

Goodwin DW (1986) Genetics factors in the development of alcoholism. Psychiatr Clin North Am 9:427–33

Goodwin DW, Guze S (1974) Heredity and alcoholism. In Kissin B, Begleiter H (eds), The biologie of alcoholism. Vol. III: clinical pathology. Plenum Press, New York, pp 37–52

Goodwin DW, Schulsinger F, Hermansen L, et al. (1973) Alcohol problems in adoptees raised apart from alcoholic biological parents. Arch Gen Psychiatry 28:238–43

Goodwin DW, Schulsinger F, Knop J, et al. (1977a) Alcoholism and depression in adopted-out daughters of alcoholics. Arch Gen Psychiatry 34:751–55

Goodwin DW, Schulsinger F, Knop J, et al. (1977b) Psychopathology in adopted and nonadopted daughters of alcoholics. Arch Gen Psychiatry 34:1005–9

Goodwin DW, Schulsinger F, Moller N (1974) Drinking problems in adopted-out and nonadopted sons of alcoholics. Arch Gen Psychiatry 31:164–69

Gorelick DA (1989) Serotonin uptake blockers and the treatment of alcoholism. In Galanter M (ed), Recent developments in alcoholism. Plenum Press, New York, vol 7, pp 267–82

Groppi A, Coutelle C, Fleury B, et al. (1991) Glutathione S transferase class μ in French alcoholic cirrhotic patients. Hum Genet 87:628–30

Gurling HMD, Murray RM (1987) Genetic influence, brain morphology and cognitive deficits in alcoholic twins. In Goedde HW, Agarwal DP (eds), Genetics and alcoholism. Allan R. Liss Inc., New York, pp 71–82

Gurling HMD, Murray RM, Clifford CA (1981) Investigations into the genetics of alcohol dependence and into its effects on brain function. In Gedda L, Parisi P, Nance WE (eds), Twin research 3. Part C. Epidemiologic and clinical studies. Alan R. Liss Inc., New York, pp 77–87

Guthrie SK, Lane EA, Linnoila M (1989) Acetylation phenotype in abstinent alcoholics. Alcohol Clin Exp Res 13:66–68

Guze S, Cloninger CR, Martin R, Clayton PJ (1986) Alcoholism as a medical disorder. Compr Psychiatry 27:501–10

Haber PS, Wilson JS, McGarity BH, et al. (1991) Alpha 1 antitrypsin phenotypes and alcoholic pancreatitis. Gut 32:945–48

Harada S, Abei M, Tanaka N, et al. (1987) Liver glutathione S-transferase polymorphism in Japanese and its pharmacogenetic importance. Hum Genet 75:322–25

Harada S, Agarwal DP, Goedde HW (1985) Aldehyde dehydrogenase polymorphism and alcohol metabolism in alcoholics. Alcohol 2:391–92

Harada S, Agarwal DP, Goedde HW, et al. (1982) Possible protective role against alcoholism for aldehyde dehydrogenase isozyme deficiency in Japan. Lancet 2:827

Harris RA, Allan AM (1989) Alcohol intoxication: ion channels and genetics. FASEB J 3:1689–95

Hayashi SI, Watanabe J, Kawajiri K (1991) Genetic polymorphism in the 5'-flanking regino change transcriptional regulation of the human cytochrome P450IIE1 gene. J Biochem 110:559–65

Heath AC, Jardine R, Martin NG (1989) Interactive effects of genotype and social environment on alcohol consumption in female twins. J Stud Alcohol 50:38–48

Heath AC, Martin NG (1988) Teenage alcohol use in the Australian twin register: genetic and social determinants of starting to drink. Alcohol Clin Exp Res 12:735–41

Heath AC, Martin NG (1991) The inheritance of alcohol sensitivity and of patterns of alcohol use. Alcohol Alcohol Suppl 1:141–45

Heath AC, Martin NG (1992) Genetic differences in psychomotor performance decrement after alcohol: a multivariate analysis J Stud Alcohol 53:262–71

Hempel J, Kaiser R, Jornvall H (1984) Human liver mitochondrial aldehyde dehydrogenase: a C-terminal segment positions and defines the structures corresponding to the one reported to differ in the Oriental enzyme variant. FEBS Lett 173:367–73

Hesselbrock V, Bauer LO, Hesselbrock MN, Gillen R (1991) Neuropsychological factors in individuals at high risk for alcoholism. In Galanter M (ed), Recent developments in alcoholism. Vol. 9: children of alcoholics. Plenum Press, New York, pp 21–40

Hesselbrock V, Meyer R, Hesselbrock M (1992) Psychopathology and addictive disorders: a specific case of antisocial personality disorder. In O'Brien J and Jaffe JH (eds), Addictive states. Raven Press, New York, pp 179–91

Higushi S, Muramatsu T, Shigemori K, et al. (1992a) The relationship between low Km aldehyde dehydrogenase phenotype and drinking behavior in Japanese. J Stud Alcohol 53:170–75

Higushi S, Parrish KM, DuFour MC, et al. (1992b) The relationship between three subtypes of the flushing response and DSM III alcohol abuse in Japanese. J Stud Alcohol 53:553–60

Hill SY (1992) Absence of paternal sociopathy in the etiology of severe alcoholism: is there a type III alcoholism? J Stud Alcohol 53:161–69

Hill SY, Aston CE, Rabin B (1988a) Suggestive evidence between alcoholism and the MNS blood group. Alcohol Clin Exp Res 12:811–14

Hill SY, Goodwin DW, Cadoret R, et al. (1975) Association and linkage between alcoholism and eleven serological markers. J Stud Alcohol 36:981–92

Hill SY, Steinhauer SR, Zubin J, et al. (1988b) Event-related potentials as markers for alcoholism risk in high density families. Alcohol Clin Exp Res 12:545–55

Hillyard SA, Picton TW, Regan D (1978) Sensation, perception and attention: analysis using ERP's. In Callaway E, Tueting P, Koslow SH (eds), Event-related brain potentials in man. Academic Press, New York, pp 223–321

Holmes RS (1988) Alcohol dehydrogenases and aldehyde dehydrogenases of anterior eye tissues from humans and others mammals. In Kuriyama K, Takada A, Ishii H (eds), Biomedical and social aspects of alcohol and alcoholism. Elsevier Science Publishers BV, Amsterdam, pp 51–57

Hrubec Z, Omenn GS (1981) Evidence of genetic predisposition to alcoholic cirrhosis and psychosis. Alcohol Clin Exp Res 5:207–15

Iron A, Richard P, Pascual de Zulueta M, et al. (1992) Genetic polymorphism of apoprotein E and alcoholic cirrhosis. Genetics and alcohol related diseases, ISBRA Satellite Symposium, Bordeaux, France, June 18–19

Johnson RC, Nagoshi CT, Schwitters SY, et al. (1984) Further investigations of racial/ethnic differences and of familial resemblances in flushing in response to alcohol. Behav Genet 14:171–78

Jonsson E, Nilsson T (1968) Alkohol konsumption hos monozygota och dizygota tvillingpar. Nord Hyg Tidskr 49:21–25

Kaij L (1960a) Alcoholism in twins. Almquist and Wiksell, Stockholm

Kaij L (1960b) Studies on the etiology and sequels of abuse of alcohol. Department of Psychiatry, University of Lund, Sweden

Kaplan RF, Hesselbrock VM, O'Connor S, Palma N (1988) Behavioral and EEG responses to alcohol in nonalcoholic men with a family history of alcoholism. Prog Neuropsychopharmacol Biol Psychiatry 12:873–85

Kaprio J, Koskenvuo M, Langinvainio H (1984) Finnish twins reared apart IV: Smoking and drinking habits. A preliminary analysis of the effect of heredity and environment. Acta Genet Med Gemeld 33:425–33

Kaprio J, Koskenvuo M, Langinvainio H, et al. (1987) Genetic influences on use and abuse of alcohol: a study of 5638 adult Finnish twin brothers. Alcohol Clin Exp Res 11:349–56

Kaprio J, Koskenvuo P, Sarna S (1981) Cigarette smoking, use of alcohol and leisure-time physical activity among same-sexed adult male twins. In Gedda L, Parisi P, Nance WE (eds), Twin research 3. Part C. Epidemiological and clinical studies. Alan R. Liss Inc., New York, pp 37–46

Kaprio J, Rose RJ, Romanov K, Koskenvuo M (1991) Genetic and environmental determinants of use and abuse of alcohol: the Finnish twin cohort studies. Alcohol Alcohol Suppl 1:131–36

Kaprio J, Viken R, Koskenvuo M, et al. (1992) Consistency and change in patterns of social drinking: a 6 year follow-up of the Finnish twin cohort. Alcohol Clin Exp Res 16:234–40

Karp RW (1992) D2 or not D2? Alcohol Clin Exp Res 16:786–87

Keller M, Doria J (1991) On defining alcoholism. Alcohol Health Res World 15:253–59

Kendler KS, Heath AC, Neale MC, et al. (1992) A population based twin study of alcoholism in women. JAMA 268:1877–82

Kiianmaa K, Tabakoff B, Saito T (eds) (1989) Genetic aspects of alcoholism. Finnish Foundation for Alcohol Studies, Helsinki, vol 37

Kopun M, Propping P (1977) The kinetics of ethanol absorption and elimination in twins and supplementary repetitive experiments in singleton subjects. Eur J Clin Pharmacol 11:337–44

Kosten TR, Rounsaville BJ, Kosten TA, Merikangas D (1991) Gender differences in the specificity of alcoholism transmission among the relatives of opioid addicts. J Nerv Ment Dis 179:392–400

Kupari, M, Eriksson CJP, Heikkila I, Ylikahri R (1983) Alcohol and the heart. Intense hemodynamic changes associated with alcohol flush in Orientals. Acta Med Scand 213:91–98

Leevy CM (1968) Cirrhosis in alcoholics. Med Clin N Am 52:1445–51

Lester D, Freed EX (1973) Theoretical review criteria for an animal model of alcoholism. Pharmacol Biochem Behav 1:103–7

Li T-K, Lumeng L, McBride WJ, Murphy JMR (1987) Rodent lines selected for factors affecting alcohol consumption. In Lindros KO, Ylikahri R, Kiianmaa K (eds), Advances in biomedical alcohol research. Alcohol Alcohol Suppl 1:91–96

Li T-K, Lumeng L, McBride WJ, Waller BM (1981) Indiana selection studies on alcohol-related behaviors. In McClearn GE, Deitrich RA, Erwin G (eds), Development of animals models as pharmacogenetic tools. NIAAA Research Monograph 6, U.S. Government Printing Office, Rockville, Maryland, pp 171–91

Lieber CS, DeCarli LM, Rubin E (1975) Sequential production of fatty liver, hepatitis and cirrhosis in subhuman primates fed ethanol with adequate diets. Proc Natl Acad Sci U S A 72:437–41

Littrell J (1988) The Swedish studies of the adopted children of alcoholics. J Stud Alcohol 49:491–509

Loehlin JC (1972) An analysis of alcohol-related questionnaire items from the National Merit Twin Study. Ann N Y Acad Sci 197:110–13

Lumeng L, Doolittle DP, Li T-K (1986) New duplicate lines of rats that differ in voluntary alcohol consumption. Alcohol Alcohol 21:A125

Mardones J (1960) Experimentally induced changes in the free selection of ethanol. Int Rev Neurobiol 2:41–76

Mardones J (1972) Experimentally induced changes in alcohol appetite. In Forsander O, Eriksson K (eds), Biological aspects of alcohol consumption. Finnish Foundation for Alcohol Studies, Helsinki, vol 20, pp 15–23

Marino MW, Fuller GM, Elder FFB (1986) Chromosomal localization of human and rat A alpha, B beta, and gamma fibrinogen genes by in situ hybridization. Cytogenet Cell Genet 42:36–41

Marshall EJ, Murray RM (1989) The contribution of twin studies to alcoholism research. In Goedde HW, Agarwal DP (eds), Alcoholism biochemical and genetic aspects. Pergamon Press, New York, pp 277–89

Marshall EJ, Murray RM (1991) The familial transmission of alcoholism. Br Med J 303:72–73

Martin NG, Oakeshott JG, Gibson JB, et al. (1985a) A twin study of psychomotor and physiological responses to an acute dose of alcohol. Behav Genet 15:305–47

Martin NG, Perl J, Oakeshott JG, et al. (1985b) A twin study of ethanol metabolism. Behav Genet 15:93–109

May DG, Thomasson HR, Martier S, et al. (1992) Ethanol metabolism in women. Relative importance of ADH genotype and intake. Alcohol Alcohol 27:41

McClearn E, Wilson JR, Petersen DR, Allen DL (1982) Selective breeding in mice for severity of ethanol withdrawal syndrome. Subst Alcohol Actions Misuse 3:135–43

McClearn GE, Deitrich RA, Erwin G (eds) (1981) Development of animal models as pharmacogenetic tools. NIAAA Research Monograph 6, U.S. Government Printing Office, Rockville, Maryland

McClearn GE, Kakihana R (1981) Selective breeding for ethanol sensitivity: short-sleep and long-sleep mice. In McClearn GE, Deitrich RA, Erwin G (eds), Development of animal models as pharmacogenetic tools. NIAAA Research Monograph 6, U.S. Government Printing Office, Rockville, Maryland, pp 147–59

McClearn GE, Rodgers DA (1959) Differences in alcohol preference among inbred strains of mice. Q J Stud Alcohol 20:691–95

McClearn GE, Wilson JR, Meredith W (1970) The use of isogenic and heterogenic mouse stocks. In Lindzey G, Thiessen DD (eds), Behavioral research in contributions to behavior-genetic analysis: the mouse as a prototype. Appleton-Century-Crofts, New York, pp 3–22

McGue M, Pickens RW, Svikis DS (1992) Sex and age effects on the inheritance of alcohol problems a twin study. J Abnorm Psychol 101:3–17

Merikangas KR (1990) The genetic epidemiology of alcoholism. Psychol Med 20:11–22

Merikangas KR, Leckman JF, Prusoff BA, et al. (1985) Familial transmission of depression and alcoholism. Arch Gen Psychiatry 42:367–72

Morin T, Martin JP, Feldman G, et al. (1975) Heterozygous alpha-1-antitrypsin deficiency and cirrhosis in adults, a fortuitous association. Lancet 1:250–51

Moss HB, Yao JK, Maddock JM (1989) Responses by sons of alcoholic fathers to alcoholic and placebo drinks: perceived mood, intoxication and plasma prolactin. Alcohol Clin Exp Res 13:252–57

Mueller GC, Fleming MF, Lemahieu MA, et al. (1988) Synthesis of phosphatidylethanol. A potential marker for adult males at risk for alcoholism. Proc Natl Acad Sci U S A 85:9778–82

Murray RM, Clifford CA, Gurling HMD (1983) Twin and adoption studies. How good is the evidence for a genetic role? In Galanter M (ed), Recent developments in alcoholism. Plenum Press, New York, pp 25–48

Myrhed M (1974) Alcohol consumption in relation to factors associated with ischemic heart disease. A cotwin control study. Acta Med Scand Suppl 567:1

Newlin DB, Thomson JB (1990) Alcohol challenge with sons of alcoholics: a critical review and analysis. Psychology Bull 108:383–402

Nixon PR, Price J, Norman Hicks M, et al. (1990) The relationship between erythrocyte transketolase activity and the "TPP effect" in Wernicke's encephalopathy and other thiamine deficiency states. Clin Chem Acta 192:89–98

O'Connor S, Hesselbrock V, Tasman A (1986) Correlates of increased risk for alcoholism in young men. Prog Neuropsychopharmacol Biol Psychiatry 10:211–18

O'Connor S, Hesselbrock V, Tasman A, et al. (1987) P3 amplitudes in two distinct tasks are decreased in young men with a history of paternal alcoholism. Alcohol 4:323–30

Ohmori T, Koyama T, Chen CC, et al. (1986) The role of aldehyde dehydrogenase isozyme variance in alcohol sensitivity, drinking habits formation and the development of alcoholism in Japan, Taiwan and the Philippines. Prog Neuropsychopharmacol Biol Psychiatry 10:229–35

Omenn GS (1988) Genetic investigation of alcohol metabolism and of alcoholism. Am J Hum Genet 43:579–81

Palmour R, Smith AJK, Parboosingh J, et al. (1992) Biochemical markers of susceptibility to familial alcoholism. Genetics and alcohol related diseases, ISBRA Satellite Symposium, Bordeaux, France, June 18–19

Park JV, Huang YH, Nagoshi CT, et al. (1984) The flushing response to alcohol use among Koreans and Taiwanese. J Stud Alcohol 45:481–85

Parsian A, Todd RD, Devor EJ, et al. (1991) Alcoholism and alleles of the human dopamine D2 receptor locus: studies of association and linkage. Arch Gen Psychiatry 48:655–63

Partanen J, Brun K, Markkanen T (1966) Inheritance of drinking behavior. Finnish Foundation for Alcohol Studies, Helsinki, pp 14–159

Pasta L, D'Amico G, Politi F, et al. (1992) C4BQ0 as a marker of genetic predisposition to liver cirrhosis. Gastroenterology 102:2183–84

Patterson BW, Williams HL, McLean GA, et al. (1987) Alcoholism and family history of alcoholism: effects on visual and auditory event-related potentials. Alcohol 4:265–74

Pederson N (1981) Twin similarity for usage of common drugs. In Gedda L, Parisi P, Nance WE (eds), Twin research 3. Part C. Epidemiological and Clinical Studies. Alan R. Liss Inc., New York, pp 53–59

Peele S (1986) The implications and limitations of genetic models of alcoholism and other addictions. J Stud Alcohol 47:63–73

Perdahl E, Wu WCS, Browning MD, et al. (1984) Protein III a neuron-specific phosphoprotein: variant forms found in human brain. Neurobehav Toxicol Teratol 6:425–31

Perry A (1973) The effect of heredity on attitudes towards alcohol, cigarettes and coffee. J Appl Psychol 58:275–77

Peters TJ, MacPherson AJS, Ward RJ, Yoshida A (1990) Acquired and genetic deficiencies of cytosolic acetaldehyde dehydrogenase. In Cloninger CR, Begleiter H (eds), Banbury Report 33. Genetics and biology of alcoholism. Cold Spring Harbor Laboratory Press, New York, pp 265–76

Peterson JB, Pihl RO, Dongier M, et al. (1992) Cardio vascular reactivity and prediction of voluntary alcohol consumption among sons of male alcoholics and controls. Genetics and alcohol related disease, ISBRA Satellite Symposium, Bordeaux, France, June 18–19

Pfefferbaum A, Ford JM, White PM, Mathalon D (1991) Event-related potential in alcoholic men: P3 amplitude reflects family history but not alcohol consumption. Alcohol 15:839–50

Pfefferbaum A, Rosenbloom M, Ford JM (1987) Late event-related potentials changes in alcoholics. Alcohol 4:275–81

Phillips TJ, Burhart-Kasch S, Terdal ES, Crabbe JC (1991) Response to selection for ethanol-induced locomotor activation: genetic analyses and selection response characterization. Psychopharmacology 103:557–66

Phillips TJ, Feller DJ, Crabbe JC (1989) Selected mouse lines, alcohol and behavior. Experientia 45:805–27

Pickens RW, Svikis DS, McGue M, et al. (1991) Heterogeneity in the inheritance of alcoholism. A study of male and female twins. Arch Gen Pschiatry 48:19–28

Polich J, Bloom FE (1987) P300 from normals and children of alcoholics. Alcohol 4:301–5

Polich J, Bloom FE (1988) Event-related potentials in individuals at high and low risk for developing alcoholism: failure to replicate. Alcohol Clin Exp Res 12:368–73

Polich J, Haier RJ, Buchsbaum M, et al. (1988) Assessment of young men at risk for alcoholism with P300 from a visual discrimination task. J Stud Alcohol 49:186–90

Polich J, Pollock V (1993) A metaanalysis of the P300 component in subjects at risk to develop alcoholism. Psychol Bull (in press)

Pollock VE, Volavka J, Mednick SA, et al. (1984) A prospective study of alcoholism: electroencephalographic finding. In Goodwin DW, Van Dusen Teilman K, Mednick SA (eds), Longitudinal research in alcoholism. Kluwer-Nijhoff Publishing, Boston, pp 125–46

Porjesz B, Begleiter H (1985) Human brain electrophysiology and alcoholism. In Tarter RD, Van Thiel D (eds), Alcohol and the brain. Plenum Press, New York, pp 139–82

Porjesz B, Begleiter H, Bihari B, Kissin B (1987) The N2 component of the event-related brain potential in abstinent alcoholics. Electroencephalogr Clin Neurophysiol 66:121–31

Porjesz B, Begleiter H (1990) Event-related potentials in individuals at risk for alcoholism. Alcohol 7:465–69

Porjesz B, Begleiter H (1991) Neurophysiological factors in individuals at risk for alcoholism. In Galanter M (ed), Recent developments in alcoholism. Vol. 9: children of alcoholics. Plenum Press, New York, pp 53–67

Porjesz B, Begleiter H (1993) Mismatch negativity and P3a in sons of alcoholic fathers (in preparation)

Poupon RE, Heintzmann F, Valette I, et al. (1991) HLA GM systems and susceptibility to alcoholic cirrhosis. A study of mixed race subjects. Alcohol Alcohol 26:417–24

Poupon RE, Nalpas B, Coutelle C, et al. and the French Group for Research on Alcohol and Liver (1992) Polymorphism of alcohol dehydrogenase, alcohol and aldehyde dehydrogenase activities: implication in alcoholic cirrhosis in white patients. Hepatology 15:1017–22

Propping P (1977a) Genetic control of ethanol action on central nervous system. Hum Genet 35:309–34

Propping P (1977b) Psycho-physiologic test performance in normal twins and in a pair of identical twins with essential tremor that is suppressed by alcohol. Hum Genet 36:321–25

Reed TE (1985) Ethnic differences in alcohol use, abuse, and sensitivity: a review with genetic interpretation. Soc Biol 32:195–209

Reed TE, Hanna JM (1986) Between and within-race variation in acute cardiovascular responses to alcohol: evidence for genetic determination in normal males in three races. Behav Genet 16:585–98

Reich T, Cloninger CR, Lewis C, Rice J (1981) Some recent findings in the study of genotype-environment interaction in alcoholism. In Meyer RE (ed), Evaluation of the alcoholic: implications for research, theory and treatment. NIAAA Research Monograph 5, U.S. Government Printing Office, Washington, DC, pp 145–66

Rex DK, Bosron WF, Smialek JE, Li TK (1985) Alcohol and aldehyde dehydrogenase isoenzymes in North American Indians. Alcohol Clin Exp Res 9:147–52

Rezvani AH, Overstreet DM, Janowsky DS (1990) Genetic serotonin deficiency and alcohol preference in the fawn hooded rats. Alcohol Alcohol 25:573–75

Ricciardi BR, Saunders JB, Williams R, Hopkinson DA (1983) Hepatic ADH and ALDH isoenzymes in different racial groups and in chronic alcoholism. Pharmacol Biochem Behav 18(suppl 1):61–65

Rodgers DA, McClearn GE (1962) Mouse strain differences in preference for various concentrations of alcohol. Q J Stud Alcohol 23:26–33

Roe A (1944) The adult adjustment of children of alcoholic parents raised in foster homes. Q J Stud Alcohol 5:378–93

Romanov K, Kaprio J, Rose RJ, Koskenvuo M (1991) Genetics of alcoholism: effects of migrations on concordance rates among male twins. Alcohol Alcohol Suppl 1:137–40

Roth WT, Tinklenberg JR, Kopell BS (1977) Ethanol and marijuana effects on event-related potentials in a memory retrieval paradigm. Electroencephalogr Clin Neurophysiol 42:381–88

Satinder KP (1970) Behavior-genetic dependent self-selection of alcohol in rats. J Comp Physiol Psychol 80:422–34

Saunders JB, Williams R (1983) The genetics of alcoholism: is there an inherited susceptibility to alcohol related problems? Alcohol Alcohol 18:189–217

Saunders JB, Wodak AD, Haines A, et al. (1982) Accelerated development of alcoholic cirrhosis in patients with HLA-B8. Lancet 1:1381–84

Schmidt AL, Neville HJ (1985) Language processing in men at risk for alcoholism: an event-related potential study. Alcohol 2:529–34

Schmidt W, Konigstedt B, Zipprich B, et al. (1987) Immunoglobulin allotypes and immuno reactivity in chronic liver disease. Hepatogastroenterology 34:206–11

Schuckit MA (1991a) Importance of subtypes in alcoholism. Alcohol Alcohol Suppl 1:511–14

Schuckit MA (1991b) A longitudinal study of children of alcoholics. In Galanter M (ed), Recent developments in alcoholism. Vol 9: children of alcoholics. Plenum Press, New York, pp 5–19

Schuckit MA (1992) Genetic factors in alcohol sensitivity. Genetics and alcohol related diseases, ISBRA Satellite Symposium Bordeaux, France, June 18–19

Schuckit MA, Gold E (1988) A simultaneous evaluation of multiple markers of ethanol/placebo challenges in sons of alcoholics and controls. Arch Gen Psychiatry 45:211–16

Schuckit MA, Gold EO, Croot K, et al. (1988) P300 latency after ethanol ingestion in sons of alcoholics and controls. Biol Psychiatry 24:310–15

Schuckit MA, Goodwin D, Winokur G (1972) A study of alcoholism in half-siblings. Am J Psych 128:122–25

Schuckit MA, Irwin M (1989) An analysis of clinical relevance of type 1 and type 2 alcoholics. Br J Addict 84:869–76

Schuckit MA, Li T-K, Cloninger CR, Deitrich RA (1985) Genetics of alcoholism. Alcohol Clin Exp Res 9:475–92

Schuckit MA, Shaskon E, Duby J (1982) Platelet MAO activities in relatives of alcoholics and controls. Arch Gen Psych 39:137–40

Searles JS (1988) The role of genetics in the pathogenesis of alcoholism. J Abnorm Psychol 97:153–67

Sher KJ (1991) Children of alcoholics. A critical appraisal of theory and research. The University of Chicago Press Ltd, London

Shibuya A, Yasunami M, Yoshida A (1989) Genotypes of alcohol dehydrogenase and aldehyde dehydrogenase loci in Japanese alcohol flushers and non flushers. Hum Genet 82:14–16

Shibuya A, Yoshida A (1988a) Frequency of the atypical aldehyde dehydrogenase 2 gene (ALDH 2/2) in Japanese and Caucasians. Am J Hum Genet 43:741–43

Shibuya A, Yoshida A (1988b) Genotypes of alcohol-metabolizing enzymes in Japanese with alcohol liver disease: a strong association of the usual Caucasian-type aldehyde dehydrogenases gene (ALPHA 2 1) with the disease. Am J Hum Genet 43:744–48

Sibert JR (1978) Hereditary pancreatitis in England and Wales. J Med Genet 15:189–201

Sinclair JD, Le AD, Kiianmaa K (1989) The AA and ANA rat lines, selected for differences in alcohol consumption. Experientia 45:798–805

Singh S, Fritze G, Fang B, et al. (1989) Inheritance of mitochondrial aldehyde dehydrogenase: genotyping in Chinese, Japanese and South Korean families reveals a dominance of the mutant allele. Hum Genet 83:119–21

Sladek NE, Manthey CL, Maki PA, et al. (1989) Xenobiotic oxidation catalyzed by aldehyde dehydrogenases. Drug Metab Rev 20:697–720

Spuhler K, Deitrich RA, Baker RC (1990) Selective breeding of rats differing in sensitivity to the hypnotic effects of acute ethanol administration. In Deitrich RA, Pawlowski AA (eds), Initial sensitivity to alcohol. NIAAA Research Monograph 20, U.S. Government Printing Office, Rockville, Maryland, pp 87–102

Steinhauer SR, Hill SY, Zubin J (1987) Event-related potentials in alcoholics and their first-degree relatives. Alcohol 4:307–14

Sullivan JL, Baenziger JC, Wagner DL, et al. (1990) Platelet MAO in subtypes of alcoholism. Biol Psychiatry 27:911–22

Suwaki H, Ohara H (1985) Alcohol-induced facial flushing and drinking behavior in Japanese men. J Stud Alcohol 46:196–98

Tabakoff BP, Hoffman PL, Lee JM, et al. (1988) Differences in platelet enzyme activity between alcoholics and non-alcoholics. N Eng J Med 318:134–39

Takase S, Takada A, Yasuhara M, Tsutsumi M (1989) Hepatic aldehyde dehydrogenase activity in liver disease, with particular emphasis on alcoholic liver disease. Hepatology 9:704–9

Tanaka F, Omata M, Ohto M (1990) ADH 2,3 and ALDH 2 gene frequency in Japanese alcoholics. Hepatology 12:926

Tanna VL, Wilson AF, Winokur G, Elston RC (1988) Possible linkage between alcoholism and esterase-D*. J Stud Alcohol 49:472–76

Thomasson HR, Edenberg HJ, Crabb DW, et al. (1991) Alcohol and aldehyde dehydrogenase genotypes and alcoholism in Chinese men. Am J Hum Genet 48:677–81

Tone S, Takikawa O, Habara-Ohkubo A, et al. (1990) Primary structure of human indoleamine 2,3 dioxygenase deduced from the nucleotide sequence of its cDNA. Nucleic Acids Res 18:367

Truitt Jr EB, Walsh MJ (1973) The role of acetaldehyde in the actions of ethanol. In Kissin H, Begleiter H (eds), Biology of alcoholism. Plenum Press, New York, vol 1, pp 161–95

Van Thiel DH (1991) Gender differences in the susceptibility and severity of alcohol induced liver disease. Alcohol Alcohol Suppl 1:9–18

Von Knorring AL, Bohman M, Von Knorring L, Oreland L (1985) Platelet MAO activity as a biological marker in subgroups of alcoholism. Acta Psychiatr Scand 72:51–58

Von Knorring AL, Hallman J, Von Knorring L, Oreland L (1991) Platelet monoamine oxidase activity in type 1 and type 2 alcoholism. Alcohol Alcohol 26:409–16

Von Olderhausen HF (1970) Alkoholische Leberschaden. Therapiewoche 20:58–73

Wall TL, Thomasson HR, Schuckit MA, Ehlers CL (1992) Subjective feelings of alcohol intoxication in Asians with genetic variations of ALDH 2 alleles. Alcohol Clin Exp Res 16:991–95

Ward RJ, Sherman D, Peters TJ (1992) Genetic basis for addiction or aversion to chronic ethanol consumption. Alcohol Alcohol 27:47

Weiner FR, Eskries DS, Compton KV, et al. (1988) Haplotype analysis of a I collagen gene and its association with alcoholic cirrhosis in man. Mol Aspects Med 10:159–68

Wermuth B, Ernst E, Von Wartburg JP, et al. (1991) Bestimmung des alkohol dehydrogenase genotyps: Keine korrelation zwischen iso enzymmuster und leberzirrhose. Schweiz Med Wochenschr 121:1880–82

Whipple SC, Berman SM, Noble EP (1991) Event-related potentials in alcoholic fathers and their sons. Alcohol 8:321–27

Whipple SC, Parker ES, Noble EP (1988) An atypical neurocognitive profile in alcoholic fathers and their sons. J Stud Alcohol 49:240–44

Wilson JR, McClearn GE, Johnson RC (1978) Ethnic variations in the use and effects of alcohol. Drug Alcohol Depend 3:147–51

Wolff PH (1972) Ethnic differences in alcohol sensitivity. Science 175:449–50

Wolff PH (1973) Vasomotor sensitivity to alcohol in diverse mongloid populations. Am J Hum Genet 25:193–99

Yamashita I, Ohmori T (1990) Biological study of alcohol dependence syndrome with reference to ethnic difference: Report of a WHO collaborative study. Jpn J Psychiatry Neurol 44:79–84

Yoshihara H, Sato N, Kamada T, Abe H (1983) Low Km ALDH isozyme and alcoholic liver injury. Pharmacol Biochem Behav 18(suppl 1):425–28

Yoshimoto K, Komura S (1987) Reexamination of the relationship between alcohol preference and brain monoamines in inbred strains of mice including senescence-accelerated mice. Pharmocol Biochem Behav 27:317–22

Zeiner AR, Girardot JM, Nichols N, et al. (1984) Isozyme deficiency among North American Indians. Alcohol Clin Exp Res 8:129